Atlas of
HEART DISEASES

CARDIOMYOPATHIES, MYOCARDITIS, AND PERICARDIAL DISEASE

Volume II

Atlas of
HEART DISEASES

CARDIOMYOPATHIES, MYOCARDITIS, AND PERICARDIAL DISEASE

Volume II

SERIES EDITOR

Eugene Braunwald, MD, MD (Hon), ScD (Hon)

Hersey Professor of the Theory and Practice of Medicine
Harvard Medical School
Chairman, Department of Medicine
Brigham and Women's Hospital
Boston, Massachusetts

VOLUME EDITOR

Walter H. Abelmann, MD

Professor Emeritus of Medicine
Harvard Medical School
Cardiovascular Division
Beth Israel Hospital
Boston, Massachusetts

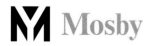 Mosby

St. Louis Baltimore Boston Carlsbad Chicago Naples New York Philadelphia Portland
London Madrid Mexico City Singapore Sydney Tokyo Toronto Wiesbaden

Developed by Current Medicine, Inc., Philadelphia

CURRENT MEDICINE

400 MARKET STREET, SUITE 700 • PHILADELPHIA, PA 19106

Development Editor .... *Maureen McNally*

Art Director .... *Paul Fennessy*

Designer .... *Lisa Caro*

Illustration Director .... *Larry Ward*

Illustrators .... *Laura Pardi Duprey,*
Wendy Jackelow,
Liz Kazanecki,
Lisa Antonucci Messina,
and Larry Ward

Production Manager .... *David Myers*

Distribution rights for North America
and territories not listed below:
MOSBY-YEAR BOOK, INC.
11830 Westline Industrial Drive
St. Louis, MO 63146

In Canada: TIMES MIRROR
PROFESSIONAL PUBLISHING LTD.
130 Flaska Drive • Markham, Ontario
Canada L6G 1B8

Distribution rights for Central and
South America: NUEVA EDITORIAL
INTERAMERICANA, SA DE CV.

Distribution rights for Japan:
NANKODO CO LTD.

Distribution rights for Indian Subcontinent
and South East Asia (except Japan):
TIMES MIRROR INTERNATIONAL
PUBLISHERS, LTD.

Cardiomyopathies, myocarditis, and pericardial disease / volume editor,
     Walter H. Abelmann.
          p. cm. – (Atlas of heart diseases; v. 2)
          Includes bibliographical references and index.
     ISBN 1-878132-24-5 (hard-cover)
     I. Abelmann, Walter H. II. Series.
     [DNLM: 1. Myocardial Diseases–atlases. 2. Pericarditis–atlases.
      WG 200 A881 1994 v. 2]
     RC682.A818 1994 vol. 2
     [RC685.M9]
     616.1′2 s–dc20
     [616.1′24]
     DNLM/DLC   94-31947
     for Library of Congress   CIP

Library of Congress Cataloging-in-Publication Data
ISBN 1-878132-24-5

Printed in Singapore by Imago Productions (FE) Ltd.

10 9 8 7 6 5 4 3 2

SERIES PREFACE

Disorders of the cardiovascular system are the most common causes of death and serious morbidity in the industrialized world. In 1991, more than 40% of all deaths in the United States were attributed to cardiac and vascular diseases. These conditions accounted for almost 5 million years of potential life lost.

Despite these sobering statistics, progress in cardiovascular medicine has been immense, and is, in fact, accelerating. Our understanding of the pathobiology of most forms of heart disease has advanced steadily and there have been enormous advances in the diagnosis, treatment, and prevention of cardiovascular disorders. For example, during just one decade, from 1981 to 1991, the overall death rates from cardiovascular disease declined by 26% and death rates from acute myocardial infarction and stroke declined by 32%. Similar progress has been made in other major cardiovascular disorders, including hypertension, valvular and congenital heart disease, congestive heart failure, and the arrhythmias.

The physician responsible for the care of patients with cardiovascular disease now has a number of vehicles available for obtaining up-to-date information, including excellent journals and textbooks of every conceivable size, scope, and depth. In developing new strategies for transmitting information about these conditions, it is important to consider that cardiovascular medicine is the most "visual" of medical specialties. Cardiovascular diagnosis is based on the recognition and understanding of a variety of graphic waveforms, images, decision trees, and microscopic sections. Treatment increasingly involves the intelligent use of algorithms, which are also most effectively portrayed visually. Likewise, mechanical correction of cardiovascular disorders, whether catheter-based or surgical, can best be described pictorially. This *Atlas of Heart Diseases* has been designed to provide a detailed and comprehensive visual exposition of all aspects of cardiovascular medicine. Several thousand images, accompanied by detailed captions, have been carefully selected by expert authors and reviewed by the 12 distinguished Volume Editors. These images are now available separately in print and slide form and also will soon be formatted for CD-ROM use.

Many people deserve credit for the successful completion of this ambitious effort. The expertise and hard work of the authors and the devoted efforts of the volume editors naturally form the foundation of the *Atlas of Heart Diseases*. Great credit is also due to Abe Krieger, President of Current Medicine, who conceived the *Atlas* series; to Maureen McNally, the extremely effective Development Editor; and to Kathryn Saxon, who coordinated the efforts in my office.

All of us who have been engaged in this project hope that each individual volume, and the entire *Atlas*, will be useful to physicians of all specialties who are responsible for the care of patients with cardiovascular disorders, to investigators and teachers of cardiovascular medicine, and ultimately to the millions of patients worldwide with disorders of the heart and circulation.

Eugene Braunwald, MD

CONTRIBUTORS

WALTER H. ABELMANN, MD
Professor Emeritus of Medicine
Harvard Medical School
Cardiovascular Division
Beth Israel Hospital
Boston, Massachusetts

HARRY ACQUATELLA, MD
Professor of Medicine
Hospital Universitario
Caracas, Venezuela

AFTAB A. ANSARI, MD
Professor
Department of Pathology and
 Laboratory Medicine
Winship Cancer Center
Emory University School of Medicine
Atlanta, Georgia

KENNETH L. BAUGHMAN, MD
Associate Professor of Medicine
Johns Hopkins University
Director, Cardiology Division
Johns Hopkins Hospital
Baltimore, Maryland

JAGDISH BUTANY, MB, MS
Associate Professor
University of Toronto
Department of Pathology
Toronto General Hospital
Toronto, Ontario

NOBLE FOWLER, MD
 Professor Emeritus of Medicine
University of Cincinnati College
 of Medicine
Cincinnati, Ohio

JAMES J. GLAZIER, MD, MRCP
Assistant Professor of Medicine
Loyola University
Chicago, Illinois
Attending Physician
Loyola University Medical Center
Maywood, Illinois
Veterans Administration Medical Center
Hines, Illinois

JUDITH K. GWATHMEY, VMD, PhD
Associate Professor of Physiology
 in Medicine
Harvard Medical School
Cardiovascular Division
Beth Israel Hospital
Boston, Massachusetts

AHVIE HERSKOWITZ, MD
Assistant Professor of Medicine and
 Immunology/Infectious Diseases
Johns Hopkins University School
 of Medicine
Baltimore, Maryland

YUZO HIROTA, MD
Associate Professor of Medicine
The Third Division
Osaka Medical College
Takatsuki City, Osaka, Japan

RALPH H. HRUBAN, MD
Department of Pathology
Johns Hopkins Hospital
Baltimore, Maryland

EDWARD K. KASPER, MD
Division of Cardiology
Johns Hopkins Hospital
Baltimore, Maryland

CHUICHI KAWAI, MD
Professor Emeritus
Department of Internal Medicine
Kyoto University
Kyoto, Japan

ALLAN D. KITCHING, MD
Clinical Scholor
Department of Medicine
 (Cardiology)
St. Joseph's Hospital
McMaster University
Hamilton, Ontario

BENEDICT F. MASSELL, MD
Director Emeritus
Rheumatic Fever Division
(House of the Good Samaritan)
Children's Hospital
Honorary Assistant Physician
Beth Israel Hospital
Boston, Massachusetts

YASUYUKI NAKAMURA, MD
First Department of
 Internal Medicine
Shiga University of
 Medical Science
Kyoto, Japan

JAGAT NARULA, MBBS, MD,
DM, PhD
Assistant Director
Center for Drug Targeting
Bouve College of Pharmacy and
 Health Sciences
Fellow, Division of Nuclear Medicine
Harvard Medical School
Massachusetts General Hospital
Boston, Massachusetts

JOSEPH K. PERLOFF, MD
Streisand/American Heart Association
Professor of Medicine and Pediatrics
UCLA School of Medicine
Los Angeles, California

HARRY RAKOWSKI, MD
Professor of Medicine
University of Toronto
Director of Clinical Cardiology
The Toronto Hospital
Toronto, Ontario

FREDERICK J. SCHOEN, MD
Associate Professor of Pathology
Harvard Medical School
Department of Pathology
Brigham and Women's Hospital
Boston, Massachusetts

E. DOUGLAS WIGLE, MD
Professor of Medicine
Division of Cardiology
The Toronto Hospital
University of Toronto
Toronto, Ontario, Canada

CONTENTS

CHAPTER 9

MYOCARDITIS
Ahvie Herskowitz and Aftab A. Ansari

CHAPTER 10

RHEUMATIC FEVER AND RHEUMATIC CARDITIS
Benedict F. Massell and Jagat Narula

CHAPTER 11

EXPERIMENTAL CARDIOMYOPATHIES
Judith K. Gwathmey

CHAPTER 12

ENDOMYOCARDIAL BIOPSY

Jagdish Butany and Frederick J. Schoen

CHAPTER 13

PERICARDIAL DISEASE

Noble Fowler

INDEX

INTRODUCTION

CHAPTER 1

Walter H. Abelmann

Cardiomyopathy, or disease of the heart muscle, has been reported in association with almost any systemic infection or disease, although it is often without clinical manifestations. Of necessity, this volume cannot be comprehensive. Instead, it is designed to present the most common forms of cardiomyopathy, as well as typical illustrative forms. Emphasis is also placed on cardiomyopathies that manifest clinically rather than rare subclinical forms. However, recognition has been given to the wide geographic variations in the incidence of cardiomyopathy, and some diseases that are largely confined to certain regions have been included.

Few of the toxic cardiomyopathies manifest as full-blown dilated cardiomyopathy or congestive heart failure. Of these, anthracycline toxicity is included in Chapter 12. Some other toxic cardiomyopathies are largely of historical interest, such as cobalt toxicity and arsenic or phosphorus poisoning. Chronic alcoholism may be associated with the manifestations of dilated cardiomyopathy, an association whose incidence markedly increases if noninvasive tests of myocardial function are applied to chronic alcoholics who exhibit no cardiovascular symptoms. Therefore, so-called alcoholic cardiomyopathy may well be the most frequent form of dilated cardiomyopathy. In its clinical manifestations, however, alcoholic cardiomyopathy is essentially different from idiopathic dilated cardiomyopathy only in the significantly better prognosis that follows total abstinence.

Chapter 11 deals with experimental models of cardiomyopathy as well as spontaneously occurring cardiomyopathies in animals. It introduces the reader to several diseases of interest from both the clinical and the experimental points of view. Much of our understanding of the pathogenesis and, more recently, the molecular biology of cardiomyopathies has been gained from such experimental models.

In keeping with the general convention, secondary references are generally omitted in this *Atlas*. A list of selected relevant monographs, however, is appended to this introduction.

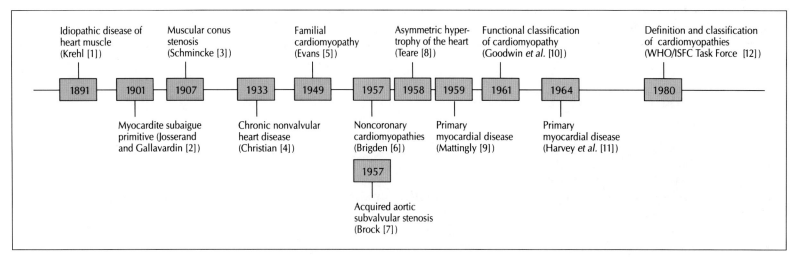

FIGURE 1-1. Milestones in the rich early history of cardiomyopathy [1–12]. Since the first published description of cardiomyopathy by Krehl in 1891 [1], study of the condition has progressed to characterization of discrete types. In 1980, after almost 90 years of study,

the World Health Organization (WHO) formally defined and classified cardiomyopathies. ISFC—International Society and Federation of Cardiology.

WHO/ISFC CLASSIFICATION OF CARDIOMYOPATHY

DILATED CARDIOMYOPATHY

Dilatation of the left, right, or both ventricles

Dilatation often severe, accompanied by hypertrophy

Impaired systolic ventricular function

CHF may/may not supervene

May present with ventricular or atrial arrhythmia

Death may occur at any stage

HYPERTROPHIC CARDIOMYOPATHY

Disproportionate hypertrophy of left, occasionally right ventricle

Involves septum more than free wall; occasionally concentric

Left ventricular volume typically normal or reduced

Systolic pressure gradients common

Inheritance by autosomal-dominant gene with incomplete penetrance

Morphologic changes, usually most severe in septum, may occur

RESTRICTIVE CARDIOMYOPATHY

May exist with or without obliteration

Includes endomyocardial fibrosis and Löffler's cardiomyopathy

Scarring affects either or both ventricles, restricts filling

Involvement of atrioventricular valves common; outflow tracts spared

Cavity obliteration characteristic of advanced cases

FIGURE 1-2. WHO/ISFC classification of cardiomyopathy. In 1980, the World Health Organization (WHO) and the International Society and Federation of Cardiology (ISFC) defined cardiomyopathies as "heart-muscle diseases of unknown cause" [12]. Although WHO/ISFC provides three distinct classifications for cardiomyopathy, a few categories do not fit readily into any group. These include some characterized by minor abnormalities in

which progression to overt cardiomyopathy may or may not occur. This has been referred to as "latent cardiomyopathy." Among the restrictive types, it has been proposed that Löffler's cardiomyopathy (endocarditis parietalis fibroplastica) should be referred to as "eosinophilic endomyocardial disease." CHF—congestive heart failure.

WHO/ISFC DEFINITION OF SPECIFIC HEART MUSCLE DISEASE, 1980

Heart muscle disease of known cause or associated with disorders of other systems

Disorders of the myocardium caused by systemic or pulmonary hypertension, coronary artery disease, valvular heart disease, or congenital cardiac anomalies have been excluded

FIGURE 1-3. The 1980 WHO/ISFC definition of specific heart muscle disease, which formerly had been known as "secondary cardiomyopathy" [12]. Although there have been objections to and reservations about this classification [13–15], it has been generally accepted.

ETIOLOGIC CLASSIFICATION OF SPECIFIC HEART MUSCLE DISEASE

A

Infections
 Bacterial
  Diphtheria*
  Tuberculosis*
  Typhoid fever*
  Rheumatic fever*
  Scarlet fever*
  Meningococcal*
  Pneumococcal
  Gonococcal
  Brucellosis
  Tetanus
  Meliodosis
  Tularemia
  Pertussis
 Spirochetal
  Syphilis
  Leptospirosis*
  Lyme disease*
 Rickettsial
  Typhus
  Rocky Mountain
   spotted fever*
  Q fever

B

Infections
 Viral
  Poliomyelitis*
  Influenza*
  Mumps*
  Rubella*
  Rubeola*
  Variola*
  Varicella*
  Epstein-Barr*
  Coxsackievirus*
  Echovirus*
  Cytomegalovirus*
  Hepatitis*
  Rabies*
  Mycoplasma*
  Psittacosis*
  Herpes
  Encephalitis
  Arboviruses*

C

Infections
 Mycotic
  Actinomycosis
  Blastomycosis
  Moniliasis
  Aspergillosis
  Histoplasmosis*
  Coccidiomycosis
  Cryptococcosis*
  Candidiasis
 Protozoal
  South American trypanosomiasis*
  African trypanosomiasis*
  Toxoplasmosis*
  Malaria

Amebiasis
Leishmaniasis
Balantidiasis
Sarcosporidiosis
Helminthic
 Trichiniasis*
 Echinococcosis
 Schistosomiasis*
 Ascariasis
 Heterophydiasis
 Filariasis
 Paragonimiasis
 Strongyloidiasis
 Cysticercosis
 Visceral larva migrans

D

Granulomatous
 Sarcoid*
 Wegener's granulomatosis*
 Granulomatous myocarditis*

Other inflammation
 Giant cell myocarditis*
 Hypersensitivity
  myocarditis*

E

Metabolic
 Endocrine
  Acromegaly*†‡
  Thyrotoxicosis*
  Hypothyroidism*†‡
  Pheochromocytoma*†‡
  Diabetes mellitus
 Familial storage diseases
  Glycogen storage diseases*‡
  Refsum disease
  Niemann-Pick disease
  Hand-Schüller-Christian
   disease
  Fabry's disease*‡
  Gangliosiderosis

Gaucher's disease*†
Sandhoff's disease*
Mucopolysaccharidosis*
 Hunter's syndrome
 Hurler's syndrome
Nutritional
 Beriberi*
 Kwashiorkor*
 Pellagra
 Selenium deficiency
  (Keshan's disease)*
Other
 Hypokalemia*
 Carnitine deficiency*
 Uremia*

F

Deposits
 Hemochromatosis*†
 Oxalosis
 Ochronosis
 Amyloid disease†
Connective tissue diseases
 Rheumatoid heart disease*
 Ankylosing spondylitis
 Systemic lupus
  erythematosus*
 Scleroderma*†
 Dermatomyositis*
 Periarteritis nodosa

Hematologic disorders
 Leukemia*
 Myeloma
 Sickle cell anemia*
 Anemia*
 Henoch-Schönlein
  purpura*
Neoplastic diseases
 Primary neoplasms†
 Metastatic neoplasms†

FIGURE 1-4. Etiologic classification of specific heart muscle disease. **A** through **H**, A comprehensive but not complete list of common as well as rare specific causes or syndromes associated with disease of heart muscle, *ie*, specific heart muscle disease. Conditions that may manifest as dilated cardiomyopathy are indicated by *asterisks*, restrictive cardiomyopathy by *daggers*, and hypertrophic cardiomyopathy by *double daggers*. These designations are neither obligatory nor exclusive. (*continued*)

G

Heredofamilial neurologic and neuromuscular diseases
  Progressive muscular dystrophy (Duchenne)*
  Limb-girdle muscular dystrophy (Erb)*
  Fascioscapulohumeral dystrophy (Landouzy-Déjerine)
  Humeroperoneal ataxia
  Friedreich's ataxia‡
  Myotonia atrophica (Steinert)*
  Myasthenia gravis
  Chronic progressive external ophthalmoplegia (Kearns-Sayre)
  Familial centronuclear myopathy
  Juvenile progressive spinal muscular atrophy (Kugelberg-
    Welander)
  Neurofibromatosis‡
Endomyocardial diseases
  Endomyocardial fibrosis*†
  Hypereosinophilic heart disease (Löffler's)†
  Endocardial fibrosis*†

H

Toxins and drugs
  Adriamycin*
  Amphetamine*
  Antimony
  Arsenic*
  Carbon monoxide
  Carbon tetrachloride
  Catecholamines*
  Cobalt*
  Cocaine*
  Cyclophosphamide
  Emetine
  Ethyl alcohol*
  Lithium
  Lead
  Methysergide

Phenothiazine drugs
Phosphorus*
Tricyclic antidepressants
Zidovudine*
Radiation*†

FIGURE 1-4. (*continued*) Many of these disorders affect the heart only rarely or late in the course of the disease. Cardiac involvement may remain subclinical and therefore detectable only by special studies or even only at postmortem examination. Although collectively these causes of heart muscle disease may account for less than 10% of all cardiomyopathies, the clinical significance of such a list lies in the fact that some of the underlying diseases or syndromes can be treated by specific therapy or are subject to secondary and even primary prevention. It should also be recognized that in many patients with heart muscle disease more than one cause or etiologic factor may play a role, *ie*, the heart muscle disease may be pluricausal [16,17]. (*Adapted from* Abelmann [13]; with permission.)

PATHOGENETIC MECHANISMS OPERATIVE IN ONE OR MORE SYNDROMES OF CARDIOMYOPATHY

Heredity	Nitric oxide
Calcium overload	Cardiotropic infectious organisms
Altered calcium handling	Immune/autoimmune processes
Endogenous catecholamines	
Hypoxia	Autonomic imbalance
Microvascular spasm	Autonomic denervation
Altered protein synthesis	Decreased coronary blood flow reserve
Altered myocardial metabolism	
Altered membrane permeability	Tachycardia
Altered myocardial receptors	Pregnancy
Altered effect on enzymes	Alterations in cardiac cytoskeleton
Oxygen free radicals	
Cytokines	

FIGURE 1-5. Pathogenetic mechanisms operative in one or more syndromes of cardiomyopathy. Many if not most of the pathogenetic mechanisms listed here owe their recognition to investigations of animal models, some of which are presented in detail in Chapter 11.

ENHANCING OR CONTRIBUTORY FACTORS IN CARDIOMYOPATHY

Myocardial hypoperfusion	Hypertension
Nutritional deficiencies	Anemia
Drugs	Exercise
Toxins	Tachycardia
Radiation	Pregnancy/puerperium
Increased afterload	Age
Increased preload	

FIGURE 1-6. Enhancing or contributory factors in myocardial disease. As stated earlier, myocardial disease is often pluricausal. In addition, certain factors are known to play contributory if not enhancing roles. The more important of these are shown here. It should be noted that a number of factors are therapeutically reversible. Among toxins, ethanol and cocaine deserve special emphasis because cardiomyopathy associated with chronic alcoholism or cocaine abuse is quite common and often responds favorably to complete withdrawal of the toxin.

REFERENCES

1. Krehl RLK: Beitrag zur Kentniss der idiopathischen Herz-muskelerkrankungen. *Dtsch Arch Klin Med* 1891, 48:413–431.

2. Josserand E, Gallavardin L: De l'asystolie progressive des jeunes sujets par myocardite subaigue primitive. *Arch Gen Med* 1901, 6:684–704.

3. Schmincke A: Ueber linksseitige muskulöse Conusstenosen. *Dtsch Med Wochenschr* 1907, 33:2082–2083.

4. Christian H: Diagnosis of chronic non-valvular heart disease (chronic myocarditis). *N Engl J Med* 1933, 208:574.

5. Evans W: Familial cardiomyopathy. *Br Heart J* 1949, 11:68–82.

6. Brigden W: Uncommon myocardial diseases: the non-coronary cardiomyopathies. *Lancet* 1957, 2:1179–1243.

7. Brock RC: Functional obstruction of the left ventricle (acquired aortic subvalvular stenosis). *Guys Hosp Rep* 1957, 106:221–238.

8. Teare D: Asymmetric hypertrophy of the heart in young adults. *Br Heart J* 1958, 20:1–8.

9. Mattingly TW: The clinical and hemodynamic features of primary myocardial disease. *Trans Am Clin Climatol Assoc* 1959, 70:132–141.

10. Goodwin JF, Gordon H, Hollman A, *et al.*: Clinical aspects of cardiomyopathy. *BMJ* 1961, 1:69–79.

11. Harvey WP, Segal JP, Gurel T: The clinical spectrum of primary myocardial disease. *Prog Cardiovasc Dis* 1964, 7:17–42.

12. WHO/ISFC: Report of the WHO/ISFC Task Force on the Definition and Classification of Cardiomyopathies. *Br Heart J* 1980, 44:672–673.

13. Abelmann WH: Classification and natural history of primary myocardial disease. *Prog Cardiovasc Dis* 1984, 27:73–94.

14. Goodwin JF: Cardiomyopathies and specific heart muscle diseases: definition, terminology and classification. In *Heart Muscle Disease.* Edited by Goodwin JF. Lancaster, UK: MTP Press; 1985:1–5.

15. Boffa GM, Thiene G, Nava A, *et al.*: Cardiomyopathy: a necessary revision of the WHO classification. *Int J Cardiol* 1991, 30:1–7.

16. Abelmann WH: The cardiomyopathies. *Hosp Pract* 1971, 6:101–112.

17. Goodwin JF: Prospects and conditions for the cardiomyopathies. *Circulation* 1974, 50:210–219.

SELECTED RELEVANT MONOGRAPHS

Bristow MR, ed: *Drug-Induced Heart Disease.* Amsterdam: Elsevier/North Holland Biomedical Press; 1980.

Cortes FM, ed: *The Pericardium and its Disorders.* Springfield, IL: CC Thomas; 1971.

Engelmeier R, O'Connell JB, eds: *Drug Therapy in Dilated Cardiomyopathy and Myocarditis.* New York: Marcel Dekker; 1988.

Fowles RE, ed: *Cardiac Biopsy.* Mt. Kisco, NY: Futura; 1992.

Giles TD, ed: *Cardiomyopathy.* Littleton, MA: PSG Publishing Co.; 1988.

Goodwin JF, ed: *Heart Muscle Disease.* Lancaster, UK: MTP Press; 1985.

Kawai C, Abelmann WH, eds: *Pathogenesis of Myocarditis and Cardiomyopathy: Recent Experimental and Clinical Studies.* Tokyo: University of Tokyo Press; 1987.

Kaye D, ed: *Infective Endocarditis.* Baltimore: University Park Press; 1976.

Kean BH, Breslau RC, eds: *Parasites of the Human Heart.* New York: Grune & Stratton; 1964.

McKinney B, ed: *Pathology of the Cardiomyopathies.* London: Butterworths; 1974.

Opie LH, Sugimoto T, eds: *Metabolic and Molecular Aspects of Cardiomyopathy.* Tokyo: University of Tokyo Press; 1991.

Perloff JD: The cardiomyopathies. *Cardiol Clin* 1988, 6:185–320.

Pomerance A, Davies MJ, eds: *The Pathology of the Heart.* Oxford: Blackwell; 1975.

Reddy PS, Leon DF, Shaver JA, eds: *Pericardial Disease.* New York: Raven Press; 1982.

Shabetai R, ed: *The Pericardium.* New York: Grune & Stratton; 1981.

Shaver JA, ed: *Cardiomyopathies: Clinical Presentation, Differential Diagnosis and Management.* Philadelphia: FA Davis; 1988.

Spodick DH, ed: *Pericardial Diseases.* Philadelphia: FA Davis; 1976.

Stimmel B, ed: *Cardiovascular Effects of Mood-Altering Drugs.* New York: Raven Press; 1979.

Ten Cate FJ, ed: *Hypertrophic Cardiomyopathy: Clinical Recognition and Management.* New York: Marcel Dekker; 1985.

Toshima H, Maron BJ, eds: *Hypertrophic Cardiomyopathy.* Tokyo: University of Tokyo Press; 1988.

Unverferth DV, ed: *Dilated Cardiomyopathy.* Mt. Kisco, NY: Futura; 1985.

Valiathan MS, Somers K, Kartha CC, eds: *Endomyocardial Fibrosis.* Delhi: Oxford University Press; 1993.

Van Stee EW, ed: *Cardiovascular Toxicology.* New York, NY: Raven Press; 1982.

HYPERTROPHIC CARDIOMYOPATHY

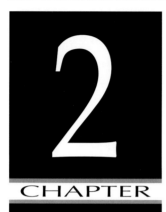

CHAPTER 2

E. Douglas Wigle, Allan D. Kitching, and Harry Rakowski

Although the pathology of hypertrophic cardiomyopathy (HCM) was described by two French pathologists in the mid-19th century [1,2] and by a German pathologist in the early 20th century [3], it remained for the virtually simultaneous reports by Brock [4] and Teare [5] some 35 years ago to bring modern attention to this fascinating entity. Subsequently, there has been an almost exponential growth in our knowledge of HCM, as well as in the number of research reports on the subject, including several reviews [6–10].

Hypertrophic cardiomyopathy may be defined as any form of left ventricular (LV) hypertrophy that is without obvious cause [6–9]. Asymmetric hypertrophy, especially of the ventricular septum, and myocardial fiber disarray are two particularly characteristic pathologic features of HCM [5,7–9]. It is important to distinguish between obstructive and nonobstructive forms of HCM. Obstructive HCM may occur at the subaortic level, where it is caused by mitral leaflet–ventricular septal contact [8–12], or at the midventricular (papillary muscle) level, where it is caused by marked midventricular hypertrophy [8,13]. In nonobstructive HCM, there is no obstruction to LV outflow at rest or on provocation. The hypertrophy is commonly septal or apical [14,15] in nonobstructive HCM and LV function may be normal (supranormal) or depressed [16]; the latter occurs in what is often termed end-stage HCM. In both obstructive and nonobstructive HCM the following may occur: diastolic dysfunction, manifested as impaired relaxation or restriction of filling [8,17]; myocardial ischemia and infarction in the presence of normal coronary arteries [18,19]; atrial and ventricular arrhythmias [20,21]; and cardiac arrest. The principal risk factors of sudden death are a history of syncope [22], a family history of sudden death [23], young age, myocardial ischemia [18], and the occurrence of ventricular arrhythmias on either ambulatory monitoring [20,21] or invasive electrophysiologic testing [24]. The annual mortality rate traditionally has been quoted as 3% to 4% [25,26] (or greater in the young), but several recent studies have reported an annual mortality of 1% [27,28].

Patients with HCM, particularly those with obstruction to LV outflow, complain of dyspnea and angina as well as presyncope and syncope on exertion. Congestive heart failure is rare except in patients with impaired systolic function (end-stage HCM) and in the presence of atrial fibrillation. There are at least seven findings on physical examination in subaortic obstructive HCM that are not found in nonobstructive forms of the disease [8].

The treatment of HCM is based on the major pathophysiologic problem presented by the particular patient. Therapy in obstructive HCM is directed at lessening the severity of the obstruction by medical means (negative inotropes) [8,9,29–32], atrioventricular sequential pacemaker therapy [33,34], or surgery (ventriculomyectomy) [35–38].

Three classes of drugs have been used in the medical therapy of obstructive HCM: β-blockers [8,29], calcium antagonists [30,31], and the negative inotropic antiarrhythmic agent disopyramide [8,32]. We have found disopyramide with or without a β blocker to be a safe and effective therapy of obstructive HCM. Although the negative inotropic effect of calcium antagonists, such as verapamil, usually lessens the obstruction, we are concerned with the potential for the vasodilating action of these drugs to worsen the obstruction. This has happened on a number of occasions, with sometimes lethal results [31]. Successful surgery (total abolition of the obstruction) provides by far the greatest symptomatic benefit to these patients and can be performed with 1% to 2% mortality [8,38]. Calcium antagonists can improve impaired relaxation in diastole [17] and are effective in relieving myocardial ischemia [18]. In patients with end-stage HCM, negative inotropes are discontinued because there is no longer any LV outflow obstruction. Such patients are subsequently treated with digoxin, afterload-reducing agents, and diuretics to improve LV function. This contrasts directly to medical therapy in cases of obstructive HCM, for which negative inotropes are indicated, and digoxin, afterload-reducing agents, and (occasionally) diuretics are contraindicated because these drugs would worsen the obstruction.

Over the past 35 years, it has been fascinating to observe how the different cardiologic investigative techniques have been applied to enhance our understanding of the pathophysiology of HCM. The 1960s and 1970s was the clinical, hemodynamic, and angiographic era, which focused mainly on obstructive HCM [6,8,39–41]. Since the 1970s, the various echocardiographic and Doppler techniques (ie, one- and two-dimensional echocardiography; and pulsed-wave, continuous-wave, and color Doppler by transthoracic and transesophageal approaches) have aided in the understanding of the obstruction, as well as systolic and diastolic function [11,12,42–46]. During this same period, nuclear techniques brought understanding and quantitation to diastolic dysfunction [17,47] and documented the occurrence of ischemia and infarction in the presence of normal epicardial coronary arteries [18]. At the same time, noninvasive and invasive electrophysiologic studies were attempting to understand the genesis and management of atrial, and particularly ventricular, arrhythmias [20–24].

In the past 5 years, we have seen the techniques of molecular biology and genetics applied to HCM with the result that we now understand that the disease is genetically heterogeneous. About 40% of familial cases are the result of missense mutations on the β myosin heavy chain gene, which is on the long arm of chromosome 14 [48–51]. More recently, abnormalities on chromosomes 1q1, 15q2, and 11q have been implicated in the familial occurrence of HCM [52,53]. The type of molecular defect in familial HCM, rather than any clinical parameter, may become the most potent predictor of natural history and outcome [49]. We have come a long way since Brock unexpectedly encountered HCM surgically in 1957, but with the ever-evolving technologies available, more is yet to come.

PATHOLOGY

TYPES OF HCM	
LEFT VENTRICULAR INVOLVEMENT	APPROXIMATE INCIDENCE, %
Asymmetric hypertrophy	95
Ventricular septal hypertrophy	90
Apical hypertrophy	3
Midventricular hypertrophy	1
Rare types	1
Symmetric (concentric) hypertrophy	5
Right ventricular involvement	

FIGURE 2-1. Definition and incidence of HCM. HCM may be defined as left or right ventricular hypertrophy of unknown cause, which is usually, but not always, asymmetric and associated with microscopic evidence of myocardial fiber disarray. Asymmetric hypertrophy of the ventricular septum, originally described by Teare [5], is by far the most common type of HCM. The incidence of the different types of HCM varies widely among centers. These data are the approximate rates taken from the Toronto Hospital. (*Adapted from* Wigle and coworkers [8]; with permission.)

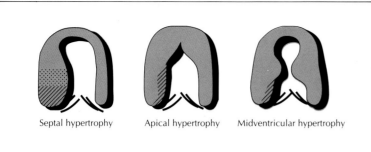

Septal hypertrophy   Apical hypertrophy   Midventricular hypertrophy

FIGURE 2-2. Three common varieties of asymmetric hypertrophy, as they would be seen in the apical four-chamber view of a two-dimensional echocardiogram. Septal hypertrophy may involve only the basal one third of the septum (subaortic area; *cross-hatched*), or it may involve the basal two thirds of the septum (down to the papillary muscles; *cross-hatched and stippled*), or the hypertrophy may extend from base to apex, involving the whole septum, in which case there is almost always anterolateral wall extension of the hypertrophy. In apical hypertrophy the principal involvement is in the apical one third of the ventricle, and there may be considerable asymmetry in this area. The apical hypertrophy rarely extends up the septum toward the base (*cross-hatched*); in this case, subaortic obstruction may occur. In midventricular hypertrophy, the maximal thickening occurs at the level of the papillary muscles. Basal septal hypertrophy (*cross-hatched*) may also occur in this variety of HCM and thus give rise to subaortic as well as midventricular obstruction (*see* Fig. 2-4). (*Adapted from* Wigle and coworkers [8]; with permission.)

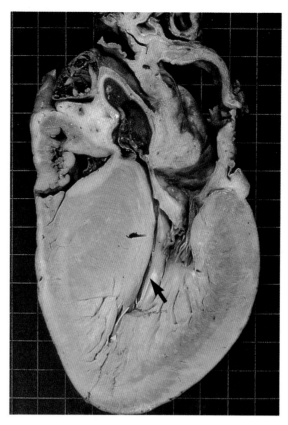

FIGURE 2-3. Asymmetric septal hypertrophy. Longitudinal section of the heart of a 32-year-old woman with subaortic obstructive HCM who died suddenly while on propranolol therapy. Hemodynamic investigation confirmed subaortic obstruction as well as mitral regurgitation. The regurgitation was partially due to an abnormal mitral valve (insertion of an anomalous papillary muscle (*arrow*) onto the ventricular surface of the anterior mitral leaflet). Note the asymmetric hypertrophy with a grossly thickened ventricular septum. A narrowed outflow tract between the upper septum and the anterior mitral leaflet, which is very thickened and fibrosed from repeated contact with the septum, can also be seen. There was microscopic evidence of extensive myocardial fiber disarray involving the septum and free wall of the left ventricle. (*Adapted from* Wigle and coworkers [8]; with permission.)

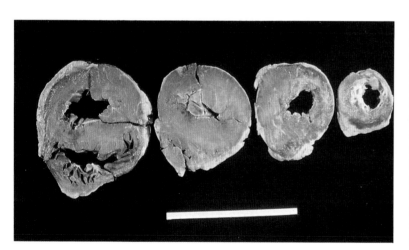

FIGURE 2-4. Midventricular hypertrophy and obstruction. Cross-sectional slices of the heart from a patient in whom midventricular obstruction had been demonstrated by hemodynamic, angiographic, and echocardiographic techniques (*see* Fig. 2-19). The site of the obstruction was at the level of the papillary muscles, where there was massive hypertrophy (second section from the left). The section at the far left is from the base of the heart, and the two sections at the right are from the apex. The apex of the left ventricle was the site of extensive myocardial infarction and aneurysm formation, which was evidenced in life by a dyskinetic apical chamber on angiography and by persistent ST segment elevation in leads V_4 to V_6 on electrocardiography. The coronary arteries were not significantly narrowed. The patient died of intractable ventricular arrhythmia. (*Adapted from* Wigle and coworkers [8]; with permission.)

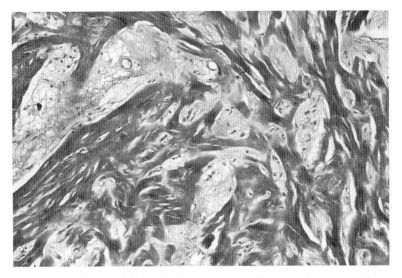

FIGURE 2-5. Myocardial fiber disarray. Microscopic section of the ventricular septum of a 28-year-old patient with HCM who died while jogging. This section shows a typical area of myocardial fiber disarray. The muscle cells are short and plump, and the nuclei are large and hyperchromatic. Note the extensive amount of loose intercellular connective tissue that may become transformed into diffuse myocardial fibrosis (*see* Fig. 2-6) late in the disease (magnification, × 100). (*Adapted from* Wigle and coworkers [8]; with permission.)

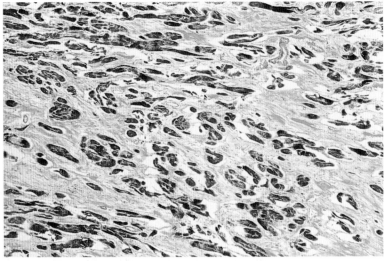

FIGURE 2-6. Myocardial fibrosis. Microscopic section of heart muscle from a patient with HCM, showing extensive interstitial fibrosis (muscle cells like islands in a sea of fibrosis). It would seem likely that this type of fibrosis develops in areas of loose intercellular connective tissue (*see* Fig. 2-5), but ischemic myocardial fibrosis may also occur in HCM as a result of small vessel disease [19] or other causes [8]. This type of myocardial fibrosis could be the cause of the diastolic dysfunction characterized by increased myocardial and chamber stiffness that is encountered in some patients with HCM. It may also contribute to the deterioration in left ventricular systolic function that is seen in some cases of end-stage HCM (magnification, × 100). (*Adapted from* Wigle and coworkers [8]; with permission.)

PATHOPHYSIOLOGY

SUBAORTIC OBSTRUCTIVE HCM

HEMODYNAMIC CLASSIFICATION OF HCM

Obstructive HCM
    Subaortic obstruction
    Midventricular obstruction
Nonobstructive HCM
    Normal (supranormal) systolic function
    Impaired systolic function (end-stage HCM)

FIGURE 2-7. Hemodynamic classification of HCM. In discussing the pathophysiology of HCM, it is important to classify it hemodynamically. In obstructive HCM, there is systolic obstruction to the outflow of blood from the left ventricle at either the subaortic level (*see* Figs. 2-3 and 2-8 through 2-15) or the midventricular level (*see* Figs. 2-4, 2-16, and 2-17). The obstruction at either level may be latent (provokable; *see* Fig. 2-12), labile (spontaneously variable), or persistent (obstruction at rest; *see* Figs. 2-8 through 2-15). In nonobstructive HCM, there is no systolic obstruction at rest or on provocation; ventricular function may be normal or impaired. The hypertrophy in nonobstructive HCM may be concentric or asymmetric, with septal and apical hypertrophy being the most common.

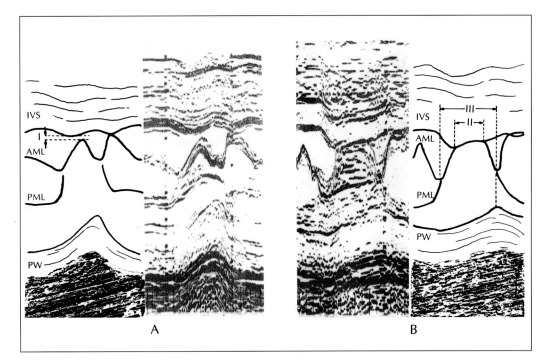

A   B

FIGURE 2-8. Determination of the degree of systolic anterior motion (SAM) of the anterior mitral leaflet (AML) in subaortic obstructive HCM. When there is no mitral leaflet–septal contact, the minimal distance between the left side of the interventricular septum (IVS) and the AML is measured (I in **A**). If that distance is 10 mm or more, the degree of mitral leaflet SAM is classified as mild. If that distance is less than 10 mm or there is brief mitral leaflet–septal contact, the degree of SAM is classified as moderate (**A**). If there is mitral leaflet–septal contact, the ratio of the duration of that contact (II in **B**) to total echocardiographic systole (III in *B*) is determined

and expressed as a percentage. When the duration of mitral leaflet–septal contact is greater than 30% of echocardiographic systole, severe SAM is said to be present (**B**). The hemodynamic state of the patient is determined by the degree of mitral leaflet SAM. Thus patients with nonobstructive HCM have no or, at most, very mild SAM. Patients with subaortic obstructive HCM have severe SAM, and patients with latent subaortic obstruction will have mild or moderate SAM, which becomes severe on provocation. PML—posterior mitral leaflet; PW—posterior wall. (*Adapted from* Gilbert and coworkers [43]; with permission.)

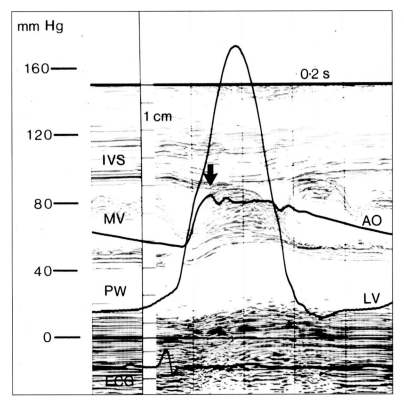

FIGURE 2-9. Simultaneous hemodynamic and echocardiographic recordings in subaortic obstructive HCM. Simultaneous left ventricular (LV) and aortic (AO) pressures and one-dimensional echocardiogram in a patient with severe subaortic obstruction (gradient = 86 mm Hg). Note the severe systolic anterior motion of the anterior mitral leaflet with early and prolonged mitral leaflet–septal contact in the presence of severe obstruction as well as the virtually simultaneous onset of both mitral leaflet–septal contact and the obstruction, defined by the peak of the aortic percussion wave (*arrow*). This association strongly suggests a cause-and-effect relationship (*ie*, mitral leaflet–septal contact is the cause of the pressure gradient). IVS—interventricular septum; MV—mitral valve; PW—posterior wall. (*Adapted from* Pollick and coworkers [54]; with permission.)

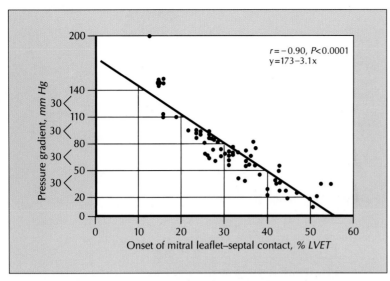

FIGURE 2-10. Correlation between the time of onset of mitral leaflet–septal contact as a percentage of the left ventricular ejection time (LVET) and the magnitude of the pressure gradient in subaortic obstructive HCM. The *vertical lines* are drawn at each 10% of the LVET. The *horizontal lines* are drawn from the intercepts of the vertical lines with the regression line to indicate the pressure gradient that corresponds with each mitral leaflet–septal contact time. For each 10% change in mitral leaflet–septal contact time, there is a 30 mm Hg change in the pressure gradient. If mitral leaflet–septal contact occurs at 20% of LVET, the pressure gradient would be 110 mm Hg. If it occurred at 40% of LVET, the pressure gradient would be only 50 mm Hg. The earlier the time of onset of mitral leaflet–septal contact, the greater the pressure gradient. Note that no pressure gradient results from mitral leaflet–septal contact after 55% of the LVET. There was a similar relationship between the onset of mitral leaflet–septal contact and the degree of prolongation of the LVET, *ie*, the earlier the mitral leaflet–septal contact occurred in systole, the greater the pressure gradient and the more prolonged the ejection time, as one would expect with an obstruction to outflow. (*Adapted from* Wigle and coworkers [8]; with permission.)

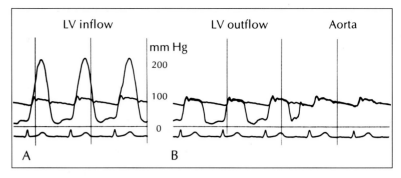

FIGURE 2-11. Subaortic obstructive HCM. Simultaneous left ventricular (LV) inflow and aortic pressures (**A**) from a 19-year-old patient with severe subaortic obstructive HCM, and withdrawal of the LV catheter to the outflow tract and aorta (**B**). Note how early in systole the pressure gradient begins in the presence of severe obstruction, as well as the characteristic spike-and-dome aortic pressure pulse that can be appreciated clinically in a significant number of patients with subaortic obstruction. Impaired relaxation in diastole is suggested by the falling LV pressure in the first half of diastole and by the elevated LV end-diastolic pressure.

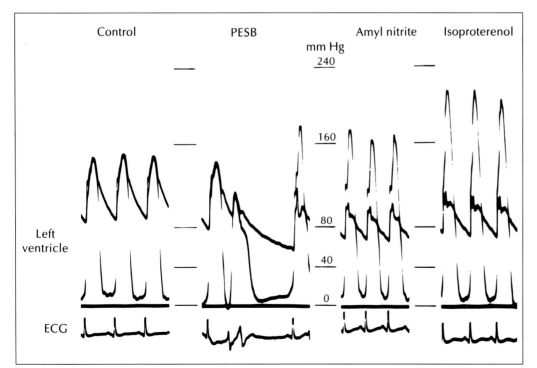

FIGURE 2-12. Latent subaortic obstructive HCM. Simultaneous left ventricular and aortic pressure tracings from a typical patient with latent obstruction show the absence of a pressure gradient under control conditions, but a pressure gradient develops in the postextrasystolic beat (PESB) and following amyl nitrite inhalation or isoproterenol infusion. Note the normal shape of the aortic pressure pulse under control conditions, and the spike-and-dome configuration of the pressure pulse following provocation of outflow obstruction. In subaortic obstructive HCM, drugs or maneuvers that decrease preload or afterload, or increase contractility, will provoke or increase the degree of obstruction to outflow. ECG—electrocardiogram. (*Adapted from* Wigle and coworkers [8]; with permission.)

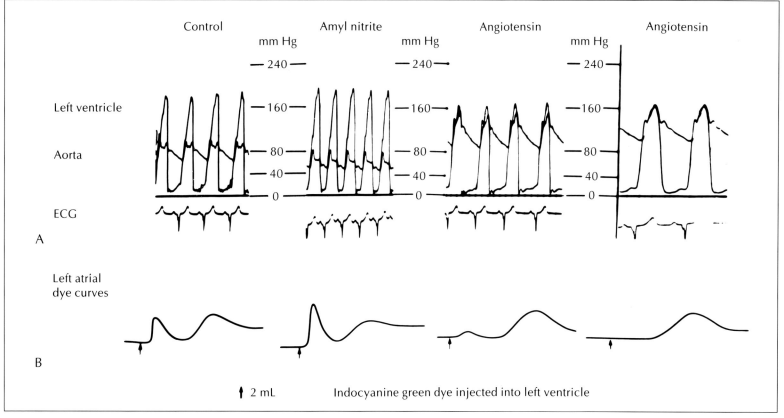

FIGURE 2-13. Relationship between pressure gradient and mitral regurgitation in subaortic obstructive HCM. Simultaneous left ventricular (LV) and aortic pressure recordings (**A**) and left atrial dye dilution curves (**B**) inscribed from left to right after LV injection of 2 mL of indocyanine green dye in a patient with subaortic obstructive HCM under control conditions, after amyl nitrite inhalation, and during angiotensin infusion. The amount of dye leaking back into the left atrium is indicated by the upward deflection of the dye curves (immediately to the right of the *arrows*), which indicates the time of LV injection of the dye. To the right of this regurgitant dye deflection is the recirculation concentration. Intensification of the outflow tract obstruction, due to inhalation of amyl nitrite, was accompanied by an increase in the amount of regurgitant dye appearing in the left atrium (*second panel*). Angiotensin infusion initially reduced (*third panel*) and eventually abolished (*fourth panel*) both the outflow tract obstruction and the

mitral regurgitation. Simultaneous one-dimensional echocardiographic recordings during these studies indicated the presence of severe systolic anterior motion (SAM) under control conditions and the abolition of SAM during angiotensin infusion, providing evidence that the abolition of the SAM abolished both the outflow obstruction and the mitral regurgitation. In 100 consecutive studies using these techniques, every patient with a pressure gradient had evidence of mitral regurgitation. In 80% of these patients, the degree of mitral regurgitation was directly related to the magnitude of the pressure gradient and the degree of SAM. In 20%, however, the degree of mitral regurgitation was independent of the pressure gradient and the degree of SAM, and there was an independent abnormality of the mitral valve (*see* Fig. 2-3) [8]. Note that an increase in afterload decreases or abolishes the pressure gradient, as would an increase in preload or a decrease in contractility. (*Adapted from* Wigle and coworkers [55]; with permission.)

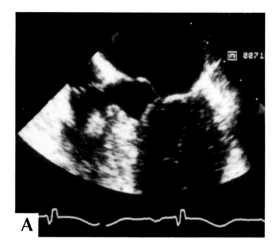

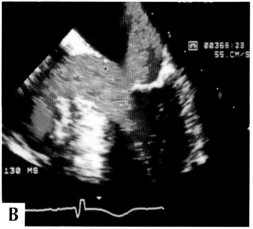

FIGURE 2-14. Echocardiographic (ECG) and color Doppler studies of subaortic obstructive HCM. **A,** Transesophageal ECG showing severe systolic anterior motion of the anterior mitral leaflet, with mitral leaflet–septal contact. Note that there is no cavity obliteration in the presence of the obstruction. **B,** Same frame with Doppler color-flow imaging demonstrating turbulent left ventricular outflow, which results from the subaortic obstruction, and a large jet of mitral regurgitation directed posteriorly into the left atrium. (*continued*)

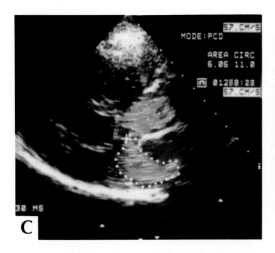
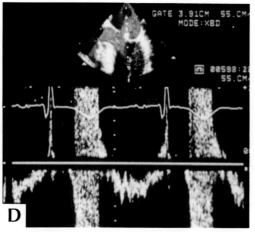

FIGURE 2-14. (continued) C, Parasternal long-axis view of an ECG/Doppler recording also showing turbulent left ventricular outflow resulting from the subaortic obstruction and a jet of mitral regurgitation directed posteriorly into the left atrium (*dotted line*). D, Pulsed-wave Doppler tracing indicating that of the mitral regurgitation occurred in the last half of systole, during inscription of the ECG T wave.

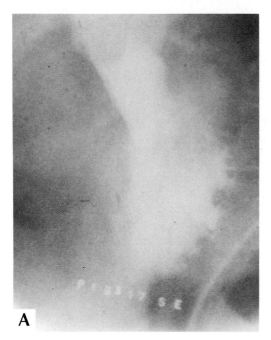
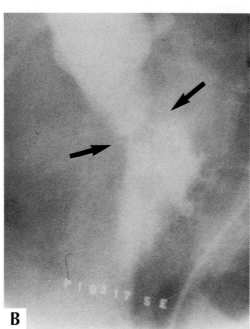
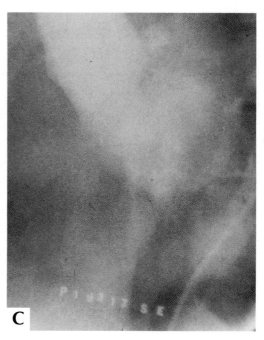

FIGURE 2-15. Eject-obstruct-leak sequence in systole in subaortic obstructive HCM. A, End-diastolic, left anterior oblique (LAO) cineangiographic frame from a patient with subaortic obstructive HCM. B, LAO left ventricular silhouette at onset of mitral leaflet–septal contact, indicated by the radiolucent line in the outflow tract (*arrows*). In early systole, there is rapid ejection into the aorta (note that the aorta is wider and more dense than in A), followed by the development of the obstruction (*arrows*), at which time there is still a large amount of angiographic dye in the left ventricle. C, End-systolic frame, showing a small end-systolic volume that is largely the result of the late systolic mitral regurgitation (note opacification of the left atrium). Thus, by both cineangiographic and ECG/Doppler (*see* Fig. 2-14) techniques, the sequence in systole of subaortic obstructive HCM is eject-obstruct-leak [8,56].

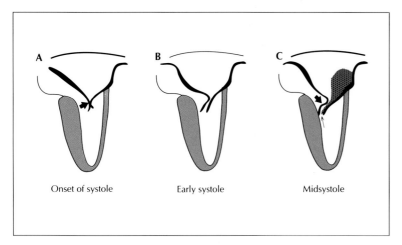

FIGURE 2-16. Functional anatomy of mitral leaflet systolic anterior motion and mitral regurgitation in subaortic obstructive HCM. Drawing of a transesophageal echocardiogram (frontal long-axis plane) demonstrating the anterior and superior motion of the anterior mitral leaflet to produce mitral leaflet–septal contact and failure of leaflet coaptation in midsystole. A, At the onset of systole, the coaptation point (*arrow*) is in the body of the anterior and posterior leaflets rather than at the tip of the leaflets, as in normal subjects [44,46]. The portion of the leaflets beyond the coaptation point is referred to as the residual length of the leaflet [44,46]. During early systole (B) and midsystole (C) there is anterior and superior movement of the residual length of the anterior mitral leaflet (*thick arrow* in C), with septal contact and failure of leaflet coaptation (*thin arrow* in C) with consequent mitral regurgitation directed posteriorly into the left atrium (*dotted area*). (*Adapted from* Grigg and coworkers [46]; with permission.)

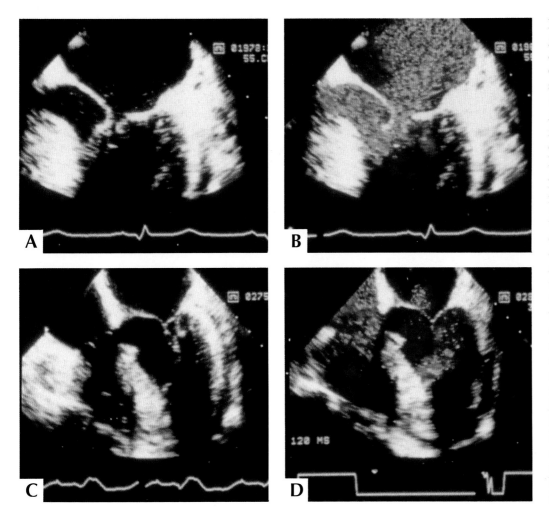

FIGURE 2-17. Obstruction and mitral regurgitation in subaortic obstructive HCM before and after myectomy. Intraoperative transesophageal echocardiographic and Doppler study (frontal long-axis plane) before (**A** and **B**) and after (**C** and **D**) myectomy. *Panel A* shows a two-dimensional systolic frame demonstrating systolic anterior motion of the residual length of the anterior mitral leaflet, with mitral leaflet–septal contact and failure of coaptation between the mitral leaflets. *Panel B* shows the same frame with Doppler color-flow imaging demonstrating turbulent left ventricular outflow as a result of the subaortic obstruction and a large jet of posteriorly directed mitral regurgitation arising from the funnel-shaped gap between the two mitral leaflets due to their failure to coapt. Note there is no evidence of left ventricular cavity obliteration at the time of subaortic obstruction and concomitant mitral regurgitation. *Panel C* is a two-dimensional systolic frame following myectomy demonstrating a widened left ventricular outflow tract and abolition of systolic anterior motion. *Panel D* is the same frame with Doppler color-flow imaging demonstrating nonturbulent left ventricular outflow with a marked reduction in the severity of the mitral regurgitation (which is now reflected only by a small residual central jet). (*Adapted from* Grigg and coworkers [46]; with permission.)

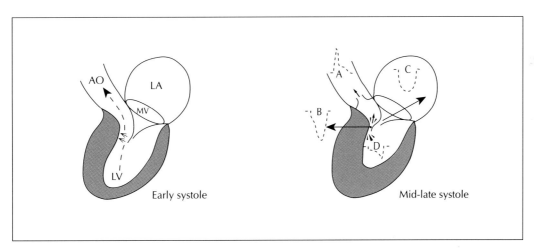

FIGURE 2-18. Pathophysiology of subaortic obstructive HCM. **Early systole**. Proposed mechanisms of mitral leaflet systolic anterior motion. The ventricular septal hypertrophy causes a narrow outflow tract, resulting in a rapid ejection velocity and a path of ejection (*dashed arrow*) that is closer to the anterior mitral leaflet than normal. These hydrodynamic and anatomic features in subaortic obstructive HCM may result in Venturi forces (*short arrows in the outflow tract*), drawing the anterior mitral leaflet toward the septum (systolic anterior motion), with subsequent development of mitral leaflet–septal contact as seen by mid-late systole [57]. Alternatively, drag forces could push this leaflet toward the septum and cause mitral leaflet–septal contact [42,58,59]. It is possible that both Venturi and drag forces play a part in the initiation and development of mitral leaflet systolic anterior motion as well as in the maintenance of mitral

leaflet–septal contact [8]. **Mid-late systole**. By midsystole, by either Venturi or drag forces, anterior mitral leaflet–septal contact causes subaortic obstruction (*converging and diverging lines*), resulting in decreased but maintained aortic flow (smaller aortic arrow than in early systole) and mitral regurgitation directed posteriorly into the left atrium through the funnel-shaped gap between the anterior and posterior mitral leaflets. A, B, C, and D indicate Doppler velocity recordings throughout systole in the ascending aorta [60] (flow toward transducer [A], at level of mitral leaflet–septal contact [B], in left atrium [C], and near the LV apex [D]). In B, C, and D, flow is away from the transducer. Peak velocities recorded at B correlate accurately with a simultaneously measured pressure gradient, whereas late peaking velocities at D do not. AO—aorta; LA—left atrium; LV—left ventricle; MV—mitral valve. (*Adapted from* Wigle [10]; with permission.)

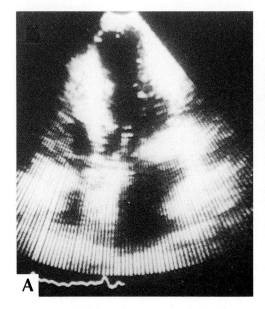
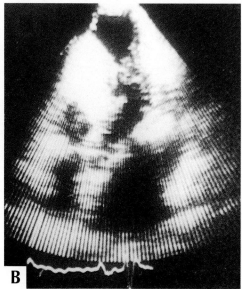

FIGURE 2-19. Midventricular obstruction. Apical four-chamber two-dimensional echocardiographic views from a patient with midventricular obstruction with apical infarction and aneurysm formation at end-diastole (**A**) and at end-systole (**B**). (For the gross pathology of the heart from this case *see* Fig. 2-4.) Note the midventricular obstruction at end-systole (*B*), and the poorly contractile, partially dyskinetic apical chamber. Cineangiography in this patient revealed midventricular occlusion at end-systole at the level of the papillary muscles. The ejection fraction of the basal chamber of the left ventricle was 91%, whereas the ejection fraction of the dyskinetic apical chamber was 16%. Apical myocardial infarction with aneurysm formation is a frequent complication of midventricular obstruction in HCM. (*Adapted from* Wigle and coworkers [8]; with permission.)

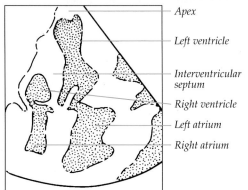
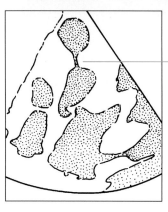

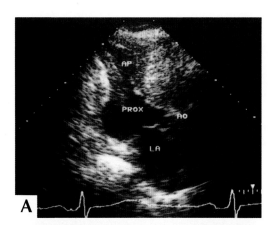
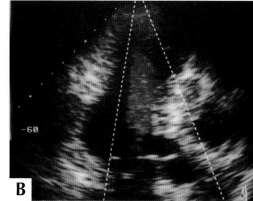
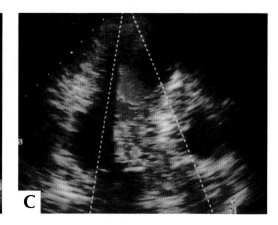

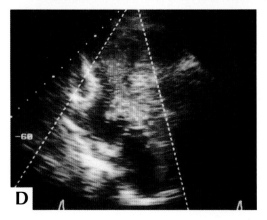

FIGURE 2-20. Midventricular obstruction. Echocardiogram–color Doppler appearance. **A,** Apical long-axis two dimensional echocardiographic appearance of midventricular hypertrophy. At the top, the apical chamber (AP) is well demonstrated. Immediately below that, the encroachment of the ventricular walls at the midventricular level can be seen. **B,** Echocardiogram–color Doppler appearance in early systole, showing no obstruction at that stage. **C,** Echocardiogram–color Doppler view later in systole, showing the beginning of turbulence at the midventricular level. **D,** The midventricular obstruction is fully developed, with marked turbulence of flow distal to the midventricular level. Ao—aorta; LA—left atrium.

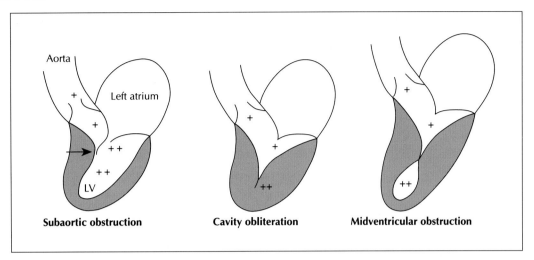

FIGURE 2-21. The left ventricular (LV) inflow tract pressure concept. This concept was initially developed to help distinguish subaortic obstructive HCM from the intraventricular pressure difference that may be encountered with cavity obliteration [41]. It is also useful in distinguishing subaortic from midventricular obstruction. In subaortic obstructive HCM, all LV pressures proximal to the outflow tract obstruction caused by mitral leaflet–septal contact (*arrow*) are elevated, including the inflow tract pressure just inside the mitral valve. In cavity obliteration, the elevated ventricular pressure is only recorded from the obliterated area of the LV and only when the catheter is trapped in that area. With cavity obliteration, the inflow tract pressure is not elevated but rather is equal to the outflow tract pressure. In midventricular obstruction, only the apical LV pressure (not inflow tract pressure) is elevated. Inflow tract pressure is equal to the outflow tract pressure. For other distinguishing features among these three causes of intraventricular pressure differences in HCM, *see* Fig. 2-22. *Two plus signs* indicate areas of increased systolic pressure; *single plus signs* indicate normal systolic pressure. (*Adapted from* Wigle [10]; with permission.)

DIFFERENTIATION OF SUBAORTIC AND MIDVENTRICULAR OBSTRUCTIVE HCM FROM CAVITY OBLITERATION

	SUBAORTIC OBSTRUCTION	MIDVENTRICULAR OBSTRUCTION	CAVITY OBLITERATION
Location	Subaortic	Midventricular	Apex
Mechanism	Mitral leaflet-septal contact*	Midventricular hypertrophy**	Apical hypertrophy
Aortic valve notch	+	-	-
Mitral regurgitation	++	-	-
Left ventricular inflow tract pressure	++	+	+
Clinical			
Spike and dome pulse	+	-	-
Double systolic apical impulse	+	-	-
Triple apical impulse	+	-	-
Apical systolic murmur	3/6	2–3/6	0–1/6
Mitral diastolic murmur	Short	Long	None

*May be recognized by angiography, echocardiography, or auscultation.
**May be recognized by angiography or echocardiography.

FIGURE 2-22. Differentiation of subaortic and midventricular obstructive HCM from cavity obliteration. In addition to the use of the left ventricular inflow tract pressure concept (*see* Fig. 2-21), there are many other differences between subaortic and midventricular obstructive HCM and cavity obliteration. This figure illustrates a number of the features of subaortic obstructive HCM that are not seen in the other two conditions. The short mitral diastolic murmur in subaortic obstruction results from increased diastolic inflow related to concomitant mitral regurgitation. On the other hand, the long mitral diastolic murmur in midventricular obstruction is related to diastolic inflow across the midventricular narrowing that is evidenced even in diastole. In addition to these three causes of intraventricular pressure difference in HCM, it is important to be aware that an early systolic impulse gradient may be exaggerated in HCM because of the rapid, early systolic ejection [61]. The impulse gradient is maximal in early systole, whereas in the other three causes of intraventricular pressure differences in HCM, the pressure difference peaks in late systole. (*Adapted from* Wigle and coworkers [8]; with permission.)

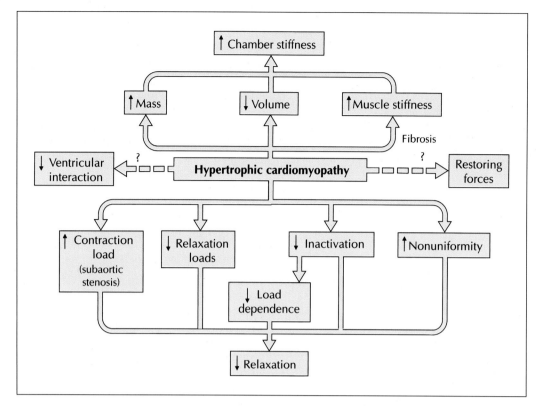

FIGURE 2-23. Diastolic dysfunction. In HCM, there is increased chamber stiffness or decreased compliance as a result of increased muscle mass and the resulting decreased ventricular volume. Increased muscle stiffness from myocardial fibrosis also occurs. Thus, all three factors that affect the stiffness or compliance of the ventricle are altered in a way that increases chamber stiffness. Left ventricular relaxation in HCM is impaired because of changes in loading conditions, decreased inactivation, and increased nonuniformity [62]. The subaortic stenosis in obstructive HCM would represent a contraction load on the ventricle, which would delay and impair relaxation. Coronary and ventricular filling loads, which aid in relaxation, are reduced in HCM because of the degree of hypertrophy and other reasons. High myoplasmic calcium would result in decreased inactivation, which would impair relaxation both directly and indirectly by reducing the load dependence of the relaxation process. Finally, there is a great deal of nonuniformity in HCM, which would also impair relaxation. Thus, all three factors that control relaxation [62] (load, inactivation, and nonuniformity) are altered in a way that relaxation would be impaired in HCM. (*Adapted from* Wigle and coworkers [8]; with permission.)

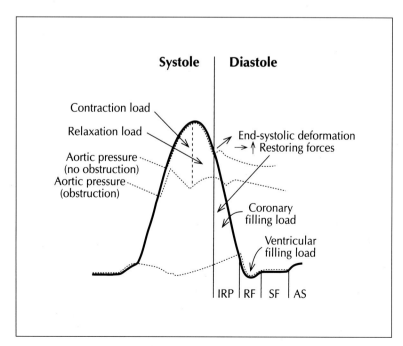

FIGURE 2-24. Hemodynamic loads affecting ventricular relaxation in HCM. Left atrial, ventricular, and aortic pressures (with and without obstruction to outflow) together with the various loads that may affect diastolic relaxation in HCM [62]. A contraction load (the subaortic obstruction) applied in the first half of systole would delay the onset and slow the rate of relaxation. The relaxation load that could be applied in the last half of systole is not believed to be important in HCM. The coronary filling load during the isovolumic relaxation period (IRP) and the ventricular filling load during rapid filling (RF) are both reduced in HCM as a result of the hypertrophy and other factors. Exaggerated end-systolic deformation, caused by extensive hypertrophy, could result in increased internal and external restoring forces. Such forces would act during the IRP to improve relaxation, off-setting other factors acting to impair relaxation. AS—atrial systole; SF—slow filling. (*Adapted from* Wigle and coworkers [8]; with permission.)

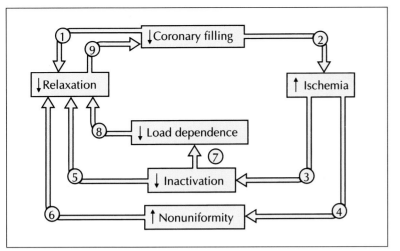

FIGURE 2-25. Vicious cycle relating myocardial ischemia and impaired relaxation in HCM. There are many causes for impaired coronary filling and myocardial ischemia in HCM, including small vessel disease, septal perforator artery compression, myocardial bridges, decreased vasodilator capacity, and reduced capillary-myocardial fiber ratio. Decreased coronary filling during the isovolumic relaxation period will impair relaxation by the decreased load (1) as well as by producing myocardial ischemia (2), which in turn decreases inactivation (3) and increases nonuniformity (4). Both of these factors act to slow the rate of relaxation (5,6). Decreased inactivation decreases load dependency (7), which further impairs relaxation (8). Finally, impaired relaxation itself reduces coronary filling (9) during the isovolumic relaxation period, and this completes the vicious cycle by further reducing the coronary filling (relaxation) load (1) and producing more myocardial ischemia (2). (*Adapted from* Wigle and coworkers [8]; with permission.)

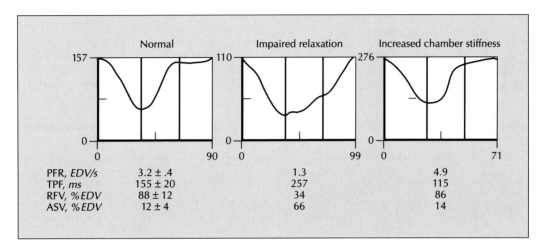

	Normal	Impaired relaxation	Increased chamber stiffness
PFR, *EDV/s*	3.2 ± .4	1.3	4.9
TPF, *ms*	155 ± 20	257	115
RFV, *%EDV*	88 ± 12	34	86
ASV, *%EDV*	12 ± 4	66	14

FIGURE 2-26. Two types of diastolic dysfunction in HCM. Nuclear diastolic function (time activity) curves in a normal subject and in two patients with HCM—one with impaired relaxation and the other with increased chamber stiffness. Impaired relaxation results in a reduced peak filling rate (PFR), a prolonged time to peak filling (TPF), and reduced rapid filling volume (RFV). In compensation, atrial systolic volume (ASV) is increased, which accounts for these patients having a loud and often palpable fourth heart sound. If these patients go into atrial fibrillation, they may become profoundly symptomatic because of the loss of atrial systole, and the rapid rate does not allow time for ventricular relaxation [10] (*see* Fig. 2-27). On the other hand, increased chamber stiffness results in an increased PFR, a shortened TPF, a normal or increased RFV, and a normal or decreased ASV. The increased RFV causes a loud third heart sound, and the normal or decreased ASV accounts for the fact that atrial fibrillation does not have profound hemodynamic consequences for these patients. EDV—end-diastolic volume. (*Adapted from* Wigle and Wilansky [63]; with permission.)

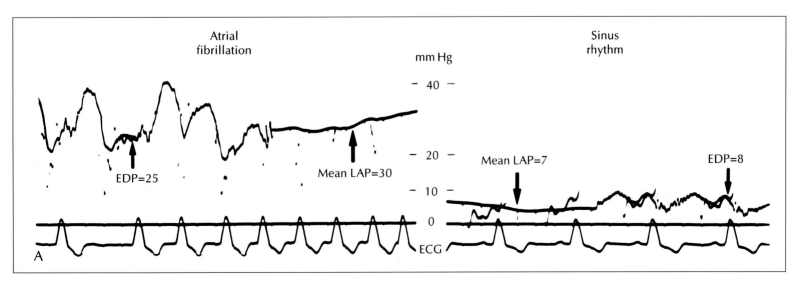

FIGURE 2-27. Hemodynamic effects of atrial fibrillation in HCM. **A,** Left atrial (LAP) and left ventricular end-diastolic (EDP) pressures in a patient with subaortic obstructive HCM in sinus rhythm (*right panel*) and atrial fibrillation (*left panel*) demonstrating a dramatic rise in mean LAP from 7 to 30 mm Hg with the onset of atrial fibrillation. Such a dramatic rise, with the onset of this arrhythmia, would be expected in a patient with impaired relaxation because 1) the rapid rate does not allow time for relaxation and 2) the loss of atrial systole deprives the patient of the most important compensatory mechanism for impaired relaxation (*see* Fig. 2-26). (*continued*)

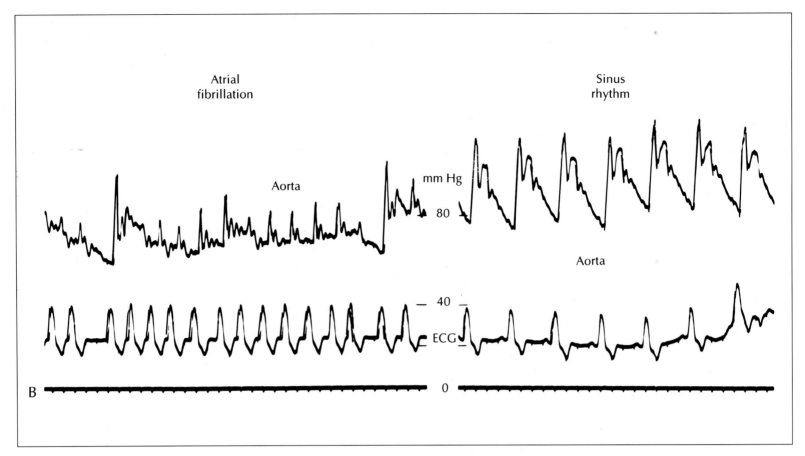

FIGURE 2-27. (*continued*) **B,** Comparison of aortic pressure in atrial fibrillation (*left panel*) and in normal sinus rhythm (*right panel*) in the same patient. Patients with impaired relaxation or subaortic obstruction in HCM will often go into acute pulmonary edema, congestive heart failure, or suffer from presyncope or syncope with the onset of atrial fibrillation. If the arrhythmia continues, patients would also be at risk for systemic and pulmonary emboli. Atrial fibrillation in HCM is usually related to an increase in atrial size (*see* Fig. 2-38). (*Adapted from* Wigle and coworkers [8]; with permission.)

APICAL HCM

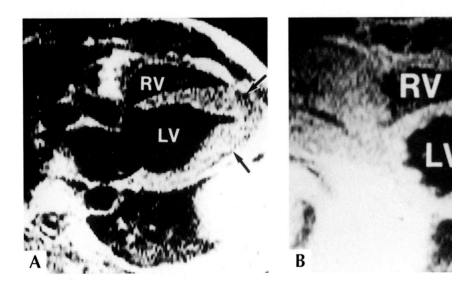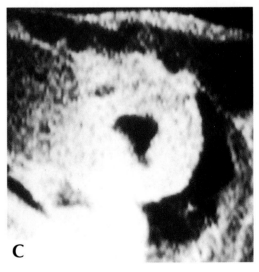

FIGURE 2-28. Apical HCM. Magnetic resonance spin-echocardiographic images from a patient with apical HCM. **A,** Long-axis, four-chamber slice demonstrates localized left ventricular (LV) hypertrophy, involving the anterior and inferior apical walls as well as the true apex (*arrows*). Note the characteristic spade-shaped LV cavity at end-diastole, an appearance originally described from cineangiographic studies by Japanese authors [14,15]. **B,** A short-axis basal slice, showing normal LV wall thickness. **C,** A short-axis apical slice, demonstrating circumferential apical hypertrophy. Recently, a nonspade type of apical HCM has been described, also by Japanese authors [64]. In these cases, the anterior and inferior apical walls, which cause the LV to be spade-shaped at end-diastole when hypertrophied, are not involved as they are in *A*. Instead, the septal and lateral walls are involved, and this can only be seen by short-axis magnetic resonance imaging, as is seen in *C*. RV—right ventricle. (*Adapted from* Webb and coworkers [65]; with permission.)

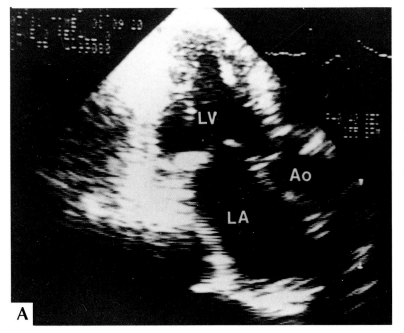

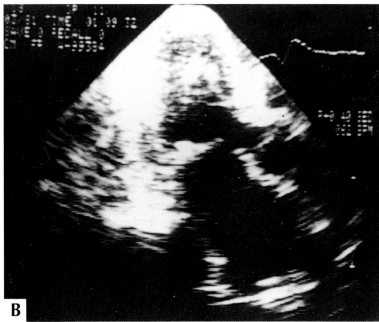

FIGURE 2-29. Apical HCM. Apical, long-axis, two-dimensional echocardiographic views from a patient with apical HCM, at end-diastole (**A**) and end-systole (**B**). Note the characteristic spade-shaped configuration of the left ventricle (LV) at end-diastole [14,15]. At end-systole there is complete obliteration of the apical portion of the LV cavity. Some authors have attributed the pressure gradient in subaortic obstructive HCM to the phenomenon of cavity obliteration or elimination. If obliteration of the LV cavity produced pressure gradients, such gradients should be seen in apical HCM, when apical cavity obliteration is greatest. However, such is not the case and apical HCM is classically a nonobstructive form. Thus, cavity obliteration (elimination) per se does not produce a pressure gradient, but one may be recorded in cavity obliteration if an LV catheter becomes trapped in the obliterated apex. This type of pressure difference may be distinguished from that encountered in subaortic or midventricular obstructive HCM (*see* Figs. 2-21 and 2-22). Note the large left atrium (LA), which was caused by impaired relaxation of the ventricle and resulted in chronic atrial fibrillation with heart failure and systemic emboli. Ao—aorta (*Adapted from* Wigle and coworkers [8]; with permission.)

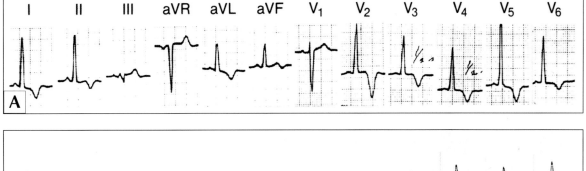

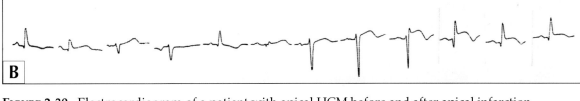

FIGURE 2-30. Electrocardiogram of a patient with apical HCM before and after apical infarction. **A,** At age 17 years, this patient had a typical spade-shaped left ventricle at end-diastole with apical cavity obliteration at end-systole. The electrocardiogram demonstrated the so-called giant T-negativity syndrome (*ie*, T waves more than 10 mV negative in precordial leads). Note that V_3 and V_4 are at half recording sensitivity. **B,** The patient presented again at age 33 years in sustained ventricular tachycardia. Following cardioversion, the electrocardiogram revealed evidence of an extensive apical infarction with aneurysm formation that was confirmed at angiography. The epicardial coronary arteries were normal. Patients with apical HCM usually have a favorable prognosis, but apical myocardial ischemia and infarction are not uncommon in the presence of severe hypertrophy. Atrial fibrillation resulting from left atrial enlargement due to impaired left ventricular relaxation is another well-recognized complication (*see* Fig. 29). (*Adapted from* Webb and coworkers [65]; with permission.)

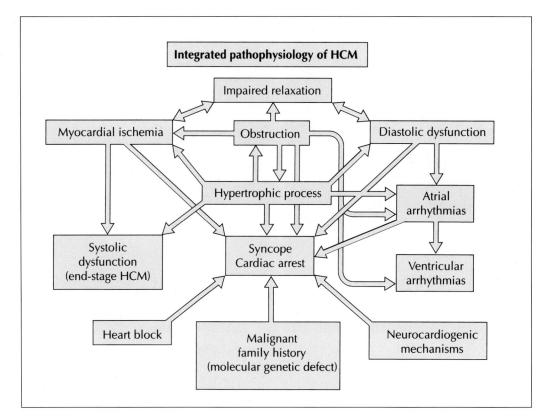

FIGURE 2-31. Myocardial ischemia, obstruction to left ventricular outflow, and diastolic dysfunction are the three principal ongoing problems in patients with HCM. These patients may also have intermittent problems, such as arrhythmias and syncope, or end-stage problems, such as HCM with impaired systolic function. The hypertrophic process may result in myocardial ischemia and/or diastolic dysfunction and either subaortic or midventricular obstruction, depending on the site of maximal hypertrophy. Both the outflow obstruction and diastolic dysfunction (ie, impaired relaxation) as well as left ventricular hypertrophy contribute to ischemia. Ischemia may, in turn, cause diastolic dysfunction by impairing relaxation (*see* Fig. 2-25), or syncope and sudden death in the young, [18] and ischemic fibrosis in end-stage HCM [19]. The obstruction to outflow may increase the degree of left ventricular hypertrophy, result in presyncope and syncope on exertion, and cause atrial arrhythmias (*see* Fig. 2-27) related to an increase in left atrial size (from the concomitant mitral regurgitation). Diastolic dysfunction is the other principal cause of increased left atrial size and atrial fibrillation in HCM (*see* Fig. 2-29). As indicated, there are a number of causes of syncope and sudden death in HCM, with myocardial ischemia being important in the young [18] and ventricular arrhythmias in older patients [24]. Obstruction to outflow is by far the most important cause of presyncope and syncope on exertion.

CLINICAL SYMPTOMS AND SIGNS

SYMPTOMS	
On exertion	Dyspnea, angina, presyncope, syncope, fatigue
On standing	Presyncope
Any time	Palpitations
At rest	Orthopnea, nocturnal dyspnea, and ankle swelling are rare in normal sinus rhythm but are encountered in end-stage HCM and with atrial fibrillation

FIGURE 2-32. Symptoms of HCM. Exertional and postural symptoms are more frequent and severe in obstructive HCM than in nonobstructive HCM. There is often a notable day-to-day variability in the severity of symptoms in subaortic obstructive HCM, which is believed to be due to variability in the obstruction. Symptoms of left or right heart failure are rare in normal sinus rhythm with normal systolic function, but may be prominent with atrial fibrillation or in the presence of impaired systolic function.

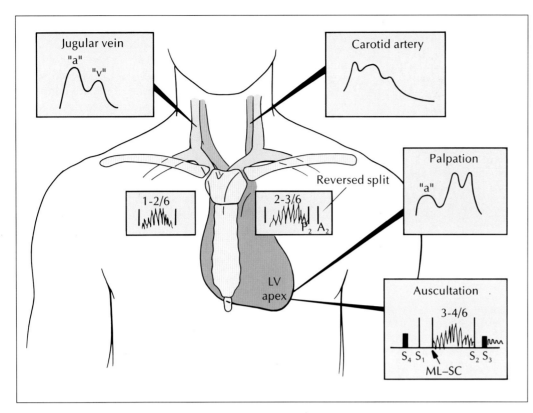

FIGURE 2-33. Physical examination in subaortic obstructive HCM. There are seven physical signs in subaortic obstructive HCM that are not found in nonobstructive HCM. On palpation, a spike-and-dome arterial pulse can often be felt in the carotid artery or in a peripheral pulse. On palpation of the left ventricular (LV) apex, there may be a triple apex beat caused by a palpable left atrial gallop and a double systolic impulse—one impulse comes before the onset of obstruction and the other after. On auscultation, at or just medial to the LV apex, there is a late onset, diamond-shaped systolic murmur of grade

3 to 4/6 in intensity. This murmur is caused by both the subaortic obstruction and the concomitant mitral regurgitation, causing the murmur to radiate to both the left sternal border and to the axilla. Because of the mitral regurgitation, there is often a short diastolic inflow murmur after the third heart sound. Rarely, a mitral leaflet–septal contact (ML–SC) sound may be heard preceding the systolic murmur at the apex. Finally, if there is severe subaortic obstruction, reversed splitting of the second heart sound may occur. In nonobstructive HCM, there is often a third or fourth heart sound at the apex, depending on the type of diastolic dysfunction (*see* Fig. 2-26). If the fourth heart sound is palpable, there will be a double apex beat, which is quite different in timing and significance from the double *systolic* apex beat that occurs in subaortic obstructive HCM. In nonobstructive HCM, there is either no apical systolic murmur or at most a grade 1 to 2/6 murmur of mitral regurgitation. In any type of HCM, a grade 1 to 3/6 systolic ejection murmur at or below the pulmonary area may be heard. This murmur may reflect obstruction to right ventricular (RV) outflow. Examining the jugular venous pulse frequently reveals a prominent a-wave that rises on inspiration, reflecting RV diastolic dysfunction. Rarely, this is accompanied by an RV fourth heart sound.

INVESTIGATION AND MANAGEMENT

TREATMENT OF OBSTRUCTIVE HCM VS NONOBSTRUCTIVE HCM WITH IMPAIRED SYSTOLIC FUNCTION (END-STAGE HCM)

	OBSTRUCTIVE HCM	END-STAGE HCM
Digoxin	-	+
Afterload reduction	-	+
Diuretics	-	+
Negative inotropes	+	-
Surgery	Myectomy	Transplant
Pacemaker	+	-

FIGURE 2-34. Treatment of obstructive HCM versus nonobstructive HCM with impaired systolic function (end-stage HCM). Medical treatment of obstructive HCM consists of administering negative inotropic agents (β-blockers, calcium antagonists, and disopyramide) to lessen the obstruction and avoiding drugs that might worsen the obstruction (digoxin, afterload-reducing agents, and diuretics). In contrast, medical therapy of end-stage HCM consists of discontinuing negative inotropic drugs (because no obstruction is present) and administering digoxin, afterload-reducing agents, and diuretics to improve ventricular function and relieve symptoms. Even the type of surgery is quite different for these different phases of the hypertrophic process.

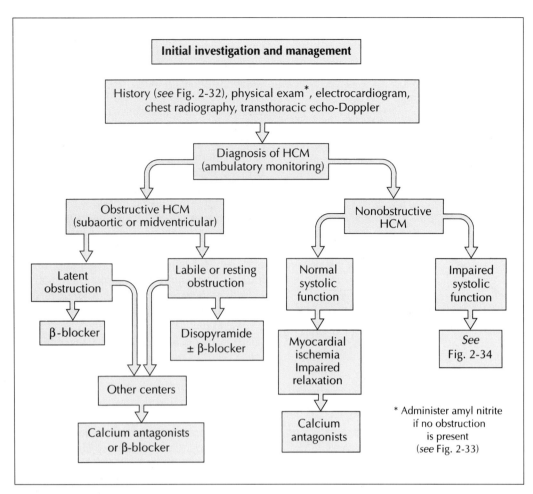

Initial investigation and management

History (*see* Fig. 2-32), physical exam*, electrocardiogram, chest radiography, transthoracic echo-Doppler

↓

Diagnosis of HCM (ambulatory monitoring)

Obstructive HCM (subaortic or midventricular)

Nonobstructive HCM

Latent obstruction → β-blocker

Labile or resting obstruction → Disopyramide ± β-blocker

Other centers → Calcium antagonists or β-blocker

Normal systolic function → Myocardial ischemia Impaired relaxation → Calcium antagonists

Impaired systolic function → *See* Fig. 2-34

* Administer amyl nitrite if no obstruction is present (*see* Fig. 2-33)

FIGURE 2-35. Initial investigation and management of HCM should include echocardiography and Doppler examination; if patients have no obstruction at rest clinically or by echocardiography, amyl nitrite should be inhaled to determine whether the patient has a latent obstruction (*see* Fig. 2-12) or no obstruction (*see* Fig. 2-7). Once HCM is diagnosed and the hemodynamic type is established, ambulatory monitoring should be used to determine if significant arrhythmias are present. Medical therapy for obstructive HCM consists of avoiding drugs that could worsen the obstruction (digoxin, afterload-reducing agents, or diuretics) and the administration of negative inotropic agents, which would act to decrease the obstruction (*see* Fig. 2-34). If the patient has latent obstruction, therapy with a β-blocker to prevent provocation of the obstruction is recommended. If the patient has a labile or resting obstruction, we would treat with disopyramide and add a β-blocker to slow the resting heart rate to 60 to 65 beats per minute, if required. Some centers treat obstructive HCM with calcium antagonists, especially verapamil, in the belief that the negative inotropic properties of the drug would lessen the obstruction. We do not use calcium antagonists for obstructive HCM because the vasodilating properties of these drugs may unpredictably worsen the obstruction, causing cardiogenic shock, pulmonary edema, and death [31]. We do, however, use calcium antagonists for the treatment of nonobstructive HCM with normal systolic function, especially when there is evidence of myocardial ischemia or impaired relaxation. The treatment of nonobstructive HCM with impaired systolic function is quite different from therapy when systolic function is normal in nonobstructive HCM, and is in direct contrast to the medical treatment of obstructive HCM (*see* Fig. 2-34).

INDICATIONS FOR SPECIAL TESTS

INDICATION	TEST
Angina pectoris	Stress thallium
Syncope or cardiac arrest	
Systolic dysfunction	Rest and exercise nuclear angiogram with
Diastolic dysfunction	diastolic function studies
Prior to or during myectomy surgery	Transesophageal echocardiogram/Doppler
Distinguish between subaortic and midventricular obstructive HCM	
Investigation of mitral regurgitation due to primary mitral valve disease in HCM	
When echocardiography fails to identify hypertrophy and HCM is strongly suspected	Magnetic resonance imaging
Considering pacemaker or surgical therapy	Hemodynamic and angiographic investigation +/- atrioventricular sequential pacing
If coronary disease is suspected	
Syncope or cardiac arrest	
Syncope or cardiac arrest	Invasive electrophysiologic testing
Sustained ventricular tachycardia	
Symptomatic nonsustained ventricular tachycardia on ambulatory monitoring	

FIGURE 2-36. Indications for special tests in HCM. After the initial investigation of HCM or after therapy has commenced (*see* Fig. 2-35) situations inevitably arise that require further investigation. This chart, although not meant to be exhaustive, indicates which tests might be appropriate in the presence of various common diagnostic and therapeutic problems.

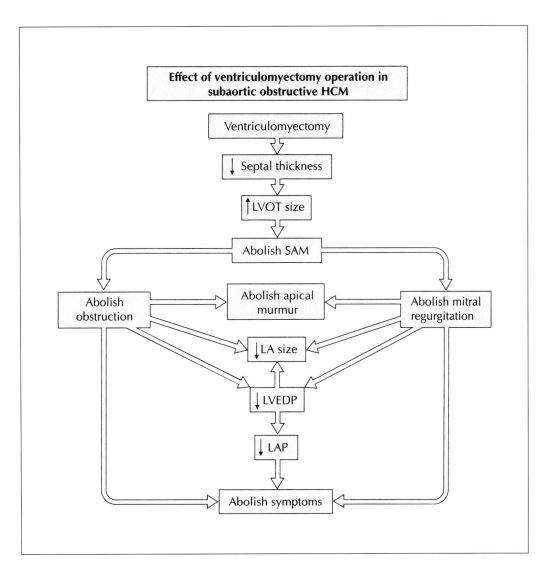

Effect of ventriculomyectomy operation in subaortic obstructive HCM

Ventriculomyectomy

↓ Septal thickness

↑ LVOT size

Abolish SAM

Abolish obstruction → Abolish apical murmur ← Abolish mitral regurgitation

↓ LA size

↓ LVEDP

↓ LAP

Abolish symptoms

FIGURE 2-37. Management of obstructive HCM that does not respond to medical therapy. When patients with obstructive HCM are unresponsive to medical therapy, or are dissatisfied by the disease-imposed limitations or the side effects of medication, atrioventricular sequential pacemaker therapy or surgery may be considered. Ventricular pacing from the right ventricular apex causes a rightward septal shift and alleviation of the subaortic obstruction with resultant symptomatic improvement in a significant number of patients. This form of therapy is not, however, effective in all patients. The obstruction is often not completely relieved, and up to 25% of patients require atrioventricular nodal ablation to achieve ventricular capture [33,34]. Ventriculomyectomy surgery, on the other hand, has been performed for over 30 years, and a number of centers have had extensive experience (and good to excellent results) [35–38]. The mechanisms of benefit of this procedure are illustrated. Myectomy thins the ventricular septum and widens the left ventricular outflow tract (LVOT), which abolishes mitral leaflet systolic anterior motion (SAM). This in turn abolishes the obstruction and mitral regurgitation. These effects eliminate the apical murmur and decrease the left ventricular end-diastolic pressure (LVEDP) as well as left atrial pressure (LAP) and size. Symptoms are dramatically relieved by these mechanisms. Myectomy is also indicated in recurrent atrial fibrillation to decrease left atrial size and restore normal sinus rhythm. The procedure should be performed in patients with obstructive HCM with unexplained syncope or cardiac arrest.

ETIOLOGY AND MANAGEMENT OF ATRIAL FIBRILLATION

Etiology	Increased left atrial size due to	
	Mitral regurgitation in subaortic obstructive HCM	
	Mitral regurgitation due to primary mitral valve disease, *eg*, mitral valve prolapse	
	Diastolic dysfunction	
	Systolic dysfunction (end-stage HCM)	
Management	Slow rate	β- or calcium blocker, digoxin
	Treat heart failure	Diuretics, *etc*
	Cardioversion	Pharmacologic or electrical
	Anticoagulation	Heparin or Coumadin
	Medical therapy	Systolic and/or diastolic dysfunction
	Surgery	Myectomy in obstructive HCM
		Mitral repair or replacement in primary mitral valve disease

FIGURE 2-38. Causes and management of atrial fibrillation. Atrial fibrillation in HCM almost always results from an increase in left atrial size. Increased left atrial size most commonly occurs in subaortic obstructive HCM, where it is related to the concomitant mitral regurgitation. There are other important causes of increased atrial size as shown. The management of atrial fibrillation in HCM involves rate slowing, treatment of heart failure, anticoagulant therapy, and pharmacologic or electrical cardioversion. If a β-blocker does not adequately slow the rate of atrial fibrillation in obstructive HCM, digoxin may be used to help slow the rate, since the β-blocker would offset the tendency of digoxin to increase the obstruction to outflow. In obstructive HCM, surgery is indicated to decrease or limit the increase of left atrial size. Successful myectomy is often effective in maintaining normal sinus rhythm in patients who have had multiple episodes of atrial fibrillation before surgery.

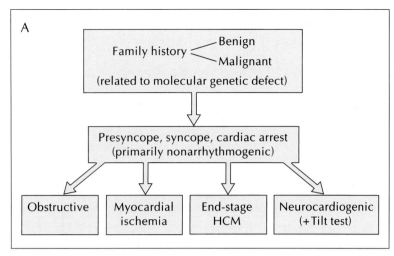

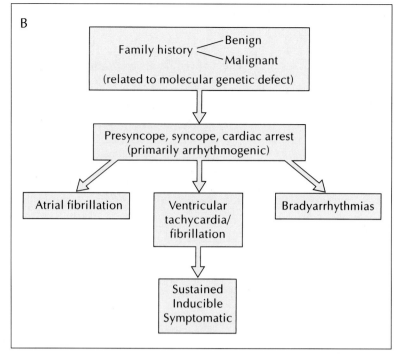

FIGURE 2-39. A and **B,** Etiology and management of syncope or resuscitated cardiac arrest in HCM. Sudden death is the commonest mode of death in HCM, making the etiology and management of presyncope, syncope, and resuscitated cardiac arrest of extreme importance. It is essential to determine whether these symptoms occur at rest or on exertion. In subaortic obstructive HCM, even minimal exertion such as standing suddenly or walking a few steps after standing or eating may occasionally result in presyncope-syncope due to the outflow tract obstruction. The management of HCM patients with syncope may be more or less aggressive, depending on whether there is a benign or malignant family history, which now appears to be related to the type of molecular genetic defect [49]. In obstructive HCM, a successful myectomy alone may suffice in the management of these symptoms [66], or antiarrhythmics or an automatic implantable cardiodefibrillator (AICD) may also be indicated. Myectomy would also be indicated in obstructive HCM if the syncope or cardiac arrest were believed to be related to myocardial ischemia, atrial fibrillation, or ventricular tachycardia. In young patients, myocardial ischemia may be associated with syncope, and medical therapy in nonobstructive cases with β- or calcium channel blockers may prevent recurrence. With cardiac arrest or positive electrophysiologic studies, antiarrhythmics and an AICD may be added to the treatment of ischemia [18]. Atrial fibrillation frequently causes presyncope or syncope and may progress to cardiac arrest. Pharmacologic or electrical cardioversion is mandatory followed by myectomy or antiarrhythmic therapy in obstructive HCM, or antiarrhythmic therapy alone in nonobstructive HCM (*see* Fig. 2-38). Ventricular tachycardia, whether nonsustained and symptomatic, sustained, or inducible at electrophysiologic studies, when associated with presyncope, syncope, or cardiac arrest, requires myectomy in obstructive HCM [25,66]. Antiarrhythmic (usually amiodarone) or AICD therapy may be an adjunct to surgery. In nonobstructive HCM, only drug therapy or an AICD is appropriate. Loss of consciousness with end-stage HCM may be best treated with a heart transplantation, and bradyarrhythmias and heart block are best treated with an atrioventricular sequential pacemaker. Neurocardiogenic syncope [67] in HCM may be treated with a β blocker in the absence of obstruction or by myectomy in obstructive HCM.

DIFFERENTIAL DIAGNOSIS

DIFFERENTIAL DIAGNOSIS OF SUBAORTIC OBSTRUCTIVE HCM

Midventricular obstruction
Mitral regurgitation
   Papillary muscle dysfunction
   Mitral valve prolapse
Combined aortic and mitral valve disease
Valvular aortic stenosis
Fibrous subaortic stenosis

Also distinguish subaortic obstruction due to HCM from subaortic obstruction in the elderly which is often associated with hypertension, a hypertrophied sigmoid septum, and/or mitral annular calcification

FIGURE 2-40. Differential diagnosis of subaortic obstructive HCM. With the availability of transthoracic and transesophageal echocardiographic and Doppler techniques, problems in the differential diagnosis of subaortic obstructive HCM are rare. Problems at the patient's bedside do arise, however, particularly in distinguishing subaortic from midventricular obstruction in HCM (*see* Fig. 2-22). Subaortic obstructive HCM must also be distinguished from different types of mitral regurgitation or mitral regurgitation combined with aortic stenosis because the murmur is maximal at or just medial to the apex. The differential diagnosis of subaortic obstructive HCM from certain types of mitral regurgitation may be particularly difficult in the emergency department, when the patient presents with atrial fibrillation and pulmonary edema. The differential diagnosis of valvular and fibrous subaortic stenoses from muscular subaortic stenosis is usually possible based on the peripheral pulse differences and the location of the maximal intensity of the murmur. It is important to distinguish idiopathic subaortic obstructive HCM from subaortic obstruction in the elderly. The latter disorder is often associated with hypertension and a sigmoid septum with or without mitral annular calcification [68–70]. A history of current hypertension, a family history of hypertension or HCM, or other manifestations of hypertension (such as retinopathy, age, and certain echocardiographic and Doppler findings) may help differentiate between these two forms of subaortic obstruction. In many cases, however, the cause of obstruction is in doubt, even at the end of a complete investigation. Screening for the molecular genetic defect in HCM may aid in this regard in the future.

REFERENCES

1. Liouville H: Retrécissement cardiaque sous aortique. *Gaz Med Paris* 1981, 24:161.

2. Hallopeau L: Retrécissement ventriculo-aortique. *Gaz Med Paris* 1869, 24:683.

3. Schmincke A: Ueber linksseitige muskulöse Conusstenosen. *Dtsch Med Wochenschr* 1907, 33:2082.

4. Brock RC: Functional obstruction of the left ventricle. *Guys Hosp Rep* 1957, 106:221–238.

5. Teare RD: Asymmetrical hypertrophy of the heart in young adults. *Br Heart J* 1958, 20:1–8.

6. Braunwald E, Lambrew C, Rockoff S, *et al.*: Idiopathic hypertrophic subaortic stenosis: I. Description of the disease based upon an analysis of 64 patients. *Circulation* 1964, 30(suppl 4):3–119.

7. Goodwin JF: Hypertrophic cardiomyopathy: a disease in search of its own identity. *Am J Cardiol* 1980, 45:177–180.

8. Wigle ED, Sasson Z, Henderson MA, *et al.*: Hypertrophic cardiomyopathy. The importance of the site and the extent of hypertrophy: a review. *Prog Cardiovasc Dis* 1985, 28:1–85.

9. Maron BJ, Bonow RO, Cannon RO, *et al.*: Hypertrophic cardiomyopathy: interrelations of clinical manifestations, pathophysiology, and therapy. *N Engl J Med* 1987, 316:780–789, 844–852.

10. Wigle ED: Hypertrophic cardiomyopathy: a 1987 viewpoint [editorial]. *Circulation* 1987, 75:311–322.

11. Shah P, Gramiak R, Kramer D: Ultrasound localization of left ventricular outflow obstruction in hypertrophic obstructive cardiomyopathy. *Circulation* 1969, 40:3–11.

12. Pollick C, Rakowski H, Wigle ED: Muscular subaortic stenosis: the quantitative relationship between systolic anterior motion and the pressure gradient. *Circulation* 1984, 69:43–49.

13. Falicov RE, Resnekov L, Bharati S, *et al.*: Midventricular obstruction: a variant of obstructive cardiomyopathy. *Am J Cardiol* 1976, 37:432–437.

14. Sakamoto T, Tei C, Murayama M, *et al.*: Giant negative T wave inversion as a manifestation of asymmetric apical hypertrophy (AAH) of the left ventricle: echocardiographic and ultrasono-cardiotomographic study. *Jpn Heart J* 1976, 17:611–629.

15. Yamaguchi H, Ishimura T, Nishiyama S, *et al.*: Hypertrophic nonobstructive cardiomyopathy with giant negative T waves (apical hypertrophy): ventriculographic and echocardiographic features in 30 patients. *Am J Cardiol* 1979, 444:401–411.

16. Oakley CM: *Hypertrophic Obstructive Cardiomyopathy: Patterns of Progression.* Edited by Wolstenholm GEW, O'Connor M. CIBA-Foundation Study Group 37, London: J & A Churchill; 1971:9–29.

17. Bonow RO, Frederick RM, Bacharach SL, *et al.*: Atrial systole and left ventricular filling in hypertrophic cardiomyopathy: effect of verapamil. *Am J Cardiol* 1983, 51:1386–1391.

18. Dilsizian V, Bonow RO, Epstein SE: Myocardial ischemia detected by thallium scintigraphy is frequently related to cardiac arrest and syncope in young patients with hypertrophic cardiomyopathy. *J Am Coll Cardiol* 1993, 22:796–804.

19. Maron BJ, Epstein SE, Roberts WC: Hypertrophic cardiomyopathy and transmural myocardial infarction without significant atherosclerosis of the extramural coronary arteries. *Am J Cardiol* 1979, 43:1086–1102.

20. Maron BJ, Savage DD, Wolfson JK, *et al.*: Prognostic significance of 24 hour ambulatory electrocardiographic monitoring in patients with hypertrophic cardiomyopathy: a prospective study. *Am J Cardiol* 1981, 48:252–257.

21. McKenna WJ, England D, Doi YL, *et al.*: Arrhythmia in hypertrophic cardiomyopathy. I: Influence on prognosis. *Br Heart J* 1981, 46:168–172.

22. McKenna W, Harris L, Deanfield J: Syncope in hypertrophic cardiomyopathy. *Br Heart J* 1982, 47:177–179.

23. Maron BJ, Lipson LC, Roberts WG, *et al.*: "Malignant" hypertrophic cardiomyopathy: identification of a subgroup of families with unusually frequent premature death. *Am J Cardiol* 1978, 41:1133–1140.

24. Fananapazir L, Chang AC, Epstein SE, *et al.*: Prognostic determinants in hypertrophic cardiomyopathy: prospective evaluation of a therapeutic strategy based on clinical, holter, hemodynamic and electrophysiological findings. *Circulation* 1992, 86:730–740.

25. Shah PM, Adelman AG, Wigle ED, *et al.*: The natural (and unnatural) history of hypertrophic obstructive cardiomyopathy. *Circ Res* 1975, 35:179–186.

26. Adelman AG, Wigle ED, Ranganathan N, *et al.*: The clinical course in muscular subaortic stenosis: a retrospective and prospective study of 60 hemodynamically proved cases. *Ann Intern Med* 1972, 77:515.

27. Spirito P, Chiarella F, Carratino L, *et al.*: Clinical course and prognosis of hypertrophic cardiomyopathy in an outpatient population. *N Engl J Med* 1989, 320:749.

28. Kofflard MJ, Waldstein DJ, Vos J, *et al.*: Prognosis in hypertrophic cardiomyopathy observed in a large clinic population. *Am J Cardiol* 1993, 72:939–943.

29. Wigle ED, Adelman AG, Felderhof CH: Medical and surgical treatment of cardiomyopathies. *Circ Res* 1974, 35:196–207.

30. Kaltenbach M, Hopf R, Kober G, *et al.*: Treatment of hypertrophic obstructive cardiomyopathy with verapamil. *Br Heart J* 1979, 42:35–42.

31. Rosing DR, Condit JR, Maron BJ, *et al.*: Verapamil therapy: a new approach to the pharmacologic treatment of hypertrophic cardiomyopathy: III. Effects of long-term administration. *Am J Cardiol* 1981, 48:545–553.

32. Pollick C: Muscular subaortic stenosis: hemodynamic and clinical improvement after disopyramide. *N Engl J Med* 1982, 307:997–999.

33. McDonald K, McWilliams E, O'Keeffe B, *et al.*: Functional assessment of patients treated with permanent dual chamber pacing as a primary treatment for hypertrophic cardiomyopathy. *Eur Heart J* 1988, 9:893–898.

34. Fananapazir L, Cannon RO, Tripodi D, *et al.*: Impact of dual-chamber permanent pacing in patients with obstructive hypertrophic and cardiomyopathy with symptoms refractory to verapamil and beta-adrenergic blocker therapy. *Circulation* 1992, 85:2149–2161.

35. Wigle ED, Chrysohou A, Bigelow W: Results of ventriculomyotomy in muscular subaortic stenosis. *Am J Cardiol* 1963, 11:572–586.

36. Maron BJ, Epstein SE, Morrow AG: Symptomatic status and prognosis of patients after operation for hypertrophic obstructive cardiomyopathy: efficacy of ventricular septal myotomy and myectomy. *Eur Heart J* 1983, 4(suppl F):175–185.

37. Beahrs MM, Tajik AJ, Seward JB, *et al.*: Hypertrophic obstructive cardiomyopathy: 10–21 year follow-up after partial septal myectomy. *Am J Cardiol* 1983, 51:1160–1166.

38. Williams WG, Wigle ED, Rakowski H, *et al.*: Results of surgery for idiopathic hypertrophic obstructive cardiomyopathy (IHSS). *Circulation* 1987, 76:V104–V108.

39. Wigle ED, Heimbecker RO, Gunton RW: Idiopathic ventricular septal hypertrophy causing muscular subaortic stenosis. *Circulation* 1962, 26:325–340.

40. Ross Jr J, Braunwald E, Gault JH, *et al.*: The mechanism of the intraventricular pressure gradient in idiopathic hypertrophic subaortic stenosis. *Circulation* 1966, 34:558–578.

41. Wigle ED, Marquis Y, Auger P: Muscular subaortic stenosis: initial left ventricular inflow tract pressure in the assessment of intraventricular pressure differences in man. *Circulation* 1967, 35:1100–1117.

42. Henry WL, Clark CE, Griffith JM, *et al.*: Mechanism of left ventricular outflow obstruction in patients with obstructive asymmetric septal hypertrophy (idiopathic hypertrophic subaortic stenosis). *Am J Cardiol* 1975, 35:337–345.

43. Gilbert BW, Pollick C, Adelman AG, *et al.*: Hypertrophic cardiomyopathy: subclassification by M-mode echocardiography. *Am J Cardiol* 1980, 45:861–872.

44. Shah PM, Taylor RD, Wong M: Abnormal mitral valve coaptation in hypertrophic obstructive cardiomyopathy: proposed role in systolic anterior motion of mitral valve. *Am J Cardiol* 1981, 48:258–262.

45. Rakowski H, Sasson Z, Wigle ED: Echocardiographic and Doppler assessment of hypertrophic cardiomyopathy. *J Am Soc Echocardiogr* 1988, 1:31–47.

46. Grigg LE, Wigle ED, Williams WG, *et al.*: Transesophageal Doppler echocardiography in obstructive hypertrophic cardiomyopathy: clarification of pathophysiology and importance in intraoperative decision making. *J Am Coll Cardiol* 1992, 20:42–52.

47. Bonow RD, Ostrow HG, Rosing DR, *et al.*: Effects of verapamil on left ventricular systolic and diastolic function in patients with hypertrophic cardiomyopathy: pressure volume analysis with a nonimaging scintillation probe. *Circulation* 1983, 68:1062–1073.

48. Jarcho JA, McKenna W, Pare JAP, *et al.*: Mapping a gene for familial hypertrophic cardiomyopathy to chromosome 14q1. *N Engl J Med* 1989, 321:1372–1378.

49. Watkins H, Rosenzweig A, Hwang DS, *et al.*: Characteristics and prognostic implications of myosin missense mutations in familial hypertrophic cardiomyopathy. *N Engl J Med* 1992, 326:1108–1114.

50. Hejtmancik JF, Brink PA, Towbin J, *et al.*: Localization of gene for familial hypertrophic cardiomyopathy to chromosome 14 q1 in a diverse US population. *Circulation* 1991, 83:1592–1597.

51. Epstein ND, Cohn GM, Cyran F, *et al.*: Differences in clinical expression of hypertrophic cardiomyopathy associated with two distinct mutations in β-myosin heavy chain gene. *Circulation* 1992, 86:345–352.

52. Watkins H, MacRae C, Thierfelder L, *et al.*: A disease locus for familial hypertrophic cardiomyopathy maps to chromosome 1q3. *Nat Genet* 1993, 3:333–337.

53. Thierfelder L, MacRae C, Watkins H, *et al.*: Two new loci for hypertrophic cardiomyopathy map to chromosome 15q2 (CMH3) and 11q (CMH4) [abstract]. *Circulation* 1993, 88:1–573.

54. Pollick C, Morgan CD, Gilbert BW, *et al.*: Muscular subaortic stenosis: the temporal relationship between systolic anterior motion of the anterior mitral leaflet and pressure gradient. *Circulation* 1982, 66:1087–1093.

55. Wigle ED, Adelman AG, Auger P, *et al.*: Mitral regurgitation in muscular subaortic stenosis. *Am J Cardiol* 1969, 24:698–706.

56. Adelman AG, McLoughlin MJ, Marquis Y, *et al.*: Left ventricular cineangiographic observations in muscular subaortic stenosis. *Am J Cardiol* 1969, 24:689–697.

57. Wigle ED, Adelman AG, Silver MD: Pathophysiological considerations in muscular subaortic stenosis. In *Hypertrophic Obstructive Cardiomyopathy*. Edited by Wolstenholme GEW, O'Connor M. Ciba Foundation Study Group 47, London: J & A Churchill; 1971: 63–70.

58. Jaing L, Levine RA, King ME, *et al.*: An integrated mechanism for systolic anterior motion of the mitral valve in hypertrophic cardiomyopathy based on echocardiographic observations. *Am Heart J* 1987, 113:633–644.

59. Sherrid MV, Chu CK, Delia E, *et al.*: An echocardiographic study of the fluid mechanics of obstruction in hypertrophic cardiomyopathy. *J Am Coll Cardiol* 1993, 22:816–825.

60. Jenni R, Ruffman K, Vieli A, *et al.*: Dynamics of aortic flow in hypertrophic cardiomyopathy. *Eur Heart J* 1985, 6:391–397.

61. Murgo JP, Alter BR, Dorethy JF, *et al.*: Dynamic aortic valve gradients in hypertrophic cardiomyopathy (HCM) [abstract]. *Circulation* 1979, 60(suppl):155.

62. Brutsaert DL, Sys SU, Gillebert TC: Diastolic failure: pathophysiology and therapeutic implications. *J Am Coll Cardiol* 1993, 22:318–325.

63. Wigle ED, Wilansky S: Diastolic dysfunction in hypertrophic cardiomyopathy. *Heart Failure* 1987, 3:82–93.

64. Suzuki J, Watanabe F, Takenaka K, *et al.*: New subtype of apical hypertrophic cardiomyopathy identified with nuclear magnetic resonance imaging as an underlying cause of markedly inverted T-waves. *J Am Coll Cardiol* 1993, 22:1175–1181.

65. Webb JG, Sasson Z, Rakowski H, *et al.*: Apical hypertrophic cardiomyopathy: clinical follow-up and diagnostic correlates. *J Am Coll Cardiol* 1990, 15:83–90.

66. Borggrefe M, Schwammenthal E, Block M, *et al.*: Pre- and post-operative electrophysiologic findings in survivors of cardiac arrest and hypertrophic obstructive cardiomyopathy undergoing myectomy [abstract]. *Circulation* 1993, 88:1–210.

67. Gilligan DM, Nihoyannopoulos P, Chan WL, *et al.*: Investigation of a hemodynamic basis for syncope in hypertrophic cardiomyopathy: use of a head-up tilt test. *Circulation* 1992, 85:2140–2148.

68. Topol EJ, Traill TA, Fortuin NJ: Hypertensive hypertrophic cardiomyopathy of the elderly. *N Engl J Med* 1985, 312:277–283.

69. Lever HM, Kuram RF, Currie PJ, *et al.*: Hypertrophic cardiomyopathy in the elderly: distinctions from the young based on cardiac shape. *Circulation* 1989, 79:580–589.

70. Lewis JF, Maron BJ: Elderly patients with hypertrophic cardiomyopathy: a subset with distinctive left ventricular morphology and progressive clinical course late in life. *J Am Coll Cardiol* 1989, 13:36–45.

IDIOPATHIC DILATED CARDIOMYOPATHY

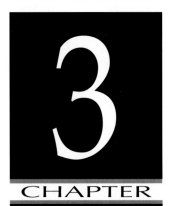

3

CHAPTER

Edward K. Kasper, Ralph H. Hruban, and Kenneth L. Baughman

Idiopathic dilated cardiomyopathy has been defined by the World Health Organization as dilatation of the left, right, or both ventricles, with impaired systolic function of unknown cause [1]. Overt congestive heart failure may or may not be present, arrhythmias are common, and the prognosis is often poor. Heart-muscle diseases of known cause, such as coronary artery disease or hypothyroidism, should be excluded. Therefore, the diagnosis of idiopathic dilated cardiomyopathy is made only after a complete evaluation for potential causes. There is a growing belief that this disorder may have multiple etiologies, with many factors potentially responsible in any single patient [2].

The usual criteria for impaired systolic function include a left ventricular ejection fraction of less than 40% to 45% calculated from echocardiography or ventriculography. Dilatation of the left ventricle is usually defined by a cardiothoracic ratio greater than 0.50 to 0.55 by chest radiography, or by a left ventricular internal diastolic dimension greater than 2.7 cm/m^2 of body surface area by echocardiography [3].

The diagnosis of idiopathic dilated cardiomyopathy can be made by many methods. Echocardiography has become a common tool for both diagnosis and follow-up of idiopathic dilated cardiomyopathy because it is readily available, relatively cost-effective, and noninvasive. Echocardiography may also be useful in predicting prognosis. The role of endomyocardial biopsy in the diagnosis of dilated cardiomyopathy remains controversial. The major role for endomyocardial biopsy may be in the exclusion of specific heart-muscle diseases, such as myocarditis and amyloidosis, which can present as dilated cardiomyopathy [3].

Treatment of idiopathic dilated cardiomyopathy is centered on symptomatic relief. The usual course is one of progressive decline, resulting in death or necessitating cardiac transplantation. The 1980s saw many advances in the treatment of congestive heart failure caused by systolic dysfunction. The mortality from idiopathic dilated cardiomyopathy, however, remains high, and our understanding of this disorder remains rudimentary.

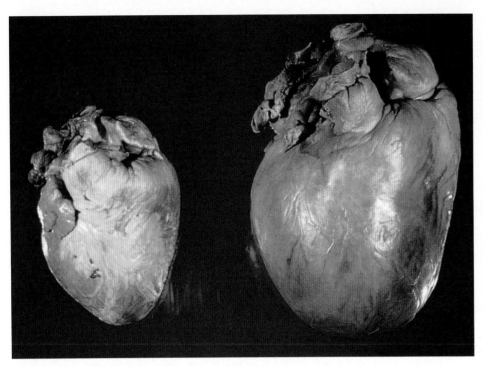 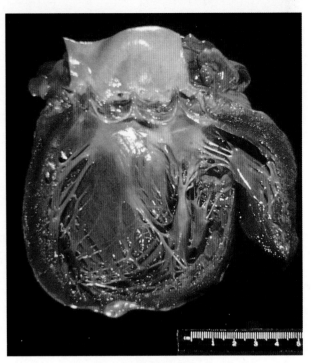

FIGURE 3-1. Gross pathology. In contrast to the normal heart (*left*), the heart in idiopathic dilated cardiomyopathy (*right*) is characterized by biventricular hypertrophy and four-chamber enlargement. The weight is often 25% to 50% above normal. Enlargement of the heart can be seen easily on chest radiography or cardiac echocardiography.

FIGURE 3-2. Gross pathology. The ventricular dilatation is even more apparent in this heart, which has been opened so that the interior of the left ventricle can be seen. Mural thrombi may develop in any cardiac chamber. Wall thickness usually remains normal, but the shape of the heart becomes globular.

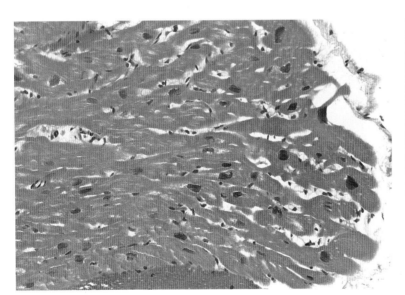 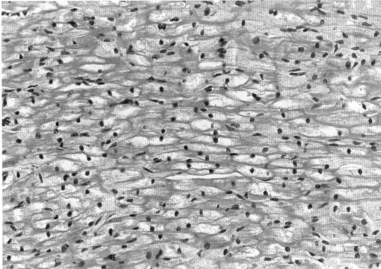

FIGURE 3-3. Endomyocardial biopsy from a patient with idiopathic cardiomyopathy. Large, irregularly shaped hyperchromatic nuclei are present, consistent with myocyte hypertrophy. The interstitium is cellular, but this should not be confused with myocarditis. These features, although nonspecific, support the diagnosis of idiopathic dilated cardiomyopathy. A completely normal endomyocardial biopsy does not support a diagnosis of idiopathic dilated cardiomyopathy and should suggest a focal cause, such as sarcoidosis, which requires further investigation [3].

FIGURE 3-4. Glycogen storage disease. Endomyocardial biopsy from a patient with a dilated heart and congestive heart failure as a result of type II glycogen storage disease. The intracytoplasmic clearing is caused by the accumulation of glycogen. Hemochromatosis, amyloidosis, sarcoidosis, adriamycin cardiotoxicity, and myocarditis are some of the potential causes of dilated cardiomyopathy that can be diagnosed by endomyocardial biopsy.

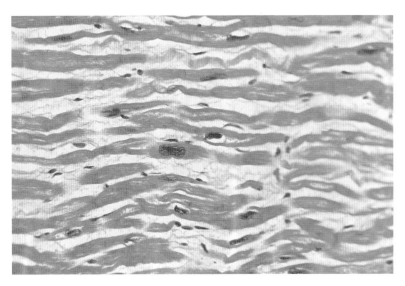

FIGURE 3-5. Dilated cardiomyopathy caused by myocarditis. This specimen is from the explanted left ventricle of a patient who underwent cardiac transplantation. The nonspecific features are similar to those seen in Fig. 3-3. The patient previously had myocarditis, diagnosed on biopsy, which did not respond to immunosuppressive therapy and resulted in dilated cardiomyopathy. Not all cases of idiopathic dilated cardiomyopathy are caused by a previous myocarditis.

DIFFERENTIAL DIAGNOSIS

EXTRAMYOCARDIAL CARDIOVASCULAR DIFFERENTIAL DIAGNOSES OF DILATED CARDIOMYOPATHY

Hypertension	Congenital heart disease
Coronary artery disease	Uncontrolled tachycardia
Valvular artery disease	Previous bypass

FIGURE 3-6. Extramyocardial causes that should be considered in the differential diagnosis of dilated cardiomyopathy. These disorders have histologic features that are indistinguishable from those of idiopathic dilated cardiomyopathy. Diagnosis can be made only by other means, such as clinical, historical, or angiographic data. Several of these disorders, such as uncontrolled tachycardia, may cause a reversible form of dilated cardiomyopathy.

SPECIFIC HEART-MUSCLE DISEASES

Heredofamilial	Sensitivities and toxic reactions
Familial cardiomyopathy	Ethanol
Muscular dystrophies	Anthracycline
Infectious	Cocaine
Bacterial	Cobalt
Viral	Catecholamines
Human immunodeficiency virus	Corticosteroids
Other	Lithium
Metabolic	Radiation
Endocrine	Heavy metal
Nutritional	Scorpion sting
Storage diseases	Other
Myocarditis	Uremia
Neoplastic	Anemia
Peripartum	Leukemia
Systemic	Obesity
Infiltrative	
Connective tissue disease	

FIGURE 3-7. Specific causes of dilated cardiomyopathy. These are also called secondary cardiomyopathies or specific heart-muscle diseases. Almost any disease process can involve cardiac muscle, as can be seen from this list. Multiple factors may actually play a causative role in any single patient. (*Adapted from* Abelmann [4]; with permission.)

EPIDEMIOLOGY OF IDIOPATHIC DILATED CARDIOMYOPATHY

STUDY	TIME PERIOD	TYPE OF STUDY	CASES, N	RATE
Dilated cardiomyopathy				
Codd et al. [5]	1975–1984	Incidence	45	6.0*
Torp [6]	1970–1979	Incidence	89	3.6
			132	5.3
			188	7.5
Bagger et al. [7]	1980–1981	Incidence	41	0.7
Codd et al. [5]	1/1/85	Prevalence	29	36.5*
Williams and Olsen [8]	1983–1984	Prevalence	76	8.3
Hypertrophic cardiomyopathy				
Codd et al. [5]	1975–1984	Incidence	19	2.5
Bagger et al. [7]	1980–1981	Incidence	20	0.4
Codd et al. [5]	1/1/85	Prevalence	15	19.7*
Bjarnason et al. [9]	1966–1977	Prevalence	11	33
Hada et al. [10]		Prevalence	22	170

FIGURE 3-8. The incidence per 100,000 person-years and prevalence per 100,000 population of both idiopathic dilated cardiomyopathy and hypertrophic cardiomyopathy are summarized from several epidemiologic studies [5–10]. Few true incidence studies are available, and estimates vary considerably. The incidence of idiopathic dilated cardiomyopathy in the Olmsted County, Minnesota study [5] increased during the study period (1975 to 1984). This may reflect improved case ascertainment. *Asterisks* indicate the overall incidence per 100,000 person-years or prevalence per 100,000 population, directly age- and sex-adjusted to the 1980 United States white population. (*Adapted from* Codd and coworkers [5]; with permission.)

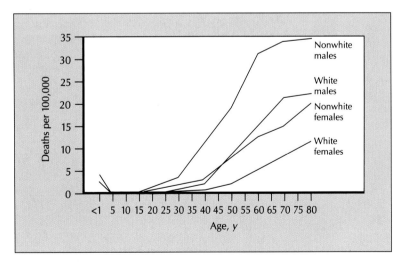

FIGURE 3-9. Deaths per 100,000 population for idiopathic cardiomyopathy in the United States from 1979 to 1983. Death certificate data from the National Center for Health Statistics show a greater death rate for affected nonwhites than whites, with nonwhite men having the greatest death rate and white women the lowest death rate. A case-controlled study from Baltimore showed a 2.7-fold increased risk of idiopathic dilated cardiomyopathy associated with the black race [11]. The increased risk in blacks was not accounted for by income, alcohol use, or body size. (*Adapted from* Gillum [12]; with permission.)

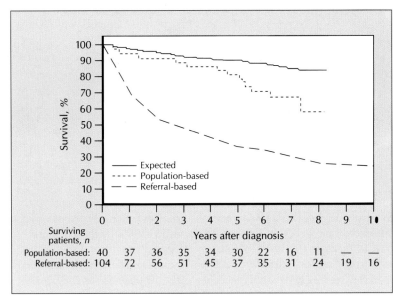

FIGURE 3-10. Survival after the initial diagnosis of idiopathic dilated cardiomyopathy. Survival among residents of Olmsted County, Minnesota, from 1975 to 1984 was poor [5]. Survival was better in a population-based rather than a referral-based cohort of patients. Not surprisingly, however, survival was still impaired compared with an age- and sex-matched cohort without idiopathic dilated cardiomyopathy (expected). (*Adapted from* Sugrue and coworkers [13]; with permission.)

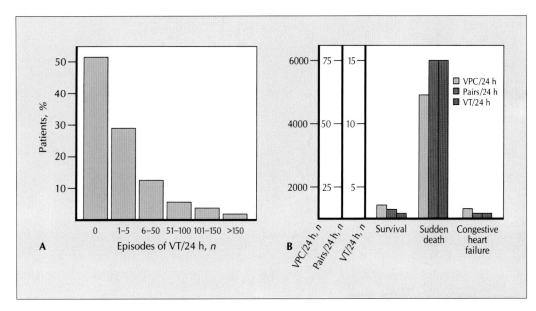

FIGURE 3-11. Ventricular arrhythmias in idiopathic dilated cardiomyopathy. **A,** The number of episodes of ventricular tachycardia (VT) during 24-hour monitoring in patients with idiopathic dilated cardiomyopathy and VT. Complex ventricular ectopy was seen in 87% and VT was seen in 49% of the patients. Ventricular arrhythmias are common in this patient population. **B,** Ventricular arrhythmias during 24-hour monitoring in patients who died suddenly, in patients who died from congestive heart failure, and in those who survived. Patients who died suddenly had a higher incidence of VT, ventricular pairs, and ventricular premature contractions (VPC). Ventricular arrhythmias are predictive of a poor prognosis in general, and in this study, of sudden death. (*Adapted from* Meinertz and coworkers [14]; with permission.)

EMBOLI ORIGINATING IN THE HEART IN IDIOPATHIC DILATED CARDIOMYOPATHY

CLINICAL DATA, N	PATIENTS WITH EMBOLI, N(%)	EXPOSURE, PATIENT-YEARS	EVENTS/100 PATIENT-YEARS
Treatment with anticoagulant agents			
Yes (n=32)	0(0)	101	0
No (n=103)	19(18)	624	3.5
Atrial fibrillation			
Yes (n=24)	8(33)	—	—
No (n=80)	11(14)	—	—

FIGURE 3-12. Patients with systemic emboli and idiopathic dilated cardiomyopathy. There is a higher incidence of systemic emboli in patients with dilated hearts from any cause. In this study of 104 patients there were no emboli in those treated with anticoagulant agents. Although 33% of the patients in atrial fibrillation had systemic emboli as compared with 14% of patients not in atrial fibrillation, this did not achieve statistical significance. (*Adapted from* Fuster and coworkers [15]; with permission.)

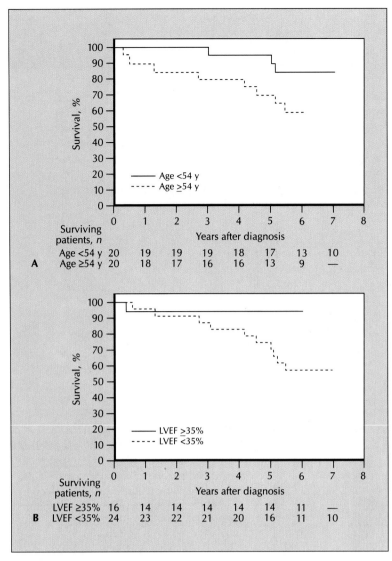

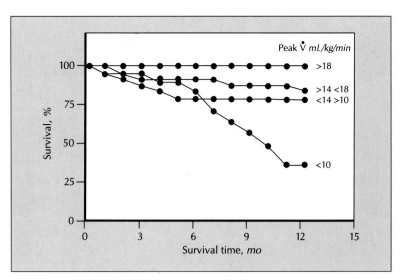

FIGURE 3-14. Peak oxygen consumption ($\dot{V}O_2$) and survival in heart failure. Peak $\dot{V}O_2$ provides an objective measure of functional capacity. In this particular study, 54% of the patients had idiopathic dilated cardiomyopathy and the other 46% had ischemic cardiomyopathy. Peak $\dot{V}O_2$, measured during maximal exercise testing with analysis of respiratory gases, was the best predictor of survival. A peak $\dot{V}O_2$ of less than 10 mL/min/kg, consistent with severe cardiopulmonary dysfunction, was associated with a significantly worse prognosis. (*Adapted from* Mancini and coworkers [16]; with permission.)

FIGURE 3-13. Effect of age (**A**) and ejection fraction (**B**) on survival after the diagnosis of idiopathic dilated cardiomyopathy. Both older age (≥54 years) and lower left ventricular ejection fraction (LVEF; <35%) were independently associated with impaired survival. (*Adapted from* Sugrue and coworkers [13]; with permission.)

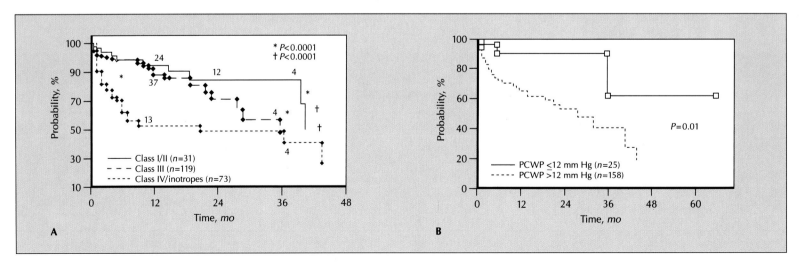

FIGURE 3-15. Effect of New York Heart Association symptom class (**A**) and pulmonary wedge pressure (PCWP; **B**) on actuarial survival in patients with either ischemic or idiopathic dilated cardiomyopathy. Numbers in parentheses indicate the number of patients at entry. Most studies have found both right heart hemodynamics and functional classification to be predictive only when they are markedly abnormal. It is often difficult to predict survival in patients with moderately severe symptoms. (*Adapted from* Keogh and coworkers [17]; with permission.)

NEUROHORMONAL STIMULATION AND PROGNOSIS IN CONGESTIVE HEART FAILURE

HORMONE	SURVIVORS (n=68)	DEATHS (n=51)	P VALUE
Angiotensin II, *pg/mL*	64±9	93±9	<0.001
Aldosterone, *pmol/L*	1108±95	1627±120	<0.001
Atrial natriuretic factor, *pg/mL*	320±95	520±61	<0.01
Norepinephrine, *pg/mL*	750±46	1188±106	<0.001
Adrenaline, *pg/mL*	119±17	239±39	<0.05

FIGURE 3-16. Multiple studies have shown a correlation between neurohormonal stimulation and mortality in congestive heart failure. The Cooperative North Scandinavian Enalapril Survival Study (CONSENSUS) compared enalapril with placebo in patients with New York Heart Association class IV symptoms of congestive heart failure. The hormones were measured at baseline in the placebo group and related to 6-month mortality. The majority of patients in the study had coronary artery disease. Neurohormonal stimulation probably plays an important pathophysiologic role in the progression of disease and clearly predicts prognosis. Values for survivors and deaths are means ± SEM. (*Adapted from* Swenberg and coworkers [18]; with permission.)

FACTORS ASSOCIATED WITH A POOR PROGNOSIS

History and physical examination
  NYHA class IV symptoms
  Prolonged symptom duration
  Low MAP
  Presence of S_3
Electrocardiography
  Left bundle branch block
  Atrial fibrillation
  Ventricular ectopy
Ventriculography
  Diffuse wall motion abnormalities
  Spherical LV geometry
  Low LVEF
  Low RVEF
  Mitral regurgitation
  Large LVEDD

Hemodynamics
  Low cardiac index
  High PCWP
  High PAS pressure
  High RA pressure
  High systemic vascular resistance
Exercise tolerance
  Low $M\dot{V}O_2$
Neurohormonal activation
  Elevated levels of
    Norepinephrine
    Epinephrine
    Angiotensin II
    Atrial natriuretic factor

FIGURE 3-17. Summary of factors associated with a poor prognosis in idiopathic dilated cardiomyopathy. Unfortunately, the prognosis in a given patient is often difficult to predict. We find peak oxygen consumption ($M\dot{V}O_2$) to be particularly useful, and use this extensively in both the timing of cardiac transplantation and the long-term follow-up of patients with dilated cardiomyopathy. LV—left ventricular; LVEDD—LV end-diastolic dimension; LVEF—LV ejection fraction; MAP—mean arterial pressure; NYHA—New York Heart Association; PAS—pulmonary artery systolic; PCWP—pulmonary capillary wedge pressure; RA—right atrial; RVEF—right ventricular ejection fraction.

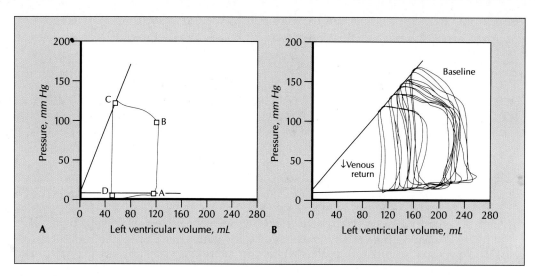

FIGURE 3-18. Pressure-volume loops from a patient with a normal heart (**A**) and a patient with idiopathic dilated cardiomyopathy (**B**). Pressure-volume loops have been useful in understanding the pathophysiology of heart failure. In a single pressure-volume loop from a patient with a normal heart (*A*), systole begins at A with the onset of isovolumic contraction. With the opening of the aortic valve (B), ventricular ejection occurs and intraventricular volume decreases. C is end-systole. Isovolumic relaxation then follows, causing a decrease in intraventricular pressure. Finally, ventricular filling (D) causes a slow rise in intraventricular volume until systole occurs again and another counterclockwise loop is formed. The area within each pressure-volume loop represents the work performed by the ventricle. Pressure-volume loops are confined between the end-systolic (*upper line*) and end-diastolic (*lower line*) relationships (*B*).

The end-systolic line represents the inotropic state of the ventricle. A decrease in contractility would be seen as a downward shift in the end-systolic pressure-volume relationship. The end-diastolic line represents the lusiotropic state of the ventricle. A decrease in compliance would shift the end-diastolic pressure-volume relationship upward. The pressure-volume loop at rest is at the far right. The other pressure-volume loops show the effects of a decrease in venous return caused by inflation of a balloon in the inferior vena cava. This patient had a 10-year history of idiopathic dilated cardiomyopathy. Blood pressure was high because he was withdrawn from all cardiac medications for 24 hours before the study. There is a marked rightward and down-ward shift in the end-systolic pressure-volume relationship (decreased contractility), moving the entire loop to the right (ventricular dilation). There is a shift upward in the end-diastolic pressure-volume relationship consistent with increased filling pressures and a decrease in left ventricular compliance. These changes are characteristic of patients with dilated cardiomyopathy.

CELLULAR AND MOLECULAR CHANGES IN THE FAILING HUMAN HEART

CELLULAR CHANGES

Decreased: β_1-adrenergic receptor
cAMP
Myofibrillar ATPase
SR calcium transport ATPase
Vasoactive intestinal peptide receptor

Increased: G_i (functional activity)
Troponin T_2 isoform
LDH_5 isoform
ADP/ATP carrier content of inner mitochondrial membrane (decreased functional activity)
Extracellular matrix

MOLECULAR CHANGES IN mRNA LEVELS

Decreased: β-adrenergic receptor
Phospholamban
SR calcium transport ATPase
SR calcium release channel

Increased: Atrial and brain natriuretic factor (from ventricular myocardium)

FIGURE 3-19. Cellular and molecular changes in the failing human heart. Multiple abnormalities of cellular function have been described in dilated cardiomyopathy. Similarly, we are beginning to understand the molecular changes that occur with a failing heart. Most of these abnormalities probably represent changes that occur with, rather than cause, a failing heart. LDH—lactate dehydrogenase; SR—sarcoplasmic reticulum.

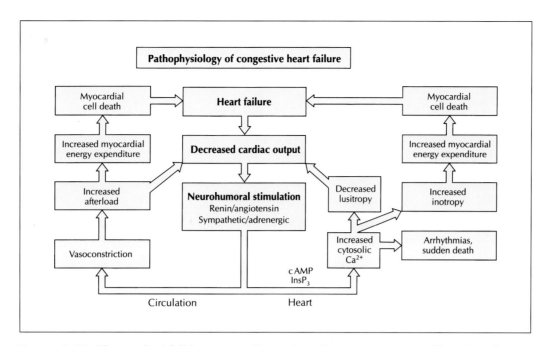

FIGURE 3-20. The marked fall in contractility and cardiac output seen in dilated cardio-myopathy eventually leads to neurohormonal stimulation, with several consequences. Within the heart, an increase in cytosolic calcium (Ca^{2+}) mediated by either cAMP or inositol-1,4,5-tris phosphate ($InsP_3$) augments contractility at the expense of increased arrhythmias and decreased lusiotropy. The increased inotropy will increase myocardial energy expenditure and potentially lead to cell death, with a concomitant fall in cardiac output. A similar negative feedback loop is found in the circulation, where an increase in $InsP_3$ causes smooth muscle contraction and vasoconstriction. The resultant increase in afterload will increase myocardial energy expenditure and potentially lead to cell death. Therefore, initial short-term adaptive responses to maintain cardiac output and blood pressure can be deleterious if maintained indefinitely. Neurohormonal stimulation is central to this schema and offers a rationale for the use of angiotensin-converting enzyme inhibitors and β-adrenergic blockers. (*Adapted from* Katz [19]; with permission.)

IMMUNOLOGIC ABNORMALITIES IN IDIOPATHIC DILATED CARDIOMYOPATHY

Defective lymphocyte activity
  Natural killer cell
  Suppressor T cell
Autoantibodies directed against
  β-adrenergic receptor
  ADP/ATP carrier
  Branch-chain ketoacid dehydrogenase complex
  Myosin heavy chain
  Laminin
  Heat shock proteins
  Unspecified heart antigens
Induction of major histocompatibility class I and class II
  antigens on myocytes
Increased frequency of HLA-DR4
Presence of enteroviral genome in ventricular myocardium

FIGURE 3-21. Immunologic abnormalities in idiopathic dilated cardiomyopathy. The myocardial damage that initiates the decrease in contractility seen in patients with this condition may be immuno-logically mediated. Several immune abnormalities have been noted in patients with idiopathic dilated cardiomyopathy. Although some patients may have a dilated cardiomyopathy caused by a previous myocarditis, with subsequent clearing of the cellular infiltrate, not all cases of idiopathic dilated cardiomyopathy are the result of healed myocarditis. The importance of the various immune abnor-malities requires further investigation.

CLINICAL MANIFESTATIONS

CLINICAL FINDINGS IN IDIOPATHIC DILATED CARDIOMYOPATHY

Physical examination	Echocardiography	Ventriculography (nuclear or contrast)	Endomyocardial biopsy
Elevated JVP with large V waves	LVEDD>2.7 cm/m^2	LVEF<40%	Myocyte hypertrophy
Venous congestion, rales, and peripheral edema	LVEF<40%	LVEDV>80 mL/m^2	Interstitial fibrosis
Diffuse apical impulse	LVFS<30%		Exclusion of specific heart-muscle diseases
Soft heart sounds	Mitral E-point septal separation>1 cm		
S$_3$, S$_4$			
Often murmurs of MR or TR			

FIGURE 3-22. Clinical findings in idiopathic dilated cardiomyopathy. The symptoms and physical examination of patients with this disorder are nonspecific. The history and physical examination should be directed at potentially reversible causes of dilated cardiomyopathy (*see* Fig. 3-29). There are multiple means of diagnosing idiopathic dilated cardiomyopathy. Echocardiography is the most widely available. Commonly used criteria are listed. The utility of endomyocardial biopsy remains controversial. However, it continues to be useful in excluding specific heart-muscle diseases that can result in dilated cardiomyopathy, such as myocarditis, amyloidosis, sarcoidosis, and hemochromatosis [3]. JVP—jugular venous pressure; LVEDD—left ventricular end-diastolic dimension; LVEDV—left ventricular end-diastolic volume; LVEF—left ventricular ejection fraction; LVFS—left ventricular fractional shortening; MR—mitral regurgitation; TR—tricuspid regurgitation. (*Adapted from* Manolio and coworkers [3]; with permission.)

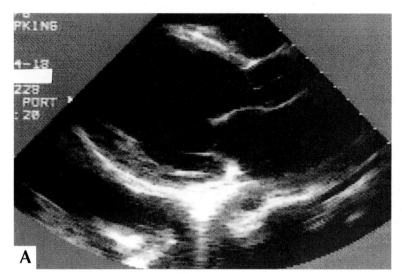

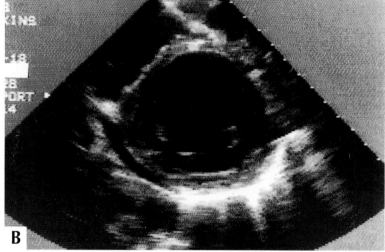

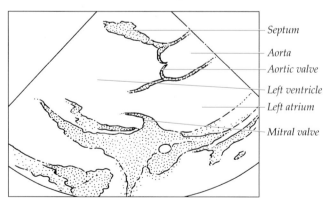

FIGURE 3-23. Echocardiographic parasternal long-axis (**A**) and short-axis (**B**) views in a 26-year-old patient with idiopathic dilated cardiomyopathy. The chambers are dilated and the walls are thin. Mitral and tricuspid regurgitation are common. The presence of a segmental wall motion abnormality does not necessarily imply the presence of coronary artery disease. In a study of 50 patients with dilated cardiomyopathy, 64% had segmental wall motion abnormalities and a better prognosis compared with those who had diffuse wall motion abnormalities [20].

ECG ABNORMALITIES SEEN IN IDIOPATHIC DILATED CARDIOMYOPATHY

ABNORMALITY	INCIDENCE, %
Rhythm	
Sinus	76
Atrial fibrillation	25
QRS axis abnormality	50
Atrial abnormality	49
Ventricular hypertrophy	44
Left only	38
Right only	5
Both	1
Conduction abnormality	
Prolonged (>0.20 s) P-R interval	23
Second degree atrioventricular block	1
Complete atrioventricular block	1
Complete bundle branch block	51
Left	41
Right	6
Indeterminant intraventricular conduction delay	4
Low voltage (sum QRS in I, II + III ≤15 mm)	22
Myocardial damage pattern	38
A. Poor R-wave progression precordial leads	22
B. Q wave II, III, aVF	7
C. Q wave I, AVL, V$_{4-6}$	2
D. Combinations A + B =	5
B + C =	2
Nonspecific ST-T wave changes	12

FIGURE 3-24. Electrocardiographic (ECG) abnormalities seen in 101 patients with idiopathic dilated cardiomyopathy [16]. In this autopsy study, ECG findings consistent with an old anteroseptal infarct were present in 22% of the patients. The ECG findings in idiopathic dilated cardiomyopathy are often confused with prior myocardial infarction until coronary arteriography shows normal coronary arteries. A variety of nonspecific ECG findings can be seen. (*Adapted from* Roberts and coworkers [21]; with permission.)

THERAPY

REVERSIBLE OR EXACERBATING CAUSES OF DILATED CARDIOMYOPATHY

Infectious causes (including sepsis)
Metabolic causes
  Endocrine
    Pheochromocytoma
    Thyroid disease
  Nutritional
    Beriberi
    Kwashiorkor
    Selenium deficiency
    (Keshan's disease)
Myocarditis
Peripartum
Sensitivities and toxic reactions
  Ethanol
  Catecholamines

Corticosteroids
Lithium
Scorpion sting
Extramyocardial cardiovascular causes
  Hypertension
  Coronary artery disease
  Valvular heart disease
  Uncontrolled tachycardia
Other causes
  Uremia
  Hypokalemia
  Hypocalcemia
  Carnitine deficiency
  Anemia
  Obesity

FIGURE 3-25. Reversible or exacerbating causes of dilated cardiomyopathy. There is no specific therapy for idiopathic dilated cardiomyopathy. Management of this disorder should include a search for potentially reversible or exacerbating causes. This can usually be accomplished with a complete history and physical examination, routine electrolyte and hematologic analysis, thyroid function tests, antinuclear antibody screening, and endomyocardial biopsy.

MANAGEMENT OF OUTPATIENTS WITH DILATED CARDIOMYOPATHY

Maximize use of angiotensin-converting enzyme inhibitors
Minimize diuretic use
  Restrict fluids
  Aim for a "dry" weight and allow patient to adjust diuretic dose
  Monitor serum potassium and magnesium
Use low-dose digoxin to avoid toxicity
Use coumadin for low-level anticoagulation
Maintain normal sinus rhythm (rather than atrial fibrillation)
Adjunctive measures
  Weight loss
  Cardiac rehabilitation, exercise
  Avoidance of cardiotoxic substances (ethanol, tobacco)
  Emotional support

FIGURE 3-26. Some basic principles of management of ambulatory patients with dilated cardiomyopathy, such as the points listed in this table, are often overlooked. Patients in New York Heart Association classes III and IV especially need close follow-up and should be seen frequently, since they have a tendency to deteriorate rapidly. It may be necessary to see some particularly ill patients on a weekly basis.

RESULTS OF VASODILATOR TRIALS IN CONGESTIVE HEART FAILURE

TRIAL	TREATMENT	NYHA CLASS	PATIENTS, n	SURVIVAL BENEFIT
V-HeFT I [22]	Hyd-Iso vs prazosin vs placebo	II,III	642	Hyd-Iso
CONSENSUS I [23]	Enalapril vs placebo	IV	253	Enalapril
V-HeFT II [24]	Hyd-Iso vs enalapril	II,III	804	Enalapril
SOLVD Treatment [25]	Enalapril vs placebo	II,III	2569	Enalapril
SOLVD Prevention [26]	Enalapril vs placebo	I	4228	No difference

FIGURE 3-27. The results of various vasodilator trials in patients with chronic heart failure. These large studies included patients with ischemic cardiomyopathy, but the results are also applicable to patients with idiopathic dilated cardiomyopathy. The SOLVD Prevention Trial, although not showing a survival benefit, did show a decrease in hospitalizations for congestive heart failure and a prolongation of the asymptomatic phase. The results of these studies suggest the use of selective vasodilators in all patients with dilated cardiomyopathy [22–26]. CONSENSUS—Cooperative North Scandinavian Enalapril Survival Study; Hyd-Iso—hydralazine-isosorbide dinitrate; NYHA—New York Heart Association; SOLVD—Studies of Left Ventricular Dysfunction; V-HeFT—Veterans Heart Failure Trial.

PRINCIPLES OF ACE INHIBITOR USE

Start drug early
Start at a low dose
Titrate to maximally tolerated dose
Tolerate low peripheral BP
  Arm BP < central BP
Decrease diuretics as needed
Decrease potassium replacement as needed

FIGURE 3-28. Principles of angiotensin-converting enzyme (ACE) inhibitor use in patients with idiopathic dilated cardiomyopathy. We use enalapril and captopril because the newer agents do not offer any substantial improvements. Captopril offers the advantage of a short half-life, making it ideal for acute titration. Cough, a common side effect of these drugs, must not be confused with the cough from pulmonary edema. An increase in serum creatinine, a side effect seen in patients with renal artery stenosis, may also be due to diuretic-induced volume depletion. Neither of these findings is necessarily a reason to withhold the drug. Angioneurotic edema, however, is a class side effect; switching to another agent within this class is contraindicated. The use of additional vasodilators may be warranted in patients with high systemic vascular resistance despite therapy with an ACE inhibitor. BP—blood pressure.

PRINCIPLES OF DIURETIC USE IN DILATED CARDIOMYOPATHY

Asymptomatic left ventricular dysfunction
  Restrict sodium intake
  Angiotensin-converting enzyme inhibitor
Mild sodium and fluid retention
  Low-dose loop diuretic
  Daily weights
  Adjustment by patient of diuretic dose to maintain "dry" weight
  Avoid use of prostaglandin inhibitors
Moderate sodium and fluid retention
  Restrict fluid intake
  Increase dose of loop diuretic
  Triamterene (aldosterone antagonist)
Severe sodium and fluid retention
  Increase dose of loop diuretic
  Add metolazone (thiazide)
  Consider admission to hospital
Refractory sodium and fluid retention
  Admission to hospital
  Intermittent intravenous loop diuretic
  Renal-dose dopamine or low-dose positive inotropic agent
  Consider ultrafiltration or dialysis
  Consider short-term infusion of loop diuretic

FIGURE 3-29. Principles of diuretic use. A loop agent is usually needed to control excessive sodium and fluid retention associated with pulmonary and systemic vascular congestion. However, use of the lowest possible dose of loop diuretic is optimal. Triamterene can be useful in conserving renal potassium and magnesium loss. The combination of an angiotensin-converting enzyme inhibitor and triamterene may lead to hyperkalemia. Careful management of electrolytes is important, aiming to keep the serum potassium greater than 4.5 mg/dL and the serum magnesium greater than 2 mg/dL.

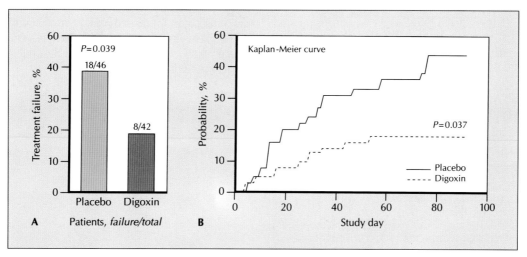

FIGURE 3-30. Use of digoxin in dilated cardiomyopathy. Several studies have shown a deterioration in exercise tolerance in patients with chronic stable heart failure who were withdrawn from digoxin. **A,** The number of patients and the cumulative incidence of treatment failure in 88 patients in normal sinus rhythm with chronic, stable, mild to moderate congestive heart failure caused by left ventricular systolic dysfunction. Digoxin was withdrawn in 46 patients (placebo group) and continued in the other 42 patients (digoxin group). There was an increased incidence of treatment failure in the group withdrawn from digoxin. **B,** Time to treatment of heart failure during the study period. The group withdrawn from digoxin required treatment for congestive heart failure sooner than did the group continued on digoxin. Exercise capacity was also worse in the placebo group. There is now strong evidence for the clinical efficacy of digoxin in patients with normal sinus rhythm and dilated cardiomyopathy with mild to moderate symptoms of congestive heart failure. We use low-dose digoxin, aiming to keep the serum digoxin level 1.0 ng/mL. The effects of digoxin on mortality are not currently known. (*Adapted from* Uretsky and coworkers [27]; with permission.)

MANAGEMENT OF VENTRICULAR ARRHYTHMIAS IN IDIOPATHIC DILATED CARDIOMYOPATHY

Drug therapy
  (amiodarone is under study)
Automatic internal cardioverter-defibrillator
  (under study)
Ablation
  Look for VT with a LBBB morphology
Treatment should be reserved for
  Patients with a history of sudden death
  Patients with symptomatic VT (hypotension-related)
  Patients with long (>20 beat) runs of VT

FIGURE 3-31. Management of ventricular arrhythmias in idiopathic dilated cardiomyopathy. The majority of patients with dilated cardiomyopathy have complex ventricular ectopy. The presence of ventricular ectopy increases as the left ventricular ejection fraction decreases and is associated with a poor prognosis. Many of the antiarrhythmics (especially type I agents) cause further worsening of left ventricular function and increase mortality. It has therefore been difficult to show that drug treatment can favorably affect the incidence of sudden death. Amiodarone or an automatic internal cardioverter-defibrillator may offer the best chance for reducing the incidence of sudden death in dilated cardiomyopathy. Ventricular tachycardia (VT) with a left bundle branch block (LBBB) morphology in patients with dilated cardiomyopathy is potentially a result of bundle branch re-entry and is curable with ablation.

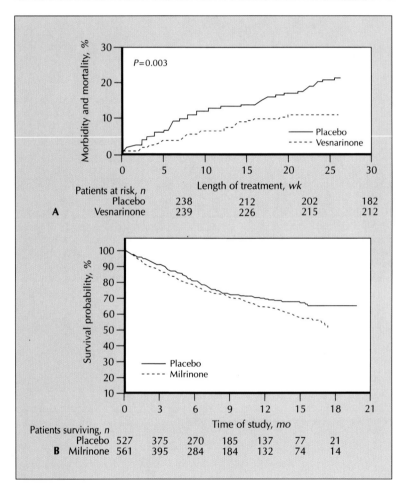

FIGURE 3-32. Oral positive inotropic agents in heart failure. There have been several large, randomized, placebo-controlled trials of oral inotropic agents in patients with congestive heart failure. The results are markedly different. **A,** Cumulative incidence of cardio-vascular morbidity or mortality from any cause in patients with symptomatic heart failure treated with vesnarinone, 60 mg/d, compared with placebo. Vesnarinone caused a decrease in mortality and morbidity. **B,** Kaplan-Meier curve showing the cumulative survival rates of patients with symptomatic heart failure treated with milrinone or placebo. Milrinone caused an increase in mortality. Both agents cause an increase in left ventricular ejection fraction greater than that seen with angiotensin-converting enzyme inhibitors. Therefore, although a low left ventricular ejection fraction is associated with a poor prognosis, an increase in ejection fraction is not necessarily associated with an improvement in mortality. This suggests that the mechanism of action may be crucial. (Part A *adapted from* Feldman and coworkers [28]; part B *adapted from* Packer and coworkers [29]; with permission.)

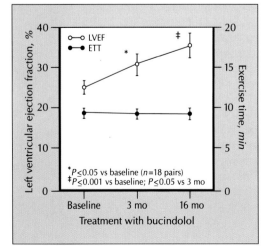

FIGURE 3-33. β-adrenergic blockade in idiopathic dilated cardiomyopathy. Although β-blockers may have adverse effects due to their negative inotropic action, they also have potentially beneficial actions. There have now been several limited studies of β-adrenergic blockade in idiopathic dilated cardiomyopathy showing beneficial effects. Bucindolol is a nonselective β-blocker with mild vasodilator properties. This study showed an improvement in left ventricular ejection fraction (LVEF) and stable exercise performance (ETT) in 20 patients with idiopathic dilated cardiomyopathy treated with bucindolol. There have been two published mortality trials to date. This first trial randomized patients in functional class III–IV to either placebo or a β-receptor agonist with partial β-blocker activity (xamoterol) and demonstrated decreased survival in the treated group [30]. The second, larger trial randomized 383 patients to metoprolol or placebo [31]. Although there was no difference in mortality, there was a statistically significant decrease in primary endpoints in the metoprolol group and fewer patients receiving metoprolol deteriorated to the point of needing cardiac transplantation. (*Adapted from* Anderson and coworkers [32]; with permission.)

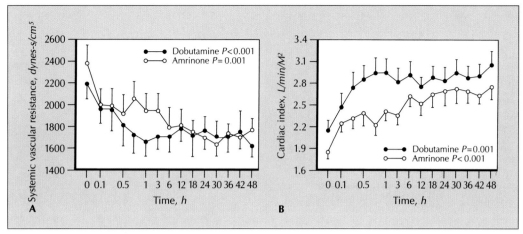

FIGURE 3-34. Short-term parenteral therapy of patients with idiopathic dilated cardiomyopathy. Parenteral dobutamine therapy is often needed in patients who prove refractory to standard oral medications. This study compared the acute hemodynamic effects of dobutamine and amrinone in 46 patients with idiopathic dilated cardiomyopathy. Both agents caused a marked improvement in hemodynamics and have an important role in the acute management of refractory pulmonary edema from idiopathic dilated cardiomyopathy. **A,** Systemic vascular resistance. **B,** Cardiac index. The use of long-term intravenous dobutamine in idiopathic dilated cardiomyopathy remains controversial. Most of the trials of home dobutamine were small, used large doses, and were without a comparable placebo arm. There may yet be a role for home dobutamine in low doses via a continuous infusion pump, especially in the management of patients awaiting cardiac transplantation. (*Adapted from* Marcus and coworkers [33]; with permission.)

EFFECTS OF IMMUNOSUPPRESSION IN IDIOPATHIC DILATED CARDIOMYOPATHY

	PATIENTS, N	BASELINE	3 mo	CHANGE	P VALUE
LVEF, %	**49**	**17.9±1.0**	**22.2±1.6**	**4.3±1.5**	0.054
	52	17.1±1.1	19.3±1.4	2.1±0.8	
NYHA functional class	**46**	**2.5±0.1**	**2.4±0.1**	**-0.1±0.1**	0.25
	51	2.4±0.1	2.4±0.1	0.0±0.1	
LVEDD, *mm*	**45**	**69.8±1.4**	**69.4±1.3**	**-0.5±0.7**	0.088
	50	67.7±1.0	68.8±1.2	1.1±1.0	
Treatment exercise performance, *METS*	**46**	**7.0±0.4**	**7.7±0.5**	**0.7±0.4**	0.44
	50	8.0±0.6	8.1±0.6	0.1±0.4	

FIGURE 3-35. Immunosuppression in idiopathic dilated cardiomyopathy. There has been one trial of prednisone in patients with this condition. In this study, 102 patients with idiopathic dilated cardiomyopathy, not myocarditis, were randomly assigned to receive either prednisone (*boldface data*) or placebo (*standard type*). There was a statistically significant but clinically insignificant improvement in left ventricular ejection fraction (LVEF) measured after 3 months of therapy in the prednisone group that was not seen after 6 months of therapy. This study effectively dampened the enthusiasm for the use of prednisone in idiopathic dilated cardiomyopathy. LVEDD—ventricular end-diastolic dimension; NYHA—New York Heart Association. (*Adapted from* Parrillo and coworkers [34]; with permission.)

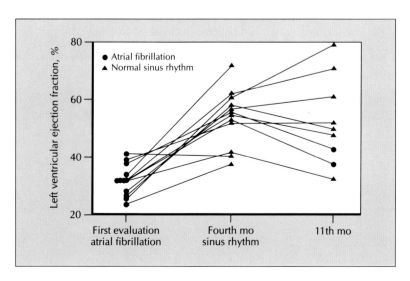

FIGURE 3-36. Atrial fibrillation and idiopathic dilated cardiomyopathy. There is increasing evidence for the importance of maintaining normal sinus rhythm in these patients. In this study of 17 patients with idiopathic dilated cardiomyopathy, conversion from atrial fibrillation to normal sinus rhythm was associated with a statistically significant improvement in left ventricular ejection fraction. Low-dose amiodarone is particularly effective, and associated with a low side effect profile, in maintaining patients in normal sinus rhythm after electrical cardioversion. (*Adapted from* Kierny and coworkers [35]; with permission.)

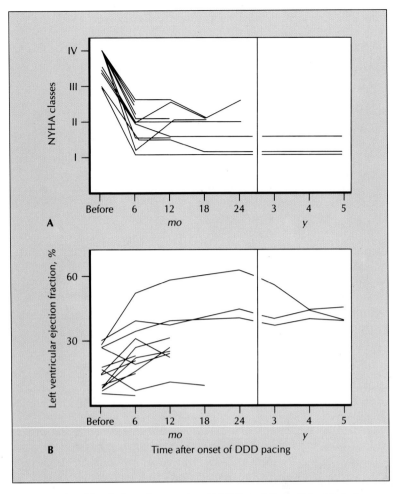

A

B

Time after onset of DDD pacing

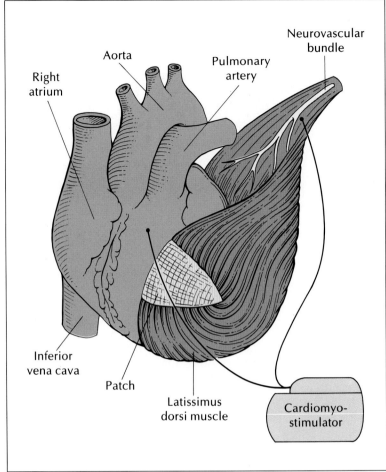

FIGURE 3-37. Dual-chamber pacing (DDD) in idiopathic dilated cardiomyopathy. In this study of 17 patients with idiopathic dilated cardiomyopathy, long-term DDD pacing at an atrioventricular delay of 100 ms produced a consistent decrease in symptoms (**A**) and an increase in left ventricular ejection fraction (**B**). This is a promising modality that requires further research. NYHA—New York Heart Association. (*Adapted from* Hochleitner and coworkers [36]; with permission.)

FIGURE 3-38. Cardiomyoplasty in idiopathic dilated cardiomyopathy. There have been several small studies of the use of the stimulated latissimus dorsi muscle to reinforce the heart muscle [37]. The latissimus dorsi is dissected free of its distal insertion, preserving the superior neurovascular pedicle. The muscle is moved into the hemithorax and wrapped around the heart. The muscle must be trained, using a progressive pacing protocol, until it is paced with every heartbeat. Currently, a phase III trial is under way comparing cardiomyoplasty with standard medical therapy. This may become a viable therapy for patients who cannot undergo cardiac transplantation and who are not symptomatic at rest.

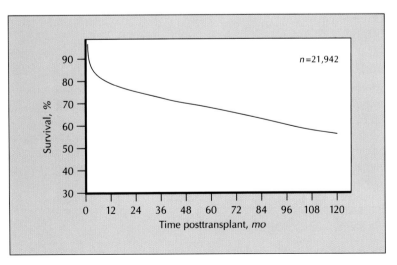

FIGURE 3-39. Survival rate for cardiac transplantation. This has become the standard therapy for end-stage heart disease. This graph shows the worldwide actuarial survival for 21,942 cardiac transplant recipients from 1967 to 1992. However, there are far more patients who could benefit from this procedure than there are potential donors. At present, one in three patients awaiting cardiac transplantation will die before a donor heart becomes available. (*Adapted from* Kaye [38]; with permission.)

INDICATIONS FOR CARDIAC TRANSPLANTATION

End-stage heart disease not amenable to other therapy

NYHA class III–IV symptoms on maximal therapy

Peak oxygen consumption <10 mL/kg/min

Age <60–65 y

Healthy apart from heart disease

Emotionally stable and compliant

Supportive social structure

FIGURE 3-40. Indications for cardiac transplantation. Not everyone can undergo cardiac transplantation, given the limited donor organ supply. However, this therapy offers the best hope for long-term survival in patients with a variety of end-stage cardiac conditions. NYHA—New York Heart Association.

POTENTIAL CONTRAINDICATIONS TO CARDIAC TRANSPLANTATION

Advancing age (>60–65 y)

Severe pulmonary hypertension

Irreversible hepatic or renal disease

Chronic obstructive pulmonary disease

Recent pulmonary infarction

Insulin-dependent diabetes mellitus

Severe cerebrovascular or peripheral vascular disease

Active peptic ulcer disease

Severe cachexia or obesity

Other systemic disease likely to limit survival or rehabilitation

Absent or inadequate external psychosocial support system

History of behavior pattern or psychiatric illness likely to interfere significantly with compliance

FIGURE 3-41. Contraindications to cardiac transplantation. Some of these contraindications are absolute, such as pulmonary hypertension. Others are only relative contraindications. The goal is optimal utilization of a scarce resource, donor hearts.

REFERENCES

1. Brandenburg RO, Chazov E, Cherian G, et al.: Report of the WHO/ISFC task force on the definition and classification of cardiomyopathies. Br Heart J 1980, 44:672–673.

2. Abelmann WH, Lorell BH: The challenge of cardiomyopathy. J Am Coll Cardiol 1989, 13:1219–1239.

3. Manolio TA, Baughman KL, Rodeheffer R, et al.: Prevalence and etiology of idiopathic dilated cardiomyopathy. Am J Cardiol 1992, 69:1458–1466.

4. Abelmann WH: Classification and natural history of primary myocardial disease. Prog Cardiovasc Dis 1985, 27:73–94.

5. Codd MB, Sugrue DD, Gersh BJ, Melton LJ: Epidemiology of idiopathic dilated and hypertrophic cardiomyopathy. Circulation 1989, 80:564–572.

6. Torp A: Incidence of congestive cardiomyopathy. Postgrad Med J 1978, 54:435–437.

7. Bagger JP, Baandrup U, Rasmussen K, et al.: Cardiomyopathy in Western Denmark. Br Heart J 1984, 52:327–331.

8. Williams DG, Olsen EGJ: Prevalence of overt dilated cardiomyopathy in two regions of England. Br Heart J 1985, 54:153–155.

9. Bjarnason I, Jonsson S, Hardarson T: Mode of inheritance of hypertrophic cardiomyopathy in Iceland: echocardiographic study. Br Heart J 1982, 47:122–129.

10. Hada Y, Sakamoto T, Amano K, et al.: Prevalence of hypertrophic cardiomyopathy in a population of adult Japanese workers as detected by echocardiographic screening. Am J Cardiol 1987, 59:183–184.

11. Coughlin SS, Szklo M, Baughman K, Pearson TA: The epidemiology of idiopathic dilated cardiomyopathy in a biracial community. Am J Epidemiol 1990, 131:48–56.

12. Gillum RF: The epidemiology of cardiomyopathy in the United States. In Progress in Cardiology 2/1. Edited by Zipes DP, Rowlands DJ. Malvern, PA: Lea and Febiger; 1989:11–21.

13. Sugrue DD, Rodeheffer RJ, Codd MB, et al.: The clinical course of idiopathic dilated cardiomyopathy. Ann Intern Med 1992, 117:117–123.

14. Meinertz T, Hofmann T, Kasper W: Significance of ventricular arrhythmias in idiopathic dilated cardiomyopathy. Am J Cardiol 1984, 53:902–907.

15. Fuster V, Gersh BJ, Giuliane ER, et al.: The natural history of idiopathic dilated cardiomyopathy. Am J Cardiol 1983, 47:525–531.

16. Mancini DM, Eisen H, Kussmaul W, et al.: Value of peak exercise oxygen consumption for optimal timing of cardiac transplantation in ambulatory patients with heart failure. Circulation 1991, 83:778–786.

17. Keogh AM, Baron DW, Hickie JB: Prognostic guides in patients with idiopathic or ischemic dilated cardiomyopathy assessed for cardiac transplantation. Am J Cardiol 1990, 65:903–908.

18. Swenberg K, Eneroth P, Kjekshus J, Wilhelmsen L: Hormones regulating cardiovascular function in patients with severe congestive heart failure and their relation to mortality. Circulation 1990, 82:1730–1736.

19. Katz AM: Heart failure. In The Heart and Cardiovascular Systems, ed 2. Edited by Fozzard HA, Jennings RB, Haber E, et al. New York: Raven Press; 1991:333–353.

20. Wallis DE, O'Connell JB, Henkin RE, et al.: Segmental wall motion abnormalities in dilated cardiomyopathy: a common finding and good prognostic sign. J Am Coll Cardiol 1984, 4:674–679.

21. Roberts WC, Siegel RJ, McManus BM: Idiopathic dilated cardiomyopathy: analysis of 152 necropsy patients. Am J Cardiol 1987, 60:1340–1355.

22. Cohn JN, Archibald DG, Ziesche S, et al.: Effect of vasodilator therapy on mortality in chronic congestive heart failure. N Engl J Med 1986, 314:1547–1552.

23. The CONSENSUS Trial Study Group: Effects of enalapril on mortality in severe congestive heart failure. *N Engl J Med* 1987, 316:1429–1435.

24. Cohn JN, Johnson GJ, Ziesche S, *et al.*: A comparison of enalapril with hydralazine-isosorbide dinitrate in the treatment of chronic congestive heart failure. *N Engl J Med* 1991, 325:303–310.

25. The SOLVD Investigators: Effect of enalapril on survival in patients with reduced left ventricular ejection fractions and congestive heart failure. *N Engl J Med* 1991, 325:293–302.

26. The SOLVD Investigators: Effect of enalapril on mortality and the development of heart failure in asymptomatic patients with reduced left ventricular ejection fractions. *N Engl J Med* 1992, 327:685–691.

27. Uretsky BF, Young JB, Shahidi FE, *et al.*: Randomized study assessing the effect of digoxin withdrawal in patients with mild to moderate chronic congestive heart failure. *J Am Coll Cardiol* 1993, 22:955–962.

28. Feldman AM, Bristow MR, Parmley WW: Effects of vesnarinone on morbidity and mortality in patients with heart failure. *N Engl J Med* 1993, 329:149–155.

29. Packer M, Carver JR, Rodeheffer RJ, *et al.*: Effect of oral milrinone on mortality in severe chronic heart failure. *N Engl J Med* 1991, 325:1468–1475.

30. The Xamoterol in Severe Heart Failure Study Group: Xamoterol in severe heart failure. *Lancet* 1990, 336:1–6.

31. Waagstein F, Bristow M, Swedberg K: Beneficial effects of metoprolol in idiopathic dilated cardiomyopathy. *Lancet* 1993, 342:1441–1446.

32. Anderson JL, Gilbert EM, O'Connell JB, *et al.*: Long-term (2 year) beneficial effects of β-adrenergic blockade with bucindolol in patients with idiopathic dilated cardiomyopathy. *J Am Coll Cardiol* 1991, 17:1373–1381.

33. Marcus RH, Raw K, Patel J, *et al.*: Comparison of intravenous amrinone and dobutamine in congestive heart failure due to idiopathic dilated cardiomyopathy. *Am J Cardiol* 1990, 66:1107–1112.

34. Parrillo JE, Cunnion RE, Epstein SE: Prospective, randomized, controlled trial of prednisone for dilated cardiomyopathy. *N Engl J Med* 1989, 321:1061–1068.

35. Kierny JR, Facello A, Arbogast R, *et al.*: Increase in radionuclide left ventricular ejection fraction after cardioversion of chronic atrial fibrillation in idiopathic dilated cardiomyopathy. *Eur Heart J* 1992, 13:1290–1295.

36. Hochleitner M, Hortnagl H, Hortnagl H, *et al.*: Long-term efficacy of physiologic dual-chamber pacing in the treatment of end-stage idiopathic dilated cardiomyopathy. *Am J Cardiol* 1992, 70:1320–1325.

37. Moreira LF, Stolf NA, Bocchi EA: Latissimus dorsi cardiomyoplasty in the treatment of patients with dilated cardiomyopathy. *Circulation* 1990, 82(suppl IV): IV257–IV263.

38. Kaye MP: The registry of the International Society for Heart and Lung Transplantation. *J Heart Lung Transplant* 1993, 12:541–548.

SPECIFIC HEART MUSCLE DISEASE

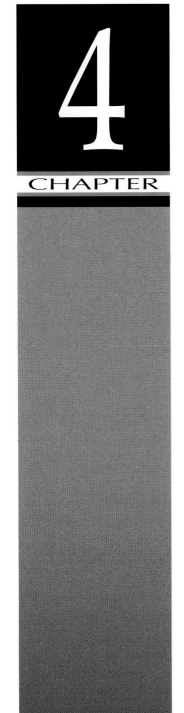

4

CHAPTER

James J. Glazier

Heart muscle involvement in a number of infectious disease processes has been a subject of particular interest in recent years. In patients with the acquired immunodeficiency syndrome (AIDS), the occurrence of dilated cardiomyopathy is a well-recognized, although apparently uncommon, clinical entity. On the basis of available information, it appears reasonable to propose that the etiology of AIDS associated cardiomyopathy is multifactorial [1]. In individual patients, factors with variable contributions to the development of such cardiomyopathy may include triggering of cell- and humoral-mediated cardiac injury by the human immunodeficiency virus (HIV) itself or by opportunistic infection, cardiotoxicity from antiretroviral and other agents, such as pentamidine and gancyclovir, which are frequently used to treat AIDS patients, and the use of cocaine and alcohol

Lyme disease is caused by a tickborne spirochete (*Borrelia burgdorferi*). About 10% of patients with Lyme disease develop evidence of transient cardiac involvement, the most common manifestation being variable degrees of atrioventricular block [2]. The demonstration of spirochetes in myocardial biopsy specimens from some patients with Lyme carditis [3] suggests that the cardiac manifestations are caused by a direct toxic effect, although there is speculation that immune-mediated mechanisms are also involved. Temporary transvenous pacing may be required in patients with high-grade block. Although they are routinely used, the efficacy of antibiotics in Lyme carditis is not established.

Myocardial involvement occurs in approximately 20% of patients with sarcoidosis [4]. Clinical manifestations include ventricular arrhythmias, conduction abnormalities, and sudden death. Although endomyocardial biopsy may provide a definitive diagnosis of myocardial sarcoidosis, normal or nonspecific findings on biopsy do not exclude the diagnosis in patients in whom this disorder is strongly suspected on clinical and other grounds. Steroids may play a useful therapeutic role; patients who do not respond to medical therapy may benefit from cardiac transplantation.

Cardiac involvement in hemochromatosis leads to a mixed dilated or restrictive cardiomyopathic presentation, with both systolic and diastolic dysfunction [5]. Cardiac involvement is usually evident from the clinical and echocardiographic features; endomyocardial biopsy may be useful to confirm (but not to exclude) the diagnosis. Repeated phlebotomies or use of the chelating agent deferoxamine may be clinically beneficial [6].

Cardiac involvement is virtually the rule in primary amyloidosis. The most common presentation is that of a restrictive cardiomyopathy. Echocardiography combined with Doppler is particularly helpful in the diagnosis of amyloidosis. Endomyocardial biopsy is valuable in establishing a definitive diagnosis. In general, the treatment of cardiac amyloidosis is unsatisfactory and ineffective.

The incidence of peripartum cardiomyopathy (PPCM) is greater in women with twin pregnancies and in women who are multiparous, over 30 years of age, or black [7]. Endomyocardial biopsy studies have revealed a greater incidence of myocarditis in PPCM compared with other forms of dilated cardiomyopathy [8]. Approximately 50% of patients show complete or near-complete recovery of cardiac function and clinical status within the first 6 months postpartum; the other 50% demonstrate continued clinical deterioration, leading to early death, or persistent left ventricular dysfunction and chronic heart failure, with high morbidity and mortality. Patients with PPCM who do not recover early should be considered for cardiac transplantation. Repeat pregnancy should be discouraged in patients with PPCM who have persistent cardiac dysfunction. Women in whom cardiac function is recovered after one episode of PPCM should be informed about the increased risk that accompanies later pregnancies.

HEART MUSCLE DISEASE ASSOCIATED WITH AIDS

CARDIAC LESIONS IN AIDS

Myocarditis
Endocarditis
Pericarditis
Dilated cardiomyopathy
Kaposi's sarcoma
Malignant lymphoma
Arteriopathy
Myocardial infarction

FIGURE 4-1. A wide spectrum of cardiac lesions may be seen in patients with AIDS [9,10]. Types of lesions involving the myocardium in AIDS include nonspecific or infectious myocarditis, inflammatory or noninflammatory myocardial necrosis, dilated cardiomyopathy, neoplastic invasion of either ventricle by Kaposi's sarcoma or lymphoma, and isolated involvement of the right ventricle as the result of pulmonary disease. Forms of pericardial involvement in AIDS patients include effusion (sterile or infective) with or without tamponade, fibrinous pericarditis, and constriction. Endocardial valvular disease may occur as a result of nonbacterial thrombotic endocarditis (NBTE, or marantic endocarditis) or infective endocarditis. In NBTE, systemic embolization may occur, resulting in myocardial infarction [9], and arteriopathy involving the small and medium-sized arteries of the heart, which may be associated with aneurysm formation, has also been described in AIDS patients [10].

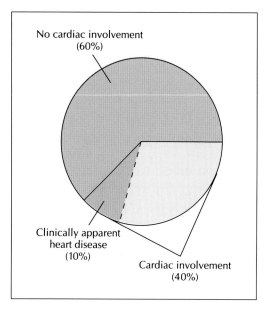

FIGURE 4-2. Frequency of cardiac involvement in patients with AIDS. Cardiac involvement, as documented by echocardiographic, endomyocardial biopsy, and autopsy studies, occurs in approximately 25% to 50% of patients with AIDS [9,10]. However, it leads to clinically apparent heart disease in only 10%. Congestive heart failure is the most common clinical manifestation of cardiac involvement in AIDS. The onset of heart failure often heralds the preterminal stages of the disease. In patients with AIDS, dyspnea is almost always presumed to be of pulmonary origin because of the development of multiple opportunistic pulmonary infections. However, cardiac dysfunction should be considered in the evaluation of patients with AIDS who have shortness of breath, especially when dyspnea or hypoxemia is out of proportion to the degree of underlying pulmonary disease [9].

THE ETIOLOGIC SPECTRUM OF MYOCARDITIS IN AIDS

Opportunistic infections
  Pneumocystis carinii
  Myocobacterium tuberculosis
  Myocobacterium avium intracellulare
  Cryptococcus neoformans
  Aspergillus fumigatus
  Candida albicans
  Histoplasma capsulatum
  Toxoplasma gondii
Viral agents
  Cytomegalovirus
  Human immunodeficiency virus
  Herpes simplex
Lymphocytic myocarditis
Noninflammatory myocardial necrosis

FIGURE 4-3. Myocarditis is the most common pathologic cardiac finding in patients with AIDS. Some cases of myocarditis appear to be caused by opportunistic viral, fungal, bacterial, or protozoal agents. However, in more than 80% of cases a clear etiologic agent is not identified. The latter cases may be related to the human immunodeficiency virus itself. Nonspecific inflammatory infiltrates without myocyte damage or necrosis are the most common histologic findings in AIDS-associated myocarditis [9]. Another common histologic finding is noninflammatory myocardial necrosis. It is postulated that the latter is a result of the long-term stress to which patients with this tragic disease are subjected [9,10], causing prolonged and excessive secretion of catecholamines. Cytomegalovirus infection can also cause necrosis without inflammation. (*Adapted from* Acierno [10]; with permission.)

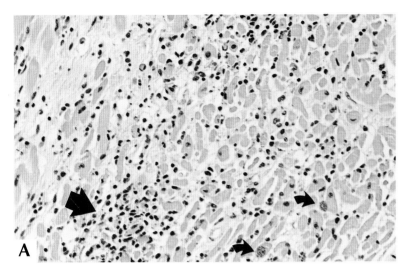

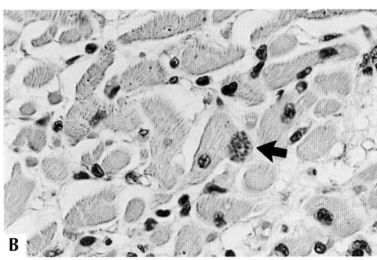

FIGURE 4-4. Toxoplasma myocarditis in a patient with AIDS. Almost any agent that can cause disseminated infection in AIDS patients may involve the myocardium. Opportunistic organisms, such as *Toxoplasma gondii*, which rarely cause myocarditis in immunocompetent patients, are common pathogens in AIDS myocarditis. This figure shows the appearance of *Toxoplasma* myocarditis in a patient with AIDS. **A,** Under low-power magni-

fication (× 412), focal nonspecific inflammation with the presence of granulocytes (*large arrow*) and several intracytoplasmic cysts filled with *T. gondii* bradyzoites (*small arrows*) are demonstrated. **B,** With high-power magnification (× 1320), these intracytoplasmic cysts (*arrows*) are shown in greater detail. (Courtesy of G.K. Haines, MD, Northwestern University, Chicago, IL.)

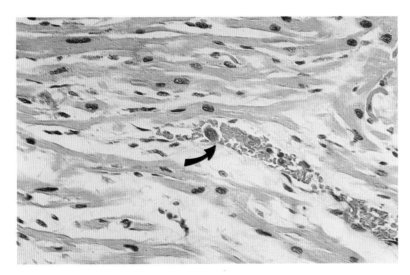

FIGURE 4-5. Cytomegalovirus (CMV) myocarditis in a patient with AIDS. Multiple common viruses, such as CMV, have also been implicated as causal agents in AIDS myocarditis. This figure shows a section through a small interfascicular vessel in a patient with AIDS and myocarditis (magnification, × 969). Demonstrated is a large endothelial cell with large intranuclear viral inclusions (*arrow*), typical for CMV infection. It is important to note that not all cells infected with CVM (as determined by in situ hybridization studies) have these inclusions. (Courtesy of G.K. Haines, Northwestern University, Chicago, IL.)

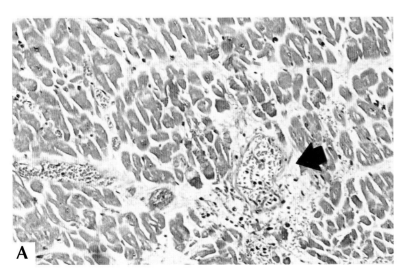

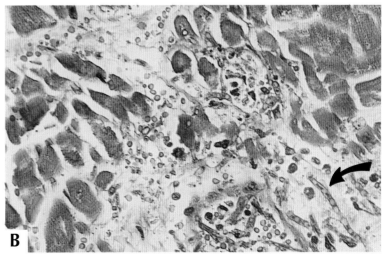

FIGURE 4-6. Aspergillus myocarditis in a patient with AIDS. Opportunistic fungal organisms, such as *Aspergillus* species, are also a cause of myocarditis in some patients with AIDS. This figure demonstrates the histologic appearances in another patient with AIDS and myocarditis. **A,** A section of heart with blood vessel and mild inflammation (*arrow*; magnification, × 330).

B, High-power examination of this area (magnification, × 825) reveals fungal hyphae invading through a blood vessel wall and into the myocardium (*arrow*). These fungal forms are marked by true septation. These appearances are suggestive of *Aspergillus* species. (Courtesy of G.K. Haines, Northwestern University, Chicago, IL.)

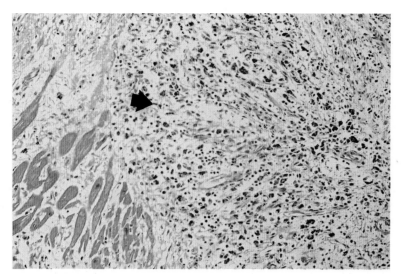

FIGURE 4-7. Nonspecific lymphocytic myocarditis in a patient with AIDS. As previously stated, in 80% of cases of AIDS associated myocarditis, no etiologic agent is identified. Such a case is well demonstrated by this illustration. In this section of myocardium, taken at autopsy of a patient with AIDS myocarditis, there is an area of myocardial necrosis with neovascularization and abundant hemosiderin-laden macrophages (*arrow*), indicating resolution of a focus of acute necrosis, which can be seen in human immunodeficiency virus myocarditis. (Courtesy of G.K. Haines, Chicago, IL.)

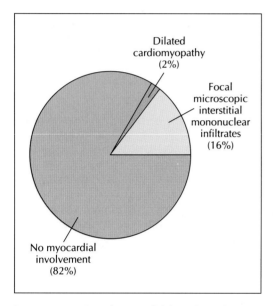

FIGURE 4-8. Incidence of dilated cardiomyopathy in AIDS afflicted patients. The incidence of AIDS associated dilated cardiomyopathy appears to be quite low. In one autopsy series reported by Lewis and Grody [11], dilated cardiomyopathy was found in only three of 128 AIDS afflicted patients. In the same series, focal microscopic interstitial mononuclear infiltrates were present in specimens from 20 autopsies (16%) after retrospective review of more than 500 histologic specimens from the 128 cases. However, given the ongoing AIDS epidemic, it appears likely that AIDS associated dilated cardiomyopathy will become increasingly recognized. This consideration has directed considerable attention toward elucidating the etiopathogenesis of this cardiomyopathy.

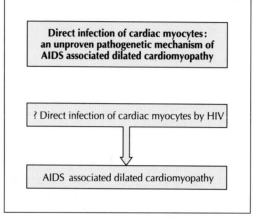

FIGURE 4-9. An intuitively appealing and often postulated mechanism for the development of AIDS associated cardiomyopathy is direct infection of cardiac myocytes by human immunodeficiency virus (HIV). However, the ability of HIV to infect and replicate within myocytes has not yet been demonstrated *in vitro*. Hybridization studies using probes against *env* (envelope), *rev* (reverse transcriptase), and *tat* have failed to demonstrate viral proteins within the myocytes of patients with HIV-associated myocarditis and cardiomyopathy [1].

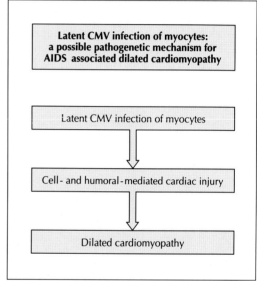

FIGURE 4-10. A second possible explanation for the occurrence of cardiomyopathy in patients infected with human immunodeficiency virus (HIV) is the role of concurrent cardiotropic viral infections common to the HIV-infected population, such as cytomegalovirus (CMV). Wu *et al.* [12] performed a series of elegant immunogenetic studies on endomyocardial biopsy samples from HIV-infected patients with cardiomyopathy. The results of their study suggest that in some, but not all, patients with AIDS associated cardiomyopathy, latent CMV infection of myocytes, triggering cell- and humoral-mediated cardiac injury, may be an important pathogenetic mechanism.

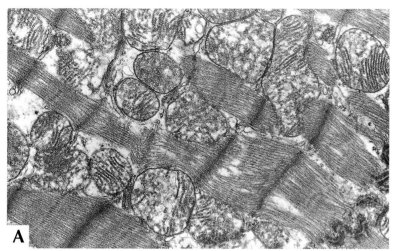

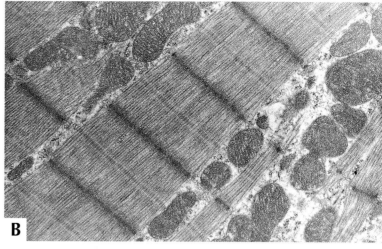

FIGURE 4-11. Mitochondrial abnormalities induced by zidovudine. Zidovudine and other antiretroviral agents may contribute to the dilated cardiomyopathy seen in some AIDS patients. Lamperth *et al.* [13] demonstrated zidovudine-induced structural and functional mitochondrial abnormalities in rat myocytes, including uncoupling of oxidative phosphorylation. **A,** Electron micrograph of rat muscle from a zidovudine-treated animal. **B,** Muscle from an untreated control. Note enlarged mitochondria with abnormal cristae in the treated animal. There is ballooning of some mitochondria, with cystlike projections and partial disappearance of the cristae and matrix. In contrast, the control tissue shows normal muscle with normal mitochondria (original magnification, × 20,000). (*Adapted from* Lamperth and coworkers [13]; with permission.)

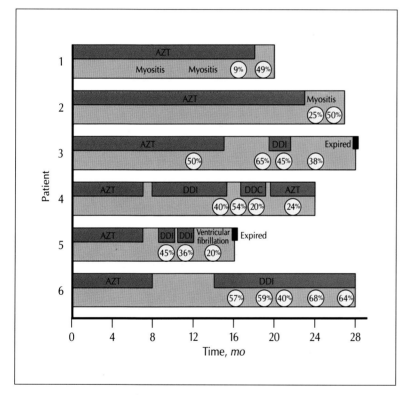

FIGURE 4-12. Temporal relation between antiretroviral therapy and changes in ventricular ejection fraction in six patients with AIDS. The above experimental observations are supported by clinical reports of an association between development of cardiac dysfunction and use of zidovudine (AZT) and dideoxycytidine (DDC) or dideoxyinosine (DDI) in patients with AIDS. Herskowitz *et al.* [14] evaluated 26 consecutive HIV-infected patients with congestive heart failure over a 2-year period. Of 13 patients who received antiretroviral therapy, six had cardiac dysfunction clinically associated with this therapy. The temporal relation between antiretroviral therapy and changes in ventricular function in each of these six patients is shown. Ejection fraction, as determined by echocardiography, is shown in *circles*. Three patients developed cardiac dysfunction during AZT therapy and improved after its discontinuation. Three patients, switched from AZT to DDI because of development of hematologic side effects attributed to AZT, and one patient switched to DDI because of apparent AZT-induced left ventricular (LV) dysfunction, developed new or further depression of LV function after being switched to this agent. The rapid improvement in cardiac function seen in four patients after discontinuation of therapy, the return of dysfunction with resumption of therapy in two patients, and the concurrent finding in two patients of myositis (a well-characterized toxic reaction to AZT), together with myocarditis, suggest a causal relation. (*Adapted from* Herskowitz and coworkers [14]; with permission.)

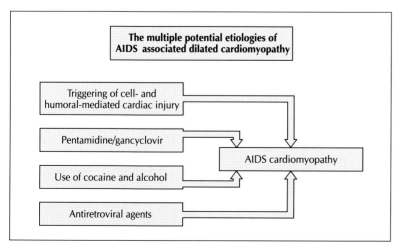

FIGURE 4-13. On the basis of available information, it appears reasonable to propose that the etiology of AIDS associated cardiomyopathy is multifactorial. In individual patients, factors with variable roles in the development of such cardiomyopathy may include triggering of cell- and humoral-mediated cardiac injury by the human immunodeficiency virus itself or by opportunistic infections, cardiotoxicity from antiretroviral and other agents such as pentamidine and gancyclovir, and the use of cocaine and alcohol.

TREATMENT OF AIDS ASSOCIATED HEART MUSCLE DISEASE

Vasodilators, diuretics, inotropes (heart failure)
Antimicrobials (infective myocarditis)
Pericardiocentesis

FIGURE 4-14. Treatment of AIDS associated heart muscle disease is aimed at providing some degree of symptomatic improvement and is, in effect, palliative. Diagnosis of dilated cardiomyopathy on echocardiography has particularly ominous implications for prognosis, with 50% of such patients dying within 6 months [9]. Despite such a poor outcome, symptoms of congestive heart failure resulting from the dilated cardiomyopathy often respond initially to conventional treatment with digoxin, diuretics, and vasodilators. Antimicrobial therapy for infective myocarditis and pericardiocentesis for relief of tamponade are the other main therapeutic options.

LYME CARDITIS

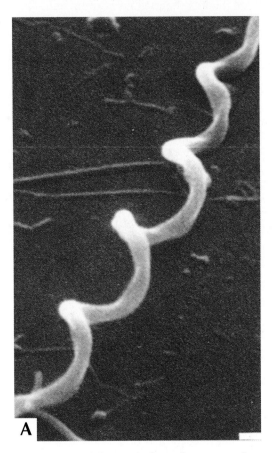

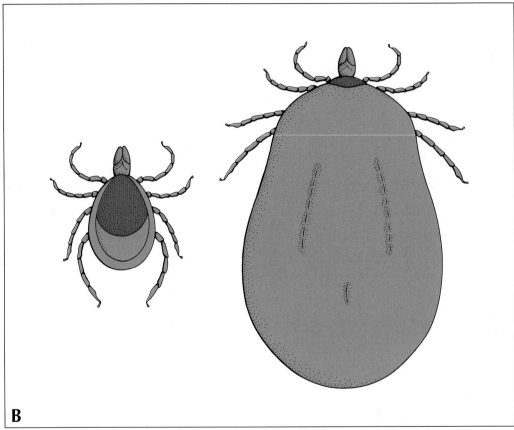

A **B**

FIGURE 4-15. The spirochete that causes Lyme disease and the tick vector. Lyme disease is the commonest vector-borne disease in the United States. It also occurs widely throughout Europe, the Soviet Union, China, Japan, and Australia [15]. **A,** This disease is caused by a spirochetal bacterium, *Borrelia burgdorferi,* which is transmitted to humans by an ixodid tick [15,16]. In the United States, the predominant tick vector of Lyme disease is *Ixodes dammini* in the East and Midwest and *I. pacificus* in the Far West. Lyme disease occurs when an infected tick (most often a nymph) feeds on a susceptible individual and transmits the causative spirochete. **B,** An *I. dammini* tick that has not recently fed (*left*) and a tick engorged by recent feeding (*right*).

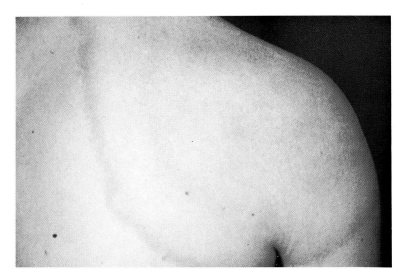

FIGURE 4-16. Erythema chronicum migrans (ECM). Lyme disease is usually contracted during the summer and is heralded by the appearance of a pathognomonic skin lesion, ECM. The appearance of ECM is generally annular, with a sharply demarcated outer border, and it is erythematous or bluish, warm to the touch, flat, and minimally tender or nontender. This unique cutaneous lesion is the best clinical marker of Lyme disease. ECM is followed in weeks to months by joint, neurologic, or cardiac involvement. However, in perhaps one third of cases, the skin lesion is absent or missed and patients present with symptoms of disseminated disease. (*Adapted from* Fitzpatrick and coworkers [16]; with permission.)

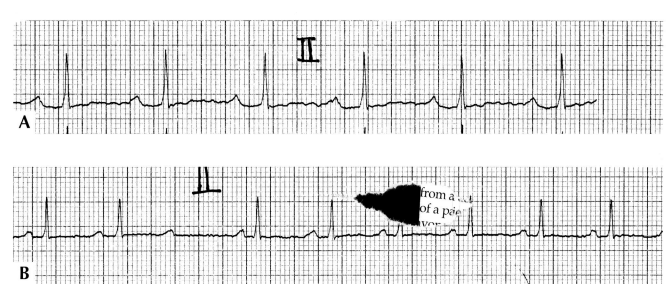

FIGURE 4-17. Development of first- and second-degree heart block in Lyme disease. About 10% of patients with Lyme disease develop evidence of transient cardiac involvement. The most common cardiac manifestation is variable degrees of atrioentricular (AV) block [2,17]. First-degree heart block (**A**) may progress to second-degree (**B**) or complete heart block over hours. According to some authorities, the risk for progression to complete heart block is much higher when the P-R interval exceeds 0.3 seconds. Syncope from complete heart block is common with cardiac involvement, as there is often associated depression of ventricular escape rhythm. McAlister *et al.* [2], in reviewing 52 reported cases of Lyme carditis, noted that 45 (87%) of these patients had documented AV block; 28 experienced either complete or high-grade AV block and were almost always symptomatic. When AV block of unknown origin develops suddenly, Lyme carditis should be considered, especially in younger patients who live in an area in which the vector is endemic [2,17].

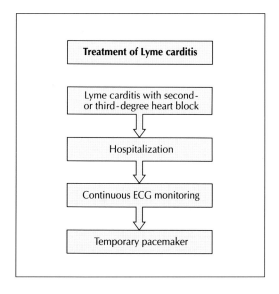

FIGURE 4-18. Several therapeutic principles of Lyme carditis are generally accepted, whereas others remain anecdotal [2]. Hospitalization and continuous electrocardiographic (ECG) monitoring are advisable for patients with second-degree or complete atrioventricular (AV) block, and for first-degree block if the P-R interval exceeds 0.3 seconds. Temporary cardiac pacing may be required for hemodynamic support. Of 26 reported cases of Lyme carditis associated with high-grade or complete AV block reviewed by McAlister *et al.* [2], temporary pacing was used in 16. Complete heart block rarely persists for more than 1 week and long-term prognosis appears to be excellent [2]. Regression from complete AV block to high-grade, then to Wenkebach second-degree, and finally to first-degree block, with subsequently decreasing P-R intervals, is a commonly observed pattern. Permanent pacemaker implantation is very rarely if ever required [2]. However, van der Linde *et al.* [17] reported a patient who, after experiencing complete heart block for more than 3 months despite treatment with antimicrobials and corticosteroids, was treated by insertion of a rate-responsive pacemaker.

FIGURE 4-19. Antibiotics are used routinely in the treatment of Lyme carditis. Suggested antimicrobial regimens are depicted. However, as there have been no controlled trials regarding the use of antibiotics in the treatment of Lyme carditis, the therapeutic efficacy of these agents is not established [15]. Similarly, the role of anti-inflammatory agents, such as corticosteroids or salicylates, in the resolution of heart block, is unknown.

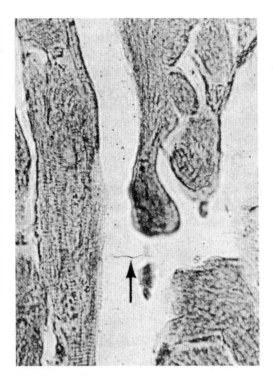

FIGURE 4-20. Isolation of *Borrelia burgdorferi* from a patient with longstanding cardiomyopathy. Recent studies suggest that Lyme borreliosis is associated with chronic heartmuscle disease. In particular, Stanek *et al.* [3] in Vienna, Austria, isolated a borrelial strain (*arrow*) [from] endomyocardial biopsy sample [from patie]nt with longstanding dilated cardiomyopathy. (*Adapted from* Stanek and coworkers [3]; with permission.)

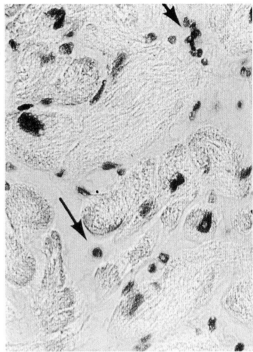

FIGURE 4-21. Endomyocardial biopsy appearance in dilated cardiomyopathy suspected to be caused by *Borrelia*. Further support for the concept of borreliosis as a cause of some cases of dilated cardiomyopathy is provided by the histopathologic observations of Klein *et al.* [18], who performed endomyocardial biopsy in two patients with heart failure from dilated cardiomyopathy. Both patients had antibodies to *Borrelia burgdorferi*, as determined by enzyme-linked immunosorbent assay. In both patients, sections stained with hematoxylin and eosin demonstrated subtle perivascular infiltration by mononuclear cells (*arrows*), moderate proliferation of connective tissue, and increased diameter of myocardial fibers. (*Adapted from* Klein and coworkers [18]; with permission.)

CARDIAC SARCOIDOSIS

INCIDENCE OF MYOCARDIAL INVOLVEMENT IN SARCOIDOSIS AS DETERMINED BY THREE LARGE AUTOPSY SERIES		
STUDY	PATIENTS WITH SARCOIDOSIS, *n*	PATIENTS WITH MYOCARDIAL INVOLVEMENT, *n(%)*
Longcope and Freiman, [19]	92	18(20)
Silverman *et al.* [20]	84	23(27)
Matsui *et al.* [21]	72	42(58)

FIGURE 4-22. Autopsy series suggest that in the United States myocardial involvement occurs in 20% to 27% of patients with sarcoidosis [19,20] and that the incidence may be as high as 58% in Japan [21]. Only 40% to 50% of patients with cardiac sarcoidosis at autopsy were diagnosed with sarcoidosis during their lifetimes [20]. Sarcoid myocardial involvement is most often limited to a small proportion of the myocardium and is clinically silent [20].

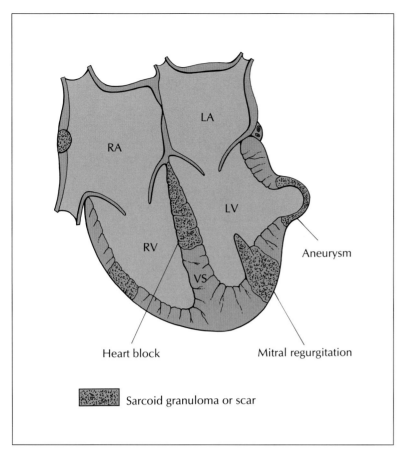

FIGURE 4-23. Distribution and consequences of sarcoid granulomas in sarcoid heart disease. In an autopsy series of 26 patients reported by Roberts *et al.* [22], cardiac granulomas were observed grossly in 25 hearts. Sarcoid granulomas were present in the left ventricular (LV) free wall of all 25 patients, in the right ventricular (RV) septum in 19, in the RV wall in 12, in the right atrial (RA) wall in three patients, and in the left atrial (LA) wall in two. Involvement of the cephalad portion of the muscular ventricular septum was associated with complete heart block. Important consequences of the involvement of the LV wall were aneurysm formation and mitral regurgitation. VS—ventricular septum. (*Adapted from* Roberts and coworkers [22]; with permission.)

CLINICAL PRESENTATIONS OF SARCOID HEART DISEASE

Complete heart block	Conduction abnormalities
Ventricular arrhythmias	Supraventricular tachycardia
Congestive heart failure	Simulated MI
Sudden death	Pericarditis

FIGURE 4-24. There is a wide range of clinical presentations of myocardial sarcoidosis. Cardiac symptoms are common in patients with sarcoidosis, but in less than 50% of cases these symptoms reflect myocardial involvement. Congestive heart failure, pericardial involvement, tamponade, valvular lesions, conduction abnormalities, ventricular arrhythmias, ventricular aneurysms, chest pain, and involvement of intramural coronary arteries have all been described [4].

FREQUENCY OF SUDDEN DEATH IN SARCOID HEART DISEASE

STUDY	PATIENTS, *n*	SUDDEN DEATH AS INITIAL PRESENTATION, *n*	TOTAL SUDDEN DEATH, *n*
Fleming and Bailey [24]	197	34	48
Roberts *et al.*, [22]	26	6	17
Total	223	40 (18%)	65 (29%)

FIGURE 4-25. On the basis of the results of a number of large series [22,24], sudden death appears to be the initial presentation of myocardial sarcoidosis in approximately 18% of patients. In addition, approximately 30% of all patients experience sudden death either as the initial clinical manifestation or after presenting with various cardiac disorders.

FREQUENCY OF VENTRICULAR TACHYCARDIA IN PATIENTS WITH SARCOID HEART DISEASE

STUDY	PATIENTS, n	PATIENTS WITH VENTRICULAR TACHYCARDIA, n(%)
Bashour et al. [25]	35	8
Roberts et al. [22]	26	6
Silverman et al. [20]	4	2
Porter [23]	33	5
Total	98	21 (21%)

FIGURE 4-26. Ventricular tachycardia has been reported in about 20% of patients with myocardial sarcoidosis [20,22,23,25]. This dysrhythmia, together with complete heart block, is presumed to be the cause of sudden death in most patients with myocardial sarcoidosis. The occurrence of ventricular tachycardia usually indicates extensive involvement of the heart by sarcoid granulomas or extensive scarring as a result of healing of the granulomas.

FREQUENCY OF COMPLETE HEART BLOCK IN PATIENTS WITH MYOCARDIAL SARCOIDOSIS

STUDY	PATIENTS, n	PATIENTS WITH COMPLETE HEART BLOCK, n (%)
Roberts et al. [22]	89	25 (28)
Bashour et al. [25]	35	8 (23)

FIGURE 4-27. Complete heart block has been reported in 20% to 30% of patients with myocardial sarcoidosis [22,25]. At autopsy, most of these patients had involvement of the basal part of the septum, particularly in the vicinity of the atrioventricular bundle. Complete heart block seems to be the result of interruption of the conduction pathways by sarcoid granulomas, scar tissue, or both.

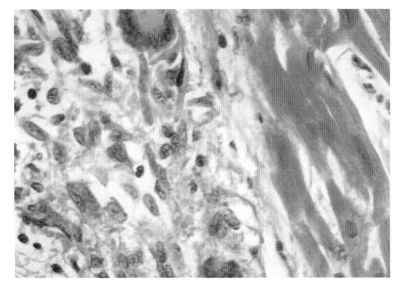

FIGURE 4-28. Endomyocardial biopsy sample demonstrating a sarcoid granuloma. Endomyocardial biopsy is the only technique that allows definitive diagnosis of myocardial sarcoidosis during life [4,26]. The depicted histologic specimen, obtained from the left ventricle, shows a typical noncaseating granuloma, that is characteristic of sarcoidosis (magnification, × 250). In some series, demonstration of sarcoid granulomas on endomyocardial biopsy is possible in only a small percentage of patients with probable myocardial sarcoidosis. This seeming discrepancy may relate to the patchy, diffuse nature of granulomatous involvement. Support for this concept is provided by the observations of Sekiguchi et al. [27], who simulated endomyocardial biopsy at different sites in both the left and right ventricles of the autopsied hearts of seven patients with fatal myocardial sarcoidosis. All seven hearts exhibited gross sarcoid involvement. Despite this, the sensitivity of biopsy was only 60% in the right ventricle and 47% in the left ventricle. Therefore, nonspecific biopsy findings do not exclude the diagnosis of myocardial sarcoidosis in clinically suspected cases. (*Adapted from* Uretsky [26]; with permission.)

TREATMENT OF MYOCARDIAL SARCOIDOSIS

Pacemaker implantation
Antiarrhythmic agents
Implantable antitachycardia device
Treatment of congestive heart failure
Corticosteroids

FIGURE 4-29. Treatment of ventricular tachycardia and high-grade conduction disturbances is a particularly important consideration in patients with sarcoidosis. The latter may necessitate insertion of a permanent pacemaker. The results of a recent study, reported by Winters et al. [28], suggest that standard antiarrhythmic therapy, even when guided with programmed ventricular stimulation, is often ineffective in preventing the recurrence of ventricular tachycardia and sudden death. This group suggests that implantation of an automatic antitachycardia device should be considered as primary therapy in some patients with myocardial sarcoidosis and ventricular tachycardia. Patients who develop congestive heart failure should be treated with conventional antifailure medication.

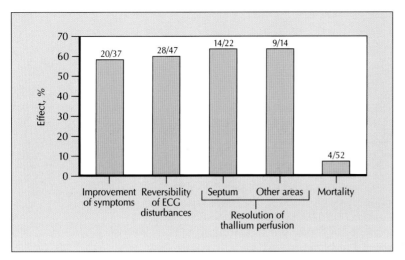

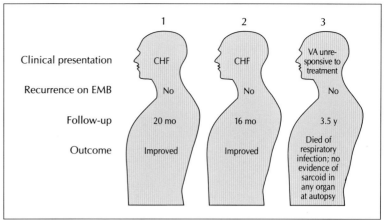

FIGURE 4-30. The apparently beneficial effect of long-term corticosteroid therapy on myocardial sarcoidosis. The general impression is that steroids are beneficial in the treatment of myocardial sarcoidosis. Schaedel *et al.* [29] reported their follow-up investigations (mean follow-up period, 6.2 years) in 52 patients with strongly suspected myocardial sarcoidosis. Steroids were given to all patients for a minimum of 1 year (mean duration of steroid therapy, 3.6 years). Twenty of the 37 patients with cardiac symptoms had improvement of these symptoms. Of 47 patients with electrocardiographic (ECG) abnormalities, 28 (60%) demonstrated reversibility of the abnormalities. In addition, the majority of documented thallium perfusion defects showed complete or partial reversibility during follow-up. The mortality rate in this series was only 8% over 6.2 years of follow-up, a much more favorable prognosis than the average 1- to 2-year survival reported in some earlier studies in which patients were not routinely treated with steroids. The observations of these studies give support to Fleming and Bailey's adage regarding treatment of myocardial sarcoidosis: "If in doubt, try steroids—you can't afford not to" [23]. (*Adapted from* Schaedel and coworkers [29]; with permission.)

FIGURE 4-31. Results of transplantation in three patients with myocardial sarcoidosis. Transplantation may be of value in patients with myocardial sarcoidosis but without pulmonary or other organ involvement who fail to respond to conventional management and steroid therapy. Valentine *et al.* [30] have reported their experience in three such patients. Two of the three patients were alive at 16 and 20 months after transplantation, with no evidence of recurrence of the disease. The third patient died of a respiratory illness 3.5 years after transplantation but without evidence of sarcoid in any organ at autopsy. It is important, before embarking on consideration for transplantation, to exclude systemic sarcoid involvement by pulmonary function tests, gallium scans of the chest and abdomen, serum angiotensin-converting enzyme levels, measurement of erythrocyte sedimentation rate, and biopsy of any lymphadenopathy. CHF—congestive heart failure; EMB—endomyocardial biopsy; VA—ventricular arrhythmias. (*Adapted from* Valentine and coworkers [30]; with permission.)

CARDIAC HEMOCHROMATOSIS

CLINICAL PROFILE OF 6 PATIENTS WITH BIOPSY-PROVEN CARDIAC HEMOCHROMATOSIS	
CLINICAL FEATURE	PATIENTS, *n*
Etiology of iron overload	
Hemochromatosis	4
Acquired sideroblastic anemia	2
Presenting symptom of dyspnea	6
Cardiomegaly on chest radiography	5
Two-dimensional echocardiography	
Left ventricular dilation and severe systolic dysfunction	5
Normal ventricular wall thickness	6
Cardiac catheterization (5 patients studied)	
Increased LVEDP	5
Left ventricular enlargement and severe hypokinesis	5
Normal coronary arteries	5

FIGURE 4-32. Patients with cardiac hemochromatosis usually present with symptoms and signs of congestive heart failure. Olson *et al.* at the Mayo Clinic [5] reported the clinical and pathologic features of this disorder, diagnosed by endomyocardial biopsy, in six male patients. Dyspnea was the presenting symptom in all six and was associated with physical signs of congestive heart failure in five. Chest roentgenograms demonstrated cardiomegaly in five patients and on two-dimensional echocardiography, left ventricular enlargement and severe systolic dysfunction were seen in five. Five of the patients studied underwent cardiac catheterization. All five had increased left ventricular end-diastolic pressures (LVEDP) and, on ventriculography, all five demonstrated left ventricular enlargement and severe hypokinesis. Although no patient in this series had the classic findings of restriction, it has been reported that early cardiac involvement by hemochromatosis may be manifested by diastolic or restrictive dysfunction [6]. (*Adapted from* Olson and coworkers [5]; with permission.)

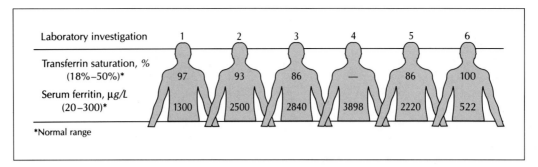

Laboratory investigation	1	2	3	4	5	6
Transferrin saturation, % (18%–50%)*	97	93	86	—	86	100
Serum ferritin, µg/L (20–300)*	1300	2500	2840	3898	2220	522

*Normal range

FIGURE 4-33. Results of screening tests for systemic iron overload in six patients with cardiac hemochromatosis. Screening for systemic iron overload in patients with suspected hemochromatosis includes determination of transferrin saturation and serum ferritin levels. The combined sensitivity and specificity of these two screening tests is approximately 95% for the detection of iron overload in patients with genetic hemochromatosis. In the series of six patients reported by Olson *et al.* [5], ferritin levels were elevated in all and percent transferrin saturation exceeded 85% in the five patients in whom it was determined. (*Adapted from* Olson and coworkers [5]; with permission.)

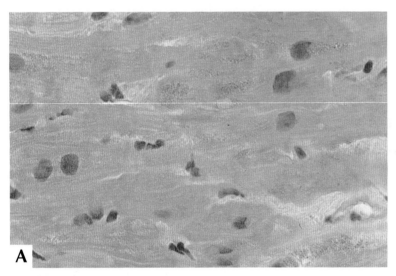

A

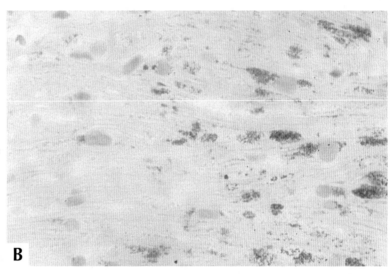

B

FIGURE 4-34. Appearance of myocardial tissue in a patient with cardiac hemochromatosis. If screening test results are consistent with iron overload, histologic confirmation of hemochromatosis is necessary [5]. In patients whose primary clinical manifestations are cardiac in origin, endomyocardial biopsy is preferred to liver biopsy and may provide a definitive diagnosis. The depicted histologic slides are those of myocardium obtained at endomyocardial biopsy in a 35-year-old man who presented to our center with progressive heart failure. **A,** Hematoxylin and eosin staining demonstrates brown-black pigmentation of the myocytes. **B,** Prussian blue staining shows the pigmentation to be iron. (Courtesy of Vijaya Reddy, MD, Loyola University Medical Center, Maywood, IL.)

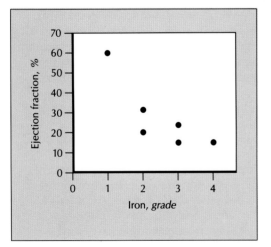

FIGURE 4-35. The inverse relationship between left ventricular ejection fraction and the quantity of stainable iron deposition in myocardial tissue. There appears to be an inverse relation between left ventricular ejection fraction and the quantity of stainable iron deposition in endomyocardial tissue. Using an iron-grading system for endomyocardial biopsy tissue (normal, 0%; grade 1, 1% to 25%; grade 2, 26% to 50%; grade 3, 51% to 75%; grade 4, > 75%), Olson *et al.* [5] plotted ejection fraction against iron grade in their six patients. As shown in this plot, there was a distinct trend for higher iron grades to be associated with lower ejection fractions. However, the small sample size precluded a demonstration of *statistical* significance (Spearman's rank correlation coefficient = -0.80; $P=0.08$). (*Adapted from* Olson and coworkers [5]; with permission.)

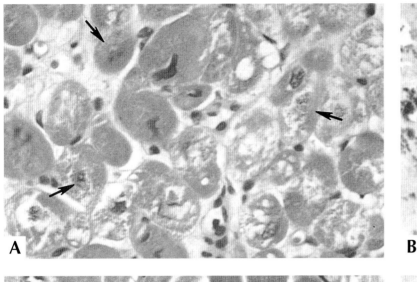

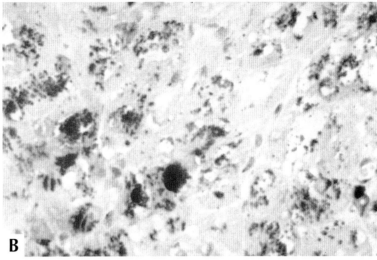

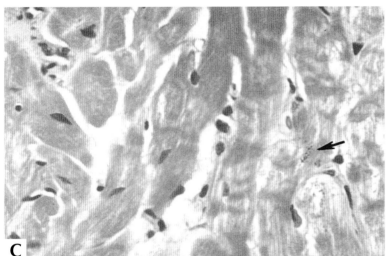

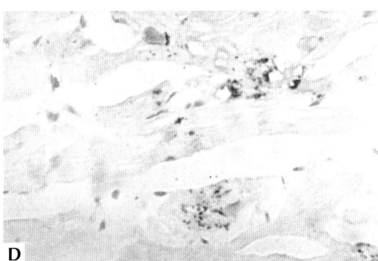

FIGURE 4-36. The ability of chelation therapy to decrease the amount of myocardial stainable iron deposition. Cardiac dysfunction associated with iron overload may be reversed after iron removal by either chelation or phlebotomy [6,26]. Serial endomyocardial biopsies may be indicated to document depletion of myocardial iron. **A,** Hematoxylin and eosin staining of a right ventricular biopsy specimen in a patient with iron-overload cardiomyopathy, before chelation therapy. Note brown-speckled intracellular material (*arrows*). These are iron deposits. **B,** In the same patient, Prussian blue staining demonstrates iron deposits in blue. After 1 year of deferoxamine therapy, the amount of iron (*arrow*) with hematoxylin and eosin (**C**) and iron (**D**) stains has considerably decreased (magnification, × 250). (*Adapted from* Uretsky [26]; with permission.)

CARDIAC AMYLOIDOSIS

CLINICAL PRESENTATIONS OF CARDIAC AMYLOIDOSIS

Restrictive cardiomyopathy
  Jugular venous distention
  Narrow pulse pressure
  Protodiastolic gallop
  Hepatomegaly
  Peripheral edema

Congestive heart failure due to
  systolic dysfunction
Orthostatic hypotension
Abnormalities of cardiac impulse
  formation and conduction
  (resulting in arrhythmias and
  conduction disturbances)

FIGURE 4-37. In amyloidosis associated with an immunocyte dyscrasia (primary amyloidosis), pathologic evidence of cardiac involvement is virtually the rule. However, clinically apparent heart disease is present in only one third to one half of patients [31,32]. The most common clinical presentation of cardiac amyloidosis is that of a restrictive cardiomyopathy, in which right-sided findings dominate the clinical picture [32]. A second common presentation is congestive heart failure due to systolic dysfunction. Much less commonly, patients may present with orthostatic hypotension or with symptoms caused by abnormalities of cardiac impulse formation and conduction.

A. ABNORMALITIES NOTED ON THE RESTING 12-LEAD ECGS OF 24 PATIENTS WITH PRIMARY AMYLOIDOSIS	
ECG ABNORMALITY	PATIENTS, n
Low voltage	15
First-degree atrioventricular block	7
Isolated left anterior hemiblock	2
Isolated left posterior hemiblock	3
Right bundle branch block	1
Bifascicular block	3
Pseudomyocardial infarction	4
Indeterminate intraventricular conduction defect	1

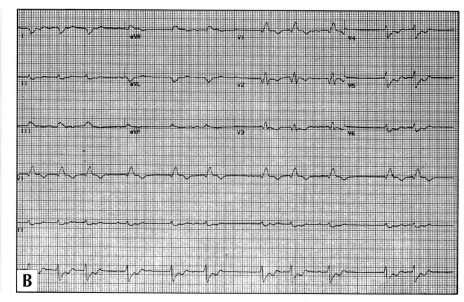

FIGURE 4-38. A, Abnormal electrocardiographic (ECG) findings are common in patients with cardiac amyloidosis. Falk *et al.* [33] reviewed the electrocardiograms of 27 patients with primary amyloidosis. Twenty-four (89%) of these patients had an abnormal resting 12-lead ECG. The single most common ECG abnormality noted was low voltage (seen in 15 patients). There was also a high incidence of conduction disturbances on standard electrocardiography, as detailed in the table. Individual patients may have more than one of the listed ECG abnormalities. **B,** The ECG shown is that of a 61-year-old man who presented to our center with progressive heart failure, anatomically normal coronary arteries, and biopsy-proven cardiac amyloidosis. It illustrates a number of the ECG abnormalities listed above, including low voltage in the limb leads, right bundle branch block, and a pseudoinfarction pattern. This man had recently developed atrial fibrillation. (Part A *adapted from* Falk and coworkers [33]; with permission.)

RESULTS OF HOLTER ECG MONITORING STUDIES IN 27 PATIENTS WITH PRIMARY AMYLOIDOSIS	
ARRHYTHMIA	PATIENTS, n
Complex ventricular arrhythmia	14
Lown grade 3 to 4b	14
Lown grade 4a to 4b	12
Sustained atrial fibrillation	2
Paroxysmal atrial fibrillation	1
Supraventricular tachycardia	7
Atrial premature beats > 20/h	6

FIGURE 4-39. Cardiac amyloidosis is associated with a strong propensity for the development of arrhythmias. Falk *et al.* [33] performed continuous 24-hour ambulatory electrocardiographic (ECG) monitoring studies in their 27 patients with primary amyloidosis. Complex ventricular arrhythmias (multiform, paired, or repetitive beats) were documented in 14 (47%) patients. Frequent premature atrial complexes and supraventricular tachycardias or atrial fibrillation, or both, were seen on Holter monitoring in 10 patients. The presence of ventricular arrhythmias correlated with heart failure and, more strongly, with an abnormal echocardiogram. There were four sudden deaths, all in patients with abnormal echocardiograms and complex ventricular arrhythmias. Prompted by these observations, Falk *et al.* have suggested that complex ventricular arrhythmias in cardiac amyloidosis may be a harbinger of subsequent sudden cardiac death (the latter event is reported to occur in about 33% of patients with cardiac amyloidosis). It is also noteworthy that patients with cardiac amyloidosis are particularly sensitive to digitalis preparations, and the use of ordinary doses may lead to serious arrhythmias. This may relate to selective binding of digoxin to amyloid fibrils in the myocardium [32]. (*Adapted from* Falk and coworkers [33]; with permission.)

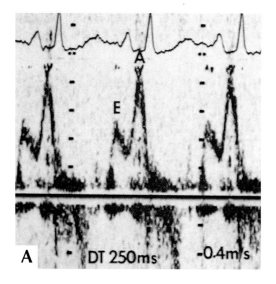

FIGURE 4-40. The spectrum of abnormal Doppler echocardiographic patterns in cardiac amyloidosis. Echocardiography is of considerable value in the diagnosis of infiltrative amyloid heart disease [34]. Typical features on two-dimensional echocardiography include a granular appearance of the myocardium and increased thickness of the myocardial walls. A number of studies have clearly shown that diastolic dysfunction in cardiac amyloidosis exhibits a spectrum of abnormalities that can be followed up serially by Doppler echocardiography. In earlier stages of amyloid heart disease, abnormal relaxation is the Doppler pattern seen (**A**). The E wave is of lower magnitude than the a-wave and the deceleration time is prolonged. (*continued*)

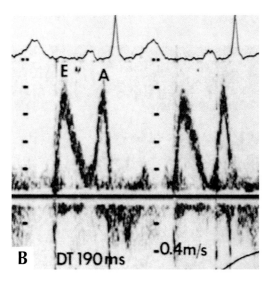

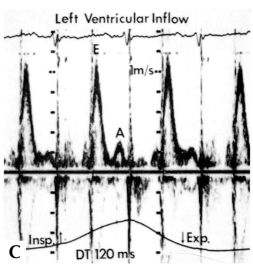

Left Ventricular Inflow

B DT 190 ms −0.4m/s

C Insp. | Exp. DT 120 m/s

FIGURE 4-40. (*continued*) As the disease progresses, a pseudonormalization Doppler pattern may emerge (**B**: the same patient as in *panel A*, taken 6 months later). Eventually, a restrictive pattern (**C**) emerges. As shown in this example (pulsed-wave Doppler recording of a left ventricular inflow profile), there is increased E/A ratio (3.7) and short deceleration time (120 ms). (*Adapted from* Klein and coworkers [34]; with permission.)

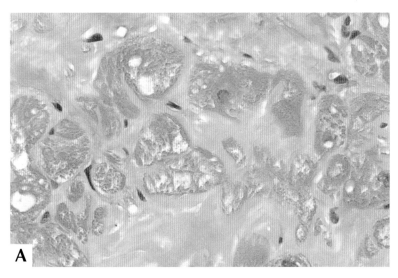

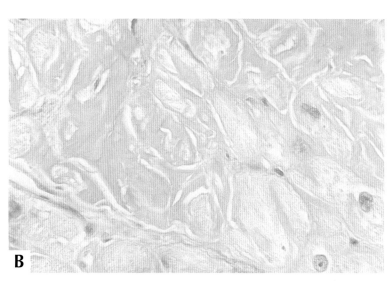

FIGURE 4-41. Appearance of myocardial tissue obtained at endomyocardial biopsy in cardiac amyloidosis. Endomyocardial biopsy may provide a definitive diagnosis in cardiac amyloidosis [32]. The depicted images are those of myocardium obtained at endomyocardial biopsy in a 53-year-old woman with rapidly progressive heart failure, in whom neither cardiac amyloidosis nor a blood dyscrasia was suspected prior to biopsy. **A,** Hematoxylin and eosin staining shows pink eosinophilic deposits of amyloid. **B,** Sulfated Alcian blue staining demonstrates apple green staining of the deposits. (Courtesy of Vijaya Reddy, Maywood, IL.)

PERIPARTUM CARDIOMYOPATHY

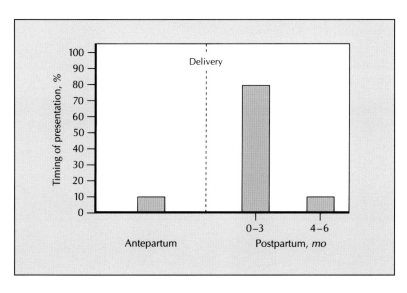

FIGURE 4-42. The timing of presentation of peripartum cardiomyopathy relative to delivery. Peripartum cardiomyopathy is defined as congestive heart failure that develops in the final 3 months of pregnancy or the first 6 months postpartum in women with no evidence of heart disease before pregnancy and no obvious cause of heart failure. Approximately 10% of cases manifest during pregnancy, 80% present in the first 3 months postpartum, and the remaining 10% up to 6 months postpartum.

INCIDENCE OF PERIPARTUM CARDIOMYOPATHY IN VARIOUS POPULATIONS

STUDY	STUDY POPULATION LOCATION	INCIDENCE OF PERIPARTUM CARDIOMYOPATHY
Davidson and Parry [35]	Nigeria (Hausa tribe)	1/100 deliveries
Meadows [36]	United States	1/1300 live births
Woolford [37]	United States	1/4000 live births
Cunningham *et al.* [38]	United States	1/15,150 deliveries

RISK FACTORS FOR PERIPARTUM CARDIOMYOPATHY

Black race
Twin births
Increased maternal age
Hypertension or toxemia
Multiparity

FIGURE 4-43. The incidence of peripartum cardiomyopathy varies with geography and race, with an incidence as high as 1% in the Hausa tribes in Nigeria [35]. The reported incidence in the United States has been one in 1300 [36] to one in 4000 live births [37]. However, in one US study, an incidence of only one in 15,150 deliveries was found when a cause for heart failure was carefully sought [38]. It is noteworthy that postpartum tribal practices are probably responsible for the high incidence of peripartum cardiomyopathy in the Hausa people [8]. For 40 days after delivery, women of this tribe lie, twice daily, on baked mud beds over a fire, splash themselves with hot water, and eat large amounts of kanwa, a dried lake salt. Postpartum hypertension is also prevalent in this group, and the combination of volume overload and pressure overload appears to be the probable mechanism responsible for the very high incidence of peripartum heart failure reported in this tribe.

FIGURE 4-44. A number of risk factors for the development of peripartum cardiomyopathy have been identified. Most studies have reported black women to be at increased risk. The increased hypertension, hemodynamic and hormonal stresses, and the nutritional demands of twin pregnancies may explain the risk associated with this condition as opposed to single pregnancies.

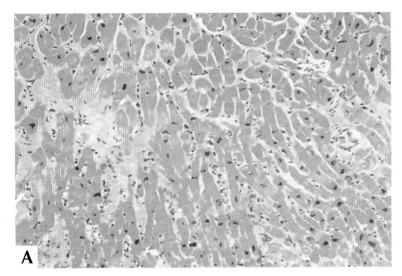

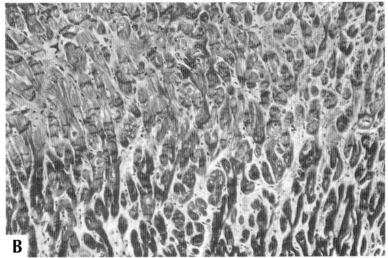

FIGURE 4-45. The nonspecific histopathologic appearances usually seen in peripartum cardiomyopathy (PPCM). Histopathologic findings in PPCM are most often nonspecific. Hematoxylin and eosin staining (**A**) and Masson's trichrome staining (**B**) of endomyocardial biopsy samples obtained from a 33-year-old multiparous black woman with PPCM are illustrated. With hematoxylin and eosin, myocyte hypertrophy and interstitial fibrosis are seen; the Masson's trichrome–stained sample better demonstrates the interstitial fibrosis. These nonspecific findings of myocyte hypertrophy and interstitial fibrosis are those most characteristically seen in PPCM. (Courtesy of Vijaya Reddy, Maywood, IL.)

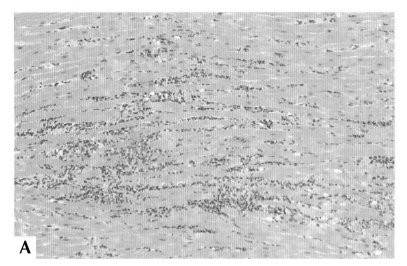

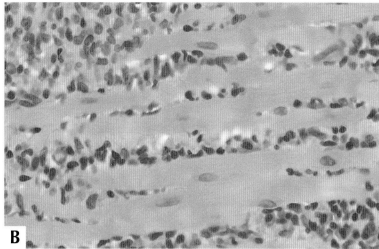

FIGURE 4-46. Histologic appearance of acute myocarditis in a patient with peripartum cardiomyopathy (PPCM). In a variably reported minority of patients with PPCM, evidence of myocarditis can be seen on endomyocardial biopsy. The likelihood of myocarditis being found is greater if biopsy is performed early after the onset of symptoms [8]. The low-power (**A**) and high-power (**B**) appearance of hematoxylin and eosin–stained myocardial tissue obtained from a 30-year-old multiparous black woman with PPCM. Under low power, diffuse infiltration of inflammatory cells can be seen. High-power examination shows myocyte necrosis. Such appearances suggest a potential etiologic role for myocarditis in some patients with PPCM. (Courtesy of Vijaya Reddy, Maywood, IL.)

SYMPTOMS IN PERIPARTUM CARDIOMYOPATHY

Malaise
Fatigue
Weakness
Exertional dyspnea

Cough (frequently nocturnal)
Paroxysmal nocturnal dyspnea
Orthopnea
Edema

FIGURE 4-47. The symptoms of peripartum cardiomyopathy are those common to heart failure from any cause. Symptoms of left ventricular failure frequently develop first, followed by symptoms of right ventricular failure. The development of hemoptysis and chest pain is not unusual, but when this occurs pulmonary embolism must be considered. Indeed, pulmonary or systemic emboli, which occur in 25% to 40% of patients, may be the presenting symptom. The incidence of emboli may be increased by the decreased fibrinogenolysis found in pregnant women.

PHYSICAL FINDINGS IN PERIPARTUM CARDIOMYOPATHY

Tachycardia, decreased pulse pressure
Increased blood pressure
Increased jugular venous pressure
Edema, ascites, hepatomegaly
Rales

Parasternal lift
Loud P_2
S_3 or S_4 gallop
Murmurs of mitral and tricuspid
   regurgitation

FIGURE 4-48. Findings on physical examination in peripartum cardiomyopathy are also similar to those of other forms of heart failure, except that the blood pressure, particularly diastolic pressure, is initially elevated. Cardiac examination frequently reveals a parasternal lift and a laterally displaced, diffuse apex beat. Murmurs of mitral and tricuspid regurgitation are not uncommon.

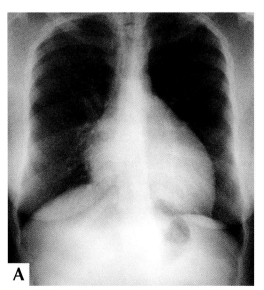

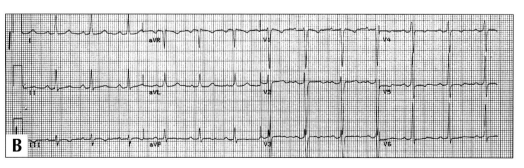

FIGURE 4-49. Chest radiographic and 12-lead electrocardiographic (ECG) appearances in a patient with peripartum cardiomyopathy. **A,** The chest radiograph reveals cardiomegaly with varying degrees of pulmonary vascular redistribution. **B,** The ECG is frequently abnormal, but the findings are nonspecific. ST-T changes and T-wave inversions are the most common abnormalities. Sinus tachycardia and voltage criteria for left ventricular hypertrophy are also common. Left and right bundle branch block are less common than with other cardiomyopathies and suggest complicating factors (*eg,* pulmonary emboli resulting in right bundle branch block).

TREATMENT OF PERIPARTUM CARDIOMYOPATHY

Oxygen
Diuretics
Positive inotropes
Vasodilators
Anticoagulants
Cardiac transplantation

FIGURE 4-50. Acute heart failure in patients with peripartum cardiomyopathy (PPCM) should be treated vigorously with oxygen, a low-salt diet, fluid restriction, diuretics, inotropic support with digitalis, and certain vasodilators [8,39]. The afterload-reducing agent hydralazine is safe for use in pregnancy. However, angiotensin-converting enzyme inhibitors have potentially deleterious effects on blood pressure control and renal function in the fetus and are therefore contraindicated for use during the antepartum period. Anticoagulation therapy is recommended. During pregnancy, subcutaneous or intravenous heparin is used to avoid the detrimental effects of coumadin on the fetus. Oral anticoagulants are used after delivery. As previously mentioned, a variable minority of patients with PPCM demonstrate evidence of myocarditis on endomyocardial biopsy. However, because no controlled studies are available, the use of immunosuppressive agents in PPCM cannot be routinely recommended [8]. For patients who remain unstable, intravenous vasodilators and insertion of an intra-aortic balloon pump should be considered. For those who remain symptomatic despite all the above measures, cardiac transplantation should be considered.

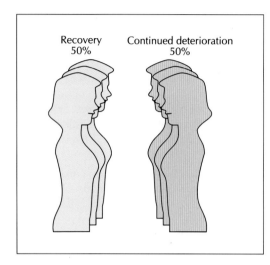

FIGURE 4-51. Prognosis for patients with peripartum cardiomyopathy. Approximately 50% of patients with peripartum cardiomyopathy demonstrate complete or near-complete recovery of cardiac function and clinical status within 6 months. Unfortunately, the remaining 50% continue to deteriorate, resulting in early death or progressive heart failure with a high incidence of morbidity and mortality.

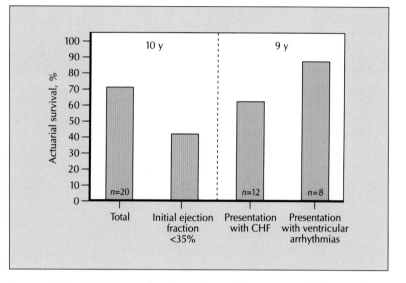

FIGURE 4-52. Predictors of outcome in peripartum cardiomyopathy. Ventricular function at presentation appears to be an important predictor of survival. Davis *et al.* [40] at the Mayo Clinic retrospectively examined the long-term outcome of 20 patients who presented with peripartum cardiomyopathy. Overall actuarial survival was 71% at 10 years. In patients with an initial ejection fraction of less than 35%, 10-year actuarial survival was only 42%. In contrast, no deaths occurred in patients with an ejection fraction of greater than 35%. Furthermore, in patients who presented with congestive heart failure (CHF), 9-year actuarial survival was 63% compared with 88% for patients who presented with ventricular arrhythmias. (*Adapted from* Davis and coworkers [40]; with permission.)

COMPARATIVE OUTCOME FOLLOWING TRANSPLANTATION FOR PERIPARTUM CARDIOMYOPATHY

	PPCM PATIENTS	OTHER WOMEN < 45 Y	P VALUE
Patients, *n*	6	10	
Follow-up, *d*	868±572	1055±911	NS
Recipient race, white/black/other, *n*	1/4/1	9/0/1	0.01
Rejection/patient/mo, *n*			
1 mo	2.2±0.8	1.2±0.9	0.05
6 mo	1.0±0.3	0.6±0.5	0.07
1 y	0.7±0.2	0.4±0.3	0.07
Total follow-up	0.6±0.7	0.4±0.4	NS
Deaths, *n(%)*	4(67)	3(30)	NS

FIGURE 4-53. The reported poor outcome after cardiac transplantation for peripartum cardiomyopathy (PPCM) has been ascribed to either hyperacute or recurrent rejection. At our center, we compared the outcomes of six women with PPCM who underwent transplantation and 10 women under 45 years of age who underwent transplantation for other indications [8]. Baseline characteristics of the two groups were similar, except for an increased number of blacks in the PPCM group. The PPCM group experienced more rejection early after transplantation, consistent with an immune cause for their original disease. Although there was a trend toward increased mortality in the PPCM patients, it did not reach statistical significance in this small series. (*Adapted from* Johnson and coworkers [8]; with permission.)

REFERENCES

1. Glazier JJ, Costanzo MR: Specific heart muscle disease. *Curr Opin Cardiol* 1993, 8:454–462.

2. McAlister HF, Klementowicz PT, Andrews C, *et al*.: Lyme carditis: an important cause of reversible heart block. *Ann Intern Med* 1989, 110:339–345.

3. Stanek G, Klein J, Bittner R, *et al*.: Isolation of *Borrelia burgdorferi* from the myocardium of a patient with long-standing cardiomyopathy. *N Engl J Med* 1990, 322:249–252.

4. Shammas RL, Movahed A: Sarcoidosis of the heart. *Clin Cardiol* 1993, 16:462–472.

5. Olson LJ, Edwards WD, Holmes DR, *et al*.: Endomyocardial biopsy in hemochromatosis: clinicopathologic correlates in six cases. *J Am Coll Cardiol* 1989, 13:116–120.

6. Rahko PS, Salerni R, Uretsky BF: Successful reversal by chelation therapy of congestive cardiomyopathy due to iron overload. *J Am Coll Cardiol* 1986, 8:436–440.

7. Lee W, Cotton DB: Peripartum cardiomyopathy: current concepts and clinical management. *Clin Obstet Gynecol* 1989, 32:54–67.

8. Johnson MR, Costanzo-Nordin MR, Gunnar RM: Peripartum cardiomyopathy. In *Progress in Cardiology* 5/2. Edited by Zipes DP, Rowlands D. Philadelphia: Lea & Febiger; 1992:145–157.

9. Kaul S, Fishbein MC, Siegel RJ: Cardiac manifestations of AIDS: a 1991 update. *Am Heart J* 1991, 122:535–544.

10. Acierno LJ: Cardiac complications in acquired immunodeficiency syndrome (AIDS): a review. *J Am Coll Cardiol* 1989, 13:1144–1154.

11. Lewis W, Grody WW: AIDS and the heart: review and consideration of pathogenetic mechanisms. *Cardiovasc Pathol* 1992, 1:53–64.

12. Wu TC, Pizzorno MC, Hayward GS, *et al*.: In situ detection of human cytomegalovirus: immediate-early gene transcripts within cardiac myocytes of patients with HIV-associated cardiomyopathy. *AIDS* 1992, 6:777–785.

13. Lamperth L, Dalakas MC, Dagani F, *et al*.: Abnormal skeletal and cardiac muscle mitochondria induced by zidovudine (AZT) in human muscle in vitro and in an animal model. *Lab Invest* 1991, 65:742–751.

14. Herskowitz A, Willoughby SB, Baughman I, *et al*.: Cardiomyopathy associated with antiretroviral therapy in patients with HIV infection: a report of six cases. *Ann Intern Med* 1992, 116:311–313.

15. Habicht GS, Beck G, Benach JL: Lyme disease. *Sci Am* 1987, 257:78–83.

16. Fitzpatrick TB, Eisen AZ, Wolff K, *et al*.: *Dermatology in General Medicine*, vol 2, ed 4. New York: McGraw-Hill; 1993:2412.

17. Van der Linde MR, Crijns HJCM, de Konig J, *et al*.: Range of atrioventricular disturbances in Lyme borreliosis: a report of four cases and review of other published reports. *Br Heart J* 1990, 63:162–168.

18. Klein J, Stanek G, Bittner R, *et al*.: Lyme borreliosis as a cause of myocarditis and heart muscle disease. *Eur Heart J* 1991, 12(suppl D):73–75.

19. Longcope WT, Freiman DG: A study of sarcoidosis based on combined investigation of 160 cases including 30 autopsies from the Johns Hopkins Hospital and Massachusetts General Hospital. *Medicine* 1952, 31:1–132.

20. Silverman KJ, Hutchins GM, Bulkley BM: Cardiac sarcoid: a clinicopathologic evaluation of 84 unselected patients with systemic sarcoidosis. *Circulation* 1978, 58:1204–1211.

21. Matsui Y, Iwai K, Tachibana T, *et al*.: Clinicopathological study in fatal myocardial sarcoidosis. *Ann NY Acad Sci* 1976, 278:455–469.

22. Roberts WC, McAlister HA, Ferrano VJ: Sarcoidosis of the heart. *Am J Med* 1977, 63:86–108.

23. Porter GM: Sarcoid heart disease. *N Engl J Med* 1960, 265:1350–1357.

24. Fleming HA, Bailey SM: Sarcoid heart disease. *J R Coll Physicians Lond* 1981, 15:245–253.

25. Bashour FA, McConnell T, Skinner W, *et al*.: Myocardial sarcoidosis. *Dis Chest* 1968, 53:413–420.

26. Uretsky BF: Diagnostic considerations in the adult patient with cardiomyopathy or congestive heart failure. In *Cardiovascular Clinics*. Edited by Shaver JA. Philadelphia: FA Davis; 1988:35–56.

27. Sekiguchi M, Numao Y, Nunoda S, *et al*.: Clinical histopathological profile of sarcoidosis of the heart and acute idiopathic myocarditis: concepts through a study employing endomyocardial biopsy. *Jpn Circ J* 1980, 44:249–263.

28. Winters SL, Cohen M, Greenberg S, *et al*.: Sustained ventricular tachycardia associated with sarcoidosis: assessment of the underlying cardiac anatomy and prospective utility of programmed ventricular stimulation drug therapy and inducible antitachycardia device. *J Am Coll Cardiol* 1991, 18:937–943.

29. Schaedel H, Kirsten D, Schmidt A, *et al*.: Sarcoid heart disease: results of follow-up investigations. *Eur Heart J* 1991, 12(suppl D):26–27.

30. Valentine HA, Tazelaar HD, Macoviak J: Cardiac sarcoidosis: response to steroids and transplantation. *J Heart Lung Transplant* 1987, 6:244–256.

31. Gertz MA, Kyle RA: Primary systemic amyloidosis: a diagnostic primer. *Mayo Clin Proc* 1989, 64:1505–1519.

32. Falk RH: Cardiac amyloidosis. In *Progress in Cardiology*. Edited by Zipes DP, Rowlands DJ. Philadelphia: Lea & Febiger; 1989:143–153.

33. Falk RH, Rubinow A, Cohen AS: Cardiac arrhythmias in systemic amyloidosis: correlation with echographic abnormalities. *J Am Coll Cardiol* 1984, 3:107–113.

34. Klein MD, Hatle LK, Burstow DJ, *et al*.: Characterization of left ventricular diastolic function in amyloidosis. *J Am Coll Cardiol* 1989, 13:1017–1026.

35. Davidson NM, Parry EHO: Peripartum cardiac failure. *Q J Med* 1978, 47:431–461.

36. Meadows WR: Idiopathic myocardial failure in the last trimester of pregnancy and the puerperium. *Circulation* 1957, 15:903–914.

37. Woolford RM: Postpartum myocardosis. *Ohio State Med J* 1952, 48:924–930.

38. Cunningham FG, Pritchard JA, Hankins GDV, *et al*.: Peripartum heart failure: idiopathic cardiomyopathy or compounding cardiovascular events? *Obstet Gynecol* 1986, 67:157–168.

39. Elkayam U: Pregnancy and cardiovascular disease. In *Heart Disease*, ed 4. Edited by Braunwald E. Philadelphia: WB Saunders; 1992:1790–1809.

40. Davis MD, Murphy JF, Olson LJ, *et al*.: Natural history and endomyocardial biopsy findings in peripartum cardiomyopathy. *Circulation* 1992, 86(suppl I):I-439.

RESTRICTIVE CARDIOMYOPATHY, CARDIAC AMYLOIDOSIS, AND HYPEREOSINOPHILIC HEART DISEASE

5

CHAPTER

Yuzo Hirota

Idiopathic restrictive cardiomyopathy is a rare disease characterized by diastolic dysfunction. There are several diseases that may be associated with restrictive physiology. It is controversial whether hypertrophic cardiomyopathy without obstruction should be included in a discussion of restrictive cardiomyopathy. In restrictive cardiomyopathy both atria are markedly enlarged without thickening of the wall or dilatation of the left ventricle. There are no specific histologic findings, and hypertrophy of the myocytes and interstitial fibrosis are the predominant features. In some cases there may be extensive disarray of the myocytes. The pathogenesis of the stiff heart remains unclear. Familial occurrence is common and association of skeletal muscle disease has been reported.

While advanced cases show pathophysiologic features similar to those of constrictive pericarditis (the strict definition of restrictive physiology), impaired relaxation and reduced compliance of the left ventricle alone (the broad definition of restrictive physiology) are characteristic in patients with less advanced disease. The natural history is long, and patients suffer from severe heart failure years after diagnosis. Because systemic thromboembolism is a common complication, patients should receive anticoagulant therapy. There is no specific treatment, and cardiac transplantation should be considered before patients are disabled from cerebral embolism or congestive cirrhosis of the liver.

Cardiac amyloidosis is caused by the accumulation of one of several amyloid proteins in the heart, among which immunoglobulin light chains (K or λ type, amyloid L) are the most common. Although patients with severe cardiac involvement have restrictive physiology with heart failure, patients with mild cardiac involvement have only early diastolic filling disturbances. Some show features of dilated cardiomyopathy, while others have features mimicking hypertrophic cardiomyopathy. Atrioventricular block, abnormal Q waves, and poor R-wave progression are common electrocardiographic findings. Diffuse left ventricular hypertrophy is commonly seen by echocardiography with peculiar sparkling echo spots. This disease should be considered when patients with unexplained heart disease also have proteinuria, gastroenteropathy, or peripheral neuropathy. The diagnosis can be established by endomyocardial biopsy. There is no specific therapy, and the prognosis is poor. Life expectancy ranges from 6 months to 2 years (after the development of heart failure).

Hypereosinophilic heart disease (Löffler's syndrome) is caused by the cytotoxicity of cationic and major basic proteins derived from eosinophilic granules. Endocarditis, myocarditis, or pericarditis are the clinical features of the acute phase. The clinical course is divided into necrotic (acute), thrombotic (subacute), and fibrotic (chronic) phases. Cavity obliteration of the ventricle with restrictive physiology is a common finding during the thrombotic and fibrotic phases in tropical regions. Valvular regurgitation and cavity dilatation with poor systolic function may be seen. This disease is associated frequently with parasitic or protozoal infections in the tropics, and with autoimmune diseases, malignancy, or allergic diseases in the temperate zone. Adequate and prolonged steroid therapy is essential for management during the necrotic phase. Progression of the disease is rapid in the tropics, and endocardial stripping is the treatment of choice for patients with severe heart failure of restrictive physiology.

IDIOPATHIC RESTRICTIVE CARDIOMYOPATHY

DEFINITION

Evidence of a stiff left ventricle

Normal or near-normal left ventricular systolic function

Absence of left ventricular dilatation or hypertrophy

Unknown etiology or association

FIGURE 5-1. Restrictive cardiomyopathy is named for its restrictive physiology. Classically, the square root sign of the ventricular diastolic pressure wave form was considered as one of the diagnostic criteria [1], but it is not required [2,3]. Restrictive cardiomyopathy predominantly affects the left ventricle, except for tropical endomyocardial fibrosis, in which the right ventricle is involved [4,5].

CONTROVERSIAL CONDITIONS FOR INCLUSION

Stiff left ventricle manifested only as elevated diastolic pressure without other heart disease (early stage of restrictive cardiomyopathy)

Heart failure with normal systolic function, or extensive myocardial disarray without left ventricular hypertrophy

Hypereosinophilic heart disease (Löffler's syndrome) and its sequel (endomyocardial fibrosis)

FIGURE 5-2. Patients in the early stage of restrictive cardiomyopathy have elevated left ventricular diastolic pressure only. The coexistence of restrictive cardiomyopathy and hypertrophic cardiomyopathy in the same family has been reported [3]. Whether these patients should be diagnosed as having restrictive cardiomyopathy or hypertrophic cardiomyopathy without hypertrophy is unknown [6,7]. Some believe Löffler's syndrome to be a classical form of restrictive cardiomyopathy [8], while others believe that this disease should be categorized as a specific heart-muscle disease [9].

HEART-MUSCLE DISEASES MANIFESTING AS RESTRICTIVE PHYSIOLOGY

Amyloidosis

Hemochromatosis

Sarcoidosis

Radiation heart disease

Glycogen storage diseases

Familial neuromuscular disorders

FIGURE 5-3. Some specific heart-muscle diseases might manifest as restrictive physiology. Amyloidosis is the most common of these. While the majority of patients with sarcoidosis have clinical features of dilated cardiomyopathy, and those with glycogen storage or neuromuscular disease have features of hypertrophic cardiomyopathy, some of these patients show restrictive cardiomyopathy. It is both important and difficult to differentiate restrictive physiology and constrictive pericarditis in patients with radiation heart disease because both types exist, and surgical cure is possible for constrictive pericarditis.

GROSS ANATOMY

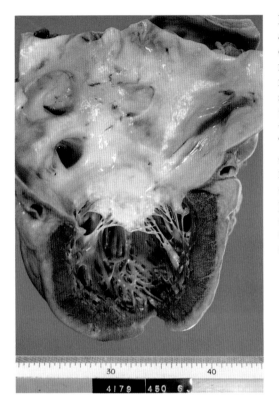

FIGURE 5-4. The left atrium is markedly dilated in idiopathic restrictive cardio-myopathy, and the size and thickness of the left ventricle are within normal limits. The left ventricular endocardium is normal, and cavity obliteration is not present [10]. In other cases (see Fig. 5-10) the endocardium is thickened.

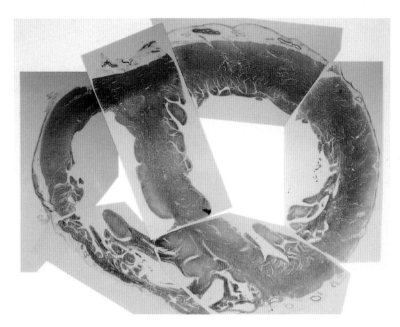

FIGURE 5-5. A cross-sectional view of the right and left ventricles with low-power magnification shows diffuse and fine interstitial fibrosis in the left ventricle without replacement fibrosis or hypertrophy of the wall. The left ventricular cavity is preserved within the normal range (Mallory-azan stain).

HISTOLOGY

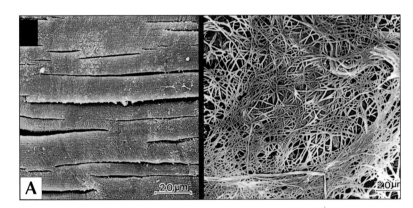

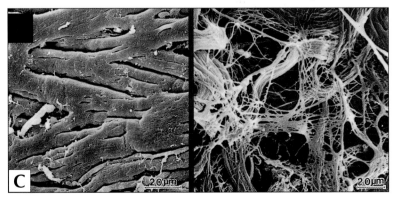

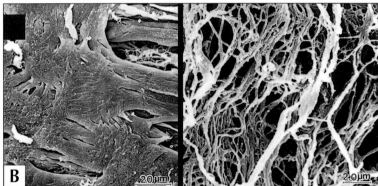

FIGURE 5-6. Scanning electron micrographs of the myocytes (left) and interstitial collagen fibers (right) of a normal heart (A), and two hearts of patients with restrictive cardiomyopathy (B and C). Hypertrophy of the myocytes is prominent in both restrictive and cardiomyopathic hearts compared with the normal heart [3,10,11]. Bizarrely shaped myocytes, frequently seen in hyper-trophic cardiomyopathy, are present in B [3,6]. The thick collagen fibers are abundant, and often form three-dimensional reticular networks in restrictive cardiomyopathy [3,9–11]. Future research into specific typing and quantitation of collagen fibers might elucidate the fundamental mechanism of the stiff ventricle, which is so characteristic of this disease.

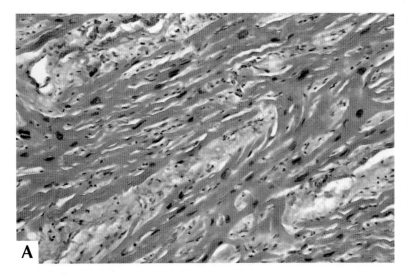

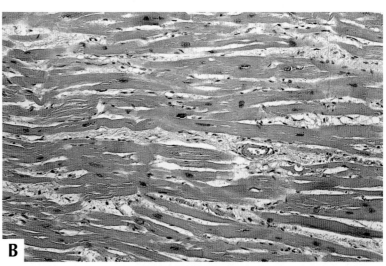

FIGURE 5-7. A, High-power view of the free wall of the left ventricle demonstrates prominent fibrosis and moderate to marked myo-cardial disarray (hematoxylin and eosin). **B,** Compared with *A,* myocyte disarray is not present, and fibrosis is not as prominent.

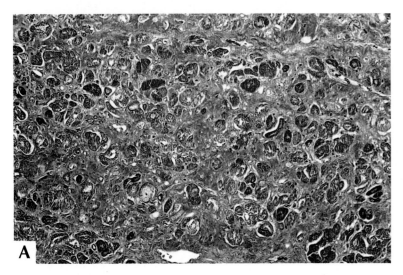

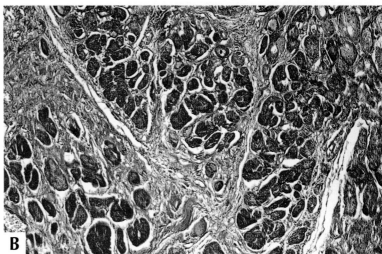

FIGURE 5-8. Cross-sectional view of myocytes surrounded by fibrous tissue (Mallory-azan stain). Whereas severe interstitial fibrosis is seen in both **A** and **B**, fibrous tissue surrounds each myocyte (predominantly endomysial fibrosis) in *A,* and fibrous tissue surrounds bundles or fascicles of the myocytes (predom-inantly perimysial fibrosis) in *B.*

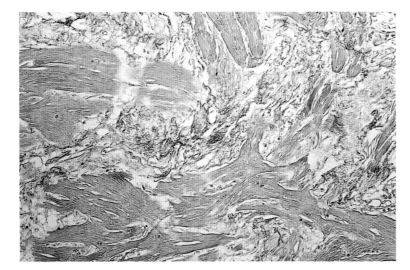

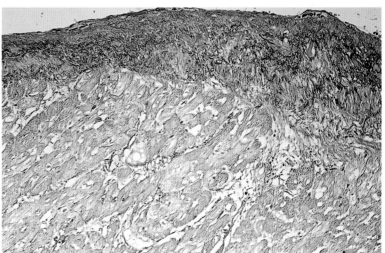

FIGURE 5-9. Myocyte disarray with elastic fiber proliferation (elastic van Gieson's stain). Surrounding the bizarrely shaped myocytes, proliferation of fine elastic fibers can be seen in the area of fibrosis.

FIGURE 5-10. The thickest part of the left ventricular endocardium (elastic van Gieson's stain). The thickening of the endocardium is nonspecific, and fine elastic filament is migrating from the endocar-dium into the subendocardial area [10–12]. The thickness of the endocardium has not exceeded 100 µm in our autopsy cases.

POSTULATED PATHOGENESIS OF STIFF VENTRICLE

MYOCYTE ABNORMALITIES

Intracellular calcium-handling abnormalities

Cytoskeletal abnormalities

Three-dimensional architectural abnormalities
(myofiber disarray)

EXTRACELLULAR MATRIX ABNORMALITIES

Proliferation of collagen fibers

Proliferation of elastic elements

FIGURE 5-11. The postulated pathogenesis of the stiff left ventricle. Prolonged relaxation is expected when calcium uptake and binding to the sarcoplasmic reticulum are impaired, and prolonged relaxation is commonly seen with restrictive cardiomyopathy [2]. The accumulation of desmin, one of the cytoskeletal components, is also reported [13]. Three-dimensional myofiber and myofibril disarray might cause less distension of the left ventricle [6]. Proliferation of interstitial collagen and elastic fibers with reticular network formation is one of the most important factors for the pathogenesis of the stiff ventricle [9].

SEQUENTIAL PATHOPHYSIOLOGY

Impaired LV relaxation and reduced LV early diastolic filling

Reduced LV compliance: elevated LV end-diastolic pressure; accentuated a-wave with E/A <1 by Doppler echocardiography; absence of square root sign

Elevation of LV diastolic and left atrial pressures: pseudonormalization of LV filling pattern by Doppler echocardiography; square root sign may be present

Development of atrial fibrillation and pulmonary congestion

Pulmonary hypertension

Elevation of right ventricular diastolic and right atrial pressures

Tricuspid regurgitation: right and left atrial pressures become equal

FIGURE 5-12. The sequential pathophysiologic changes in restrictive cardiomyopathy. The differences between the early and late stages are well documented in amyloid heart disease [14,15]. Pseudonormalization of transmitral flow by Doppler echocardiography is seen when left atrial pressure is elevated [15–17]. Elevation of right atrial pressure with severe tricuspid regurgitation is seen in patients in advanced stages [3]. E/A—ratio of the peak early diastolic (E) to atrial (A) contraction transmitral flow velocities; LV—left ventricular.

SIGNS AND SYMPTOMS

SYMPTOMS	CAUSATIVE MECHANISMS
Palpitation	Atrial tachyarrhythmias
Syncope	High-degree atrioventricular block and cerebral thromboembolism
Dyspnea on exertion, paroxysmal nocturnal dyspnea, orthopnea	Pulmonary congestion and pleural effusion
Weakness and exercise intolerance	Low cardiac output
Peripheral edema, abdominal distension, loss of appetite	Right ventricular failure
Atypical chest pain	Arrhythmias? pulmonary hypertension? pulmonary embolism?

SIGNS

S_4 in patients with normal sinus rhythm

S_3 either from left or right ventricular origin

Moist rales in the lung fields

Jugular venous distension, hepatosplenomegaly, ascites, pretibial edema, jaundice

FIGURE 5-13. Although there are no specific signs or symptoms of restrictive cardiomyopathy, this condition is manifested principally as congestive heart failure, pulmonary hypertension, thromboembolism, and arrhythmias.

FIGURE 5-14. The clinical manifestations in restrictive cardio-myopathy differ from one patient to another according to the disease process. Signs and symptoms (*see* Fig. 5-13) are easily understood when the sequential pathophysiologic changes are considered. For a better understanding of the disease, these changes are divided into four stages. LAP—left atrial pressure; RAP—right atrial pressure.

ECHOCARDIOGRAPHY

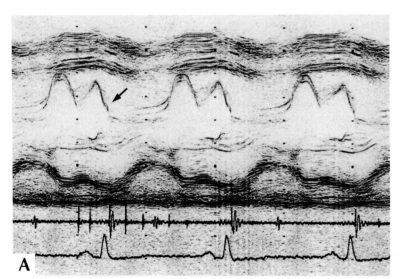

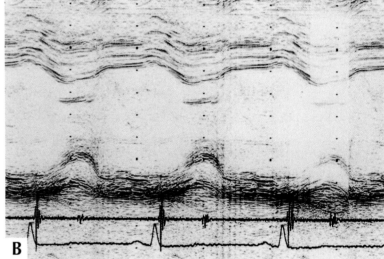

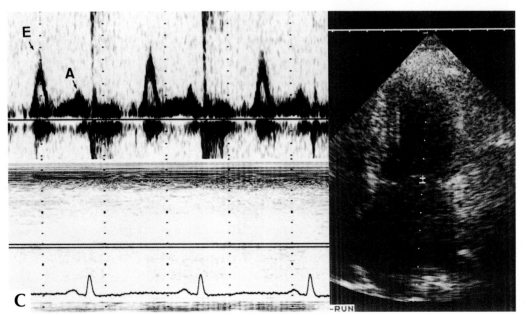

FIGURE 5-15. A, M-mode echocardiogram of the mitral valve. The B bump formation of the mitral valve at end-diastole (*arrow*) suggests an elevated end-diastolic pressure. **B,** M-mode echocardiogram of the left ventricle at the tip of the mitral valve. The left ventricle is contracting normally with normal cavity size, and prominent left ventricular hypertrophy is absent. **C,** Transmitral flow pattern (*left*) of Doppler echocardiography sampled at the tip of the mitral valve (*right*). Transmitral flow suggests a normal pattern with prominent E waves (E) and small a-waves (A), but the deceleration rate of the E wave is rapid. Considering B bump formation, this pattern is interpreted as "pseudonormalization" [16].

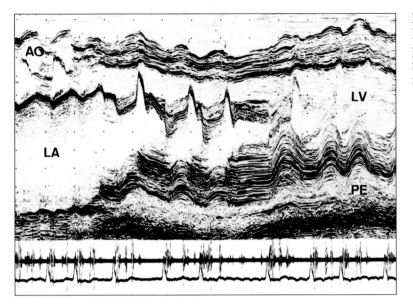

FIGURE 5-16. M-mode scan echocardiogram (same patient as in Fig. 5-4) indicates a markedly enlarged left atrium (LA). A large pericardial effusion (PE) can be seen, which is a common finding in patients with restrictive cardiomyopathy and severe heart failure. AO—aorta; LV—left ventricle.

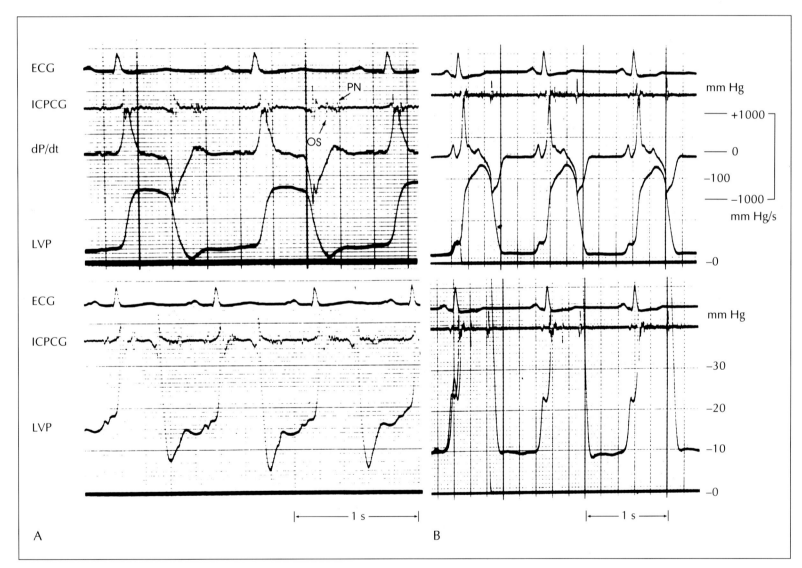

FIGURE 5-17. Differences of left ventricular pressure wave form between constrictive pericarditis (**A**) and restrictive cardiomyopathy (**B**). Both pressures were recorded with the catheter-tipped manometer system. While high-gain left ventricular pressure (LVP) of constrictive pericarditis shows the typical square root sign in the lower panel (*A*), small peak negative dP/dt and high a-wave with the absence of the square root sign are characteristic of restrictive cardiomyopathy (*B*). ECG—electrocardiogram; dP/dt—first derivative of the pressure; ICPCG—intracardiac phonocardiogram.

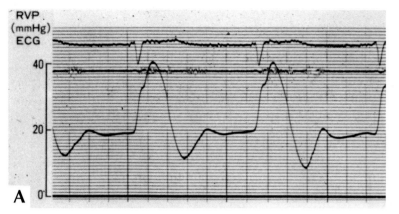

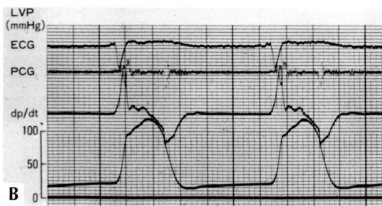

FIGURE 5-18. Right (**A**) and left (**B**) ventricular pressures recorded with a catheter-tipped manometer in a patient with restrictive cardiomyopathy. The typical square root sign of the diastolic pressure wave form is seen in the right ventricle, but not in the left ventricle. Right (RVP) and left (LVP) diastolic pressures are equal, which is commonly seen in association with severe tricuspid regurgitation. This patient also had sick sinus syndrome, and pressures were recorded during ventricular pacemaker rhythm; therefore, atrial contraction is absent. dp/dt—first derivative of the pressure; ECG—electrocardiogram; PCG—phonocardiogram.

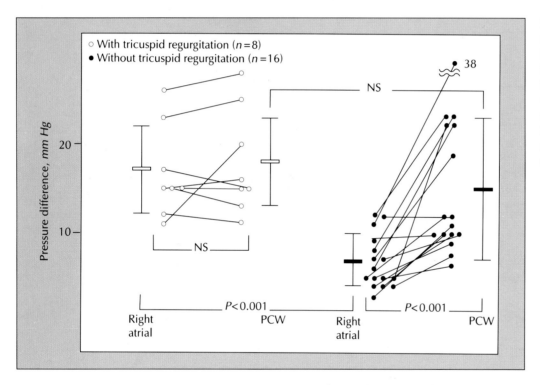

FIGURE 5-19. Right and left atrial pressure differences with and without severe tricuspid regurgitation. In patients without tricuspid regurgitation left atrial pressure is elevated above right atrial pressure, but with tricuspid regurgitation no significant differences are observed between right and left atrial pressures. PCW—pulmonary capillary wedge. (*Adapted from* Hirota and coworkers [3]; with permission.)

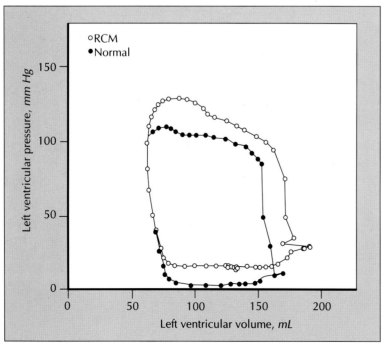

FIGURE 5-20. Pressure-volume loop of a normal heart and the heart of a patient with restrictive cardiomyopathy (RCM). The pressure-volume loops were obtained by frame-by-frame analysis of left ventricular cineangiograms and the simultaneous recording of left ventricular pressure with an 8F pigtail catheter-tipped manometer angiocatheter. The diastolic pressure-volume slope is flat until atrial contraction begins, which is against the concept of "reduced compliance" of the ventricle [18]. The flat slope during the early to mid-diastole suggests that slow and active relaxation continues until this phase. Abnormalities of intracellular calcium handling could be postulated from this observation.

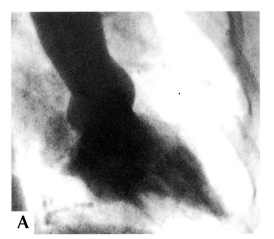 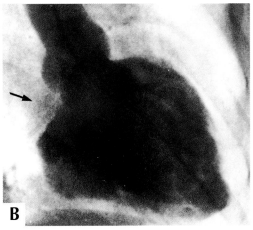

FIGURE 5-21. Left ventricular cineangiograms. **A,** End systole. **B,** End diastole. There are no diagnostic characteristics of restrictive cardiomyopathy with a normal-sized cavity, and normal or near-normal systolic function without severe hypertrophy. The leakage of contrast material into the left atrium during diastole is a common finding because of the stiff left ventricle (*arrow* in *B*).

RESTRICTIVE CARDIOMYOPATHY vs CONSTRICTIVE PERICARDITIS: NONINVASIVE DIFFERENTIAL DIAGNOSIS

History

Physical examination

Chest radiography

Echocardiography

Atrioventricular flow pattern with Doppler
echocardiography

Computed tomography or magnetic
resonance imaging

FIGURE 5-22. Restrictive cardiomyopathy is likely if there is a family history of heart disease or if symptoms of left ventricular failure are predominant. Constrictive pericarditis is likely if the patient has a past history of pericarditis (*eg*, tuberculosis, autoimmune diseases, or open-heart surgery) or if symptoms of right ventricular failure are predominant. The presence of S$_3$ and mitral or tricuspid regurgitation are associated with restrictive cardiomyopathy, while pericardial knock is diagnostic of constrictive pericarditis. Small heart with pulmonary congestion or pleural effusion suggests constrictive pericarditis, and diagnosis is established with the presence of pericardial calcification. An enlarged heart may be seen on chest radiography with restrictive cardiomyopathy. Restrictive cardiomyopathy is likely if echocardiography reveals an enlarged left atrium, pericardial effusion, low E and high a-waves, and pulmonary hypertension (>40 mm Hg). The diagnosis of constrictive pericarditis is established when pericardial thickening (≥4 mm) or calcification is observed with echocardiography, computed tomography, or magnetic resonance imaging [19].

RESTRICTIVE CARDIOMYOPATHY vs CONSTRICTIVE PERICARDITIS: INVASIVE STRATEGY FOR DIFFERENTIAL DIAGNOSIS

Left and right atrial pressure differences
Equal without tricuspid regurgitation—CP likely
Equal with massive tricuspid regurgitation—RCM likely
LAP-RAP≥5 mm Hg—RCM likely

Right ventricular systolic pressure ≤40 mm Hg with end-
diastolic pressure ≥1/3 of systolic pressure—CP likely

Square root sign of left ventricular pressure—CP likely

Square root sign of right ventricular pressure—of no
diagnostic value

Angiography—of no diagnostic value

Endomyocardial biopsy
With some histologic abnormalities—RCM likely
Without histologic abnormalities—CP likely

FIGURE 5-23. The invasive strategy for the differential diagnosis between restrictive cardiomyopathy (RCM) and constrictive pericarditis (CP) is based on right and left ventricular diastolic pressure levels and endomyocardial biopsy findings. In CP, the right and left ventricles are equally affected, thus the filling pressures are always equal. In RCM because the left ventricle is less compliant than the right, the left ventricular filling pressure is usually higher than that of the right ventricle, but in the advanced stage, both right and left ventricular filling pressures may become equal with the development of tricuspid regurgitation. Because of the reduction of cardiac output, right ventricular systolic pressure does not exceed 40 mm Hg in CP. While CP is a disease of the pericardium, and the myocardium is free of disease, left ventricular relaxation is preserved, and the square root sign is present in both ventricles. This square root sign may be absent in the left ventricle of RCM when relaxation disturbance is prominent [2]. Although there is no specific histologic finding, there are some abnormalities consistent with the stiff ventricle in RCM [3,9,12]. In CP, the pathologic process does not extend to the endocardium, and myocardial histology is normal.

PROGNOSIS, NATURAL HISTORY, AND TREATMENT

PROGNOSIS
Poor for children with heart failure
Prolonged course in adults with heart failure

TREATMENT (NO SPECIFIC TREATMENT)
Diuretics
Digitalis
Vasodilators
Anticoagulation with warfarin
Cardiac transplantation

FIGURE 5-24. The natural history of restrictive cardiomyopathy is poor in children with heart failure [20], and the disease course is often prolonged in adults [1,3,21]. Adults suffer from severe symptoms of heart failure for a long period, and die of low cardiac output. Cardiac cirrhosis and thromboembolism are common complications. Because there is no specific treatment, cardiac transplantation should be considered when the patient becomes resistant to the conventional medical therapy for heart failure and before serious complications develop. Digitalis glycosides should be used with caution.

CARDIAC AMYLOIDOSIS

CLINICAL RECOGNITION OF CARDIAC AMYLOIDOSIS

In asymptomatic patients with unexplained electrocardiographic abnormalities

In patients with heart failure with one of the following findings without obvious causes:

Proteinuria

Gastroenteropathy

Anemia

Plasmacytosis

Peripheral neuropathy

Bone pain

WORK-UP FOR CARDIAC AMYLOIDOSIS

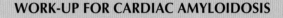

Echocardiography

Urine for Bence Jones protein

Serum for immunoelectrophoresis

Bone survey

Bone marrow aspiration

Biopsy
  Endomyocardial
  Abdominal subcutaneous fat
  Rectal
  Gingival

FIGURE 5-25. Cardiac amyloidosis can be diagnosed easily with endomyocardial biopsy. Physicians should consider amyloidosis in the differential diagnoses in asymptomatic patients with unexplained electrocardiographic abnormalities such as sick sinus syndrome, atrioventricular block, poor R-wave progression, abnormal Q waves, or ST-T abnormalities, especially when these findings have developed recently. Evidence of other organ involvements is also very common in cardiac amyloidosis.

FIGURE 5-26. When considering cardiac amyloidosis in the differential diagnosis, the echocardiogram is especially important (see Fig. 5-29). The cardinal manifestations of plasma cell dyscrasia must be examined at the same time. Histologic evidence is mandatory in order to establish the diagnosis. Biopsy of the abdominal subcutaneous fat tissue is most easily obtained [22], but endomyocardial biopsy is necessary for the diagnosis of cardiac amyloidosis.

FIGURE 5-27. Histologic demonstration of the amyloid protein. Viewed under cross-polaroid light, amyloid gives an apple-green fluorescence. The accumulation of amyloid protein is predominant in the interstitium and perivascular area, and only a few myocytes show positive apple-green fluorescence. This specimen was taken by endomyocardial biopsy (Congo red stain).

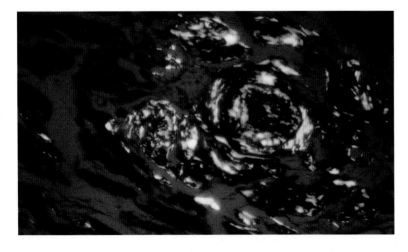

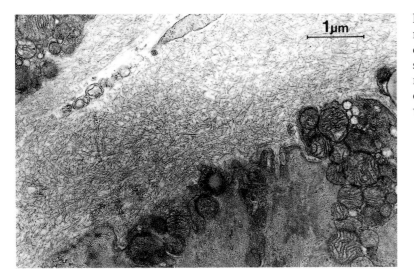

FIGURE 5-28. Electron micrograph of amyloid fibrils in the myocardium. In the extracellular matrix, amyloid presents as a collection of unbranched, usually straight or slightly bent fibrillar structures that are approximately 10 nm in diameter, but can measure up to about 40 nm in diameter. Amyloid fibrils are often oriented randomly and surround the myocytes. (Double-stained with uranyl acetate and lead citrate.)

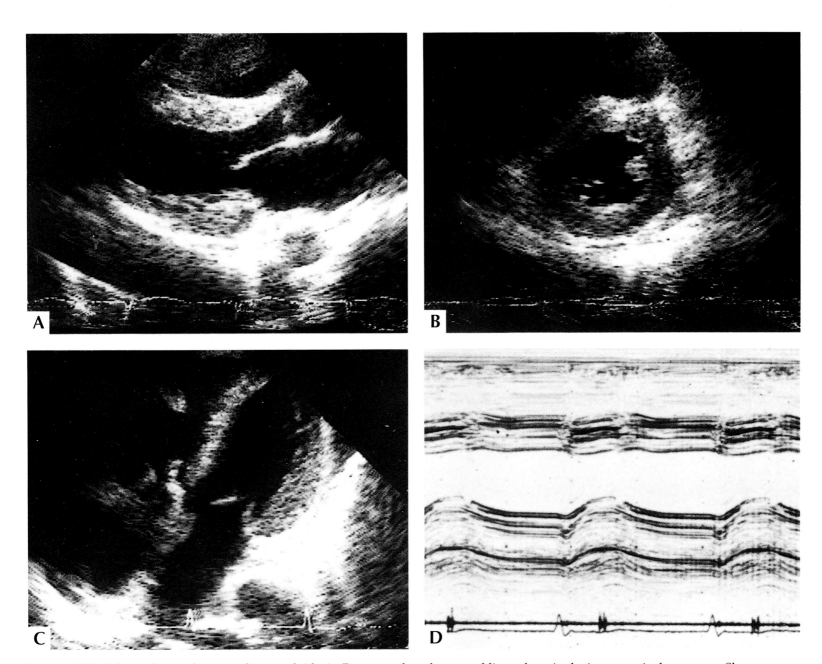

FIGURE 5-29. Echocardiography in cardiac amyloidosis. Parasternal long axis (**A**), short axis (**B**), and apical four-chamber (**C**) views of two-dimensional and left ventricular M-mode (**D**) echocardiograms show sparkling echoes in the interventricular septum. Slow deceleration of the posterior wall during early diastole suggests impairment of left ventricular relaxation and early diastolic filling.

PROGNOSIS, TREATMENT, AND SURVIVAL	
PROGNOSIS	SURVIVAL
With electro- or echocar- diographic abnormalities	<2 years
With heart failure	<6 months

FIGURE 5-30. Prognosis is poor for cardiac amyloidosis [15,22]. There is no specific treatment. Asymptomatic patients with electrocardiographic or echocardiographic abnormalities usually die within 2 years after diagnosis, and the life expectancy for symptomatic patients is less than 6 months. Because this is a systemic disease, cardiac transplantation is not appropriate for primary amyloidosis.

HYPEREOSINOPHILIC HEART DISEASE (LÖFFLER'S SYNDROME)

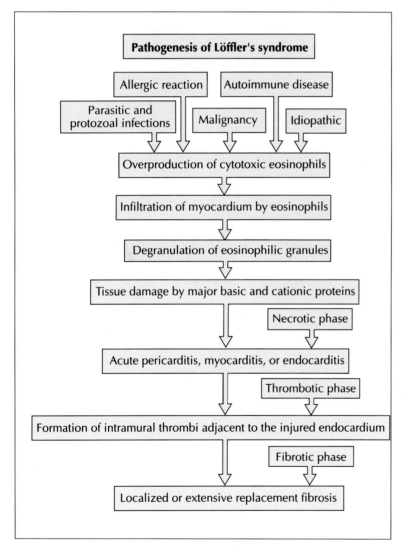

FIGURE 5-31. The pathogenesis of Löffler's syndrome. Tissue damage is caused by major basic and cationic proteins derived from cytotoxic eosinophils [4,5,23–25]. These cytotoxic proteins may stay in the myocardium for a prolonged period and produce continuous tissue damage. At the fibrotic phase, various types of heart diseases, such as endomyocardial fibrosis, dilated cardiomyopathy, atrioventricular block, or valvular regurgitation can be seen according to the difference of the most dominantly involved site.

CLINICAL MANIFESTATIONS

Necrotic phase

Manifestations of acute endo-, myo-, or pericarditis with hypereosinophilia

Thrombotic phase

Cavity obliteration with intramural thrombi with or without hypereosinophilia (common in the tropics and rare in the temperate zone)

Fibrotic phase

Atrioventricular block

Valvular regurgitation

Heart failure with restrictive physiology (ranging from diastolic dysfunction to endomyocardial fibrosis) or systolic dysfunction

Absence of hypereosinophilia

FIGURE 5-32. The clinical manifestations of Löffler's syndrome and endomyocardial fibrosis [4,24]. The necrotic phase is acute, lasting for months. The thrombotic phase is subacute, lasting for months to 2 years. The fibrotic phase is chronic, and lasts for years.

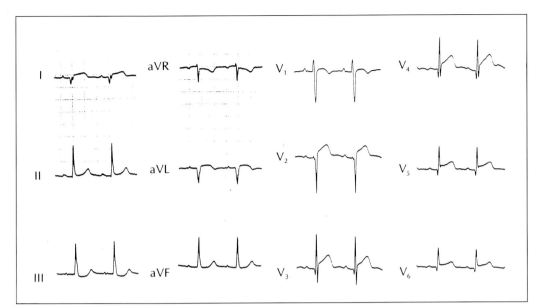

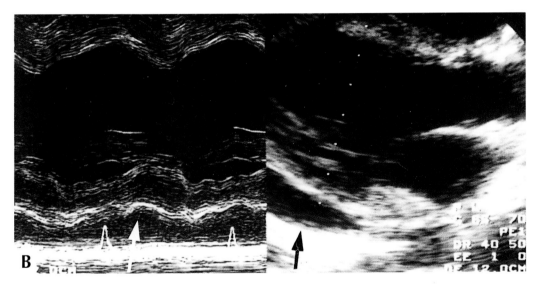

FIGURE 5-33. A 13-year-old boy was admitted with chest pain and orthopnea of 2 days' duration. **A,** The admission electrocardiogram suggested acute myocardial infarction. **B,** M-mode (*left*) and two-dimensional (*right*) echocardiograms showed a normally contracting left ventricle with a moderate pericardial effusion (*arrows*). Emergency coronary cineangiograms were normal. Endomyocardial biopsy was performed. The eosinophil count was 1440/mm^3, and the serum creatine phosphokinase MB level was 25 U/L (normal is <16 U/L). The tentative diagnosis was acute perimyocarditis.

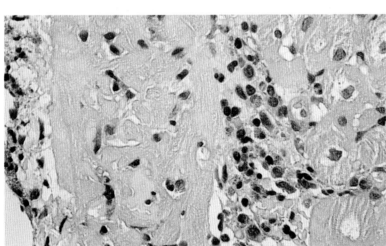

FIGURE 5-34. Histologic view of the biopsy specimen (same patient as in Fig. 5-33) showed massive infiltration of eosinophils in the myocardium as well as in the endocardium (hematoxylin and eosin).

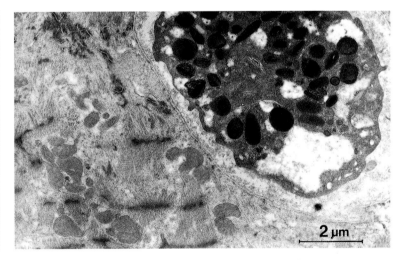

FIGURE 5-35. An eosinophil is seen in the vicinity of a myocyte in this electron photomicrograph (same patient as in Fig. 5-33). The eosinophil contains granules with reversed density, which is a characteristic finding of the activated eosinophils by electron microscopy [23]. Many vacuoles in the cytoplasm of the eosinophil suggest that degranulation has occurred. From these biopsy findings and hypereosinophilia, the diagnosis of hypereosinophilic heart disease was established, and prednisolone, 50 mg/d, was started.

DIAGNOSIS

NECROTIC PHASE

Demonstration of eosinophilic infiltration of the heart
with endomyocardial biopsy

THROMBOTIC AND FIBROTIC PHASES

Demonstration of thick endocardium with thrombus
formation detected by echocardiography, magnetic
resonance imaging, or computed tomography

Demonstration of thick and fibrous endocardium by
endomyocardial biopsy

Difficult or impossible to differentiate from idiopathic,
restrictive, or dilated cardiomyopathy in the absence of
hypereosinophilia, and endomyocardial fibrosis

FIGURE 5-36. During the necrotic phase, other organ involvement
such as dermatitis, pleuropneumonitis, and hepatitis may be
present. The clinical diagnosis of hypereosinophilic heart disease
can be established by the documentation of such inflammatory
processes with hypereosinophilia and elevation of serum major
basic and cationic proteins. Hypereosinophilia is usually not
present during the fibrotic phase, and it is impossible to establish
the diagnosis of hypereosinophilic heart disease in many patients
unless they have been followed from the necrotic phase.

TREATMENT

NECROTIC PHASE

Corticosteroids

Anticoagulation with warfarin

Supportive care for heart failure,
atrioventricular block, and tachyarrhythmias

THROMBOTIC AND FIBROTIC PHASES

Anticoagulation with warfarin

Supportive care

Surgical treatment

FIGURE 5-37. Treatment of hypereosinophilic heart disease. In the
necrotic phase. The initial dose of corticosteroid is prednisolone,
1 to 2 mg/kg/d, and the maintenance dose is 0.25 to 0.5 mg/kg/d.
How long corticosteroid treatment should be continued is unknown.
It may be necessary to continue the maintenance dose until major
basic and cationic proteins disappear from the myocardium on
repeat endomyocardial biopsy. Surgical treatment, consisting of
endocardial stripping with or without pacemaker implantation and
valve replacement, is indicated for patients with severe heart failure
secondary to endomyocardial fibrosis in tropical areas [26].

REFERENCES

1. Benotti JR, Grossman W, Cohn PF: Clinical profile of restrictive cardiomyopathy. *Circulation* 1980, 61:1206–1212.

2. Hirota Y, Kohriyama T, Hayashi T, *et al.*: Idiopathic restrictive cardiomyopathy: differences of left ventricular diastolic relaxation and diastolic wave forms from constrictive pericarditis. *Am J Cardiol* 1983, 52:421–423.

3. Hirota Y, Shimizu G, Kita Y, *et al.*: Spectrum of restrictive cardiomyopathy: report of the national survey in Japan. *Am Heart J* 1990, 120:188–194.

4. Spry CJF, Tai PC: Clinical studies on endomyocardial fibrosis in patients with hypereosinophilia: a historical review. In *Cardiomyopathy Update 3. Restrictive Cardiomyopathy and Arrhythmias.* Edited by Olsen EGJ, Sekiguchi M. Tokyo: University of Tokyo Press; 1990:81–98.

5. Vijayaraghavan G, Sadanandan S, Cherian G: Endomyocardial fibrosis in India: an overview. In *Cardiomyopathy Update 3. Restrictive Cardiomyopathy and Arrhythmias.* Edited by Olsen EGJ, Sekiguchi M. Tokyo: University of Tokyo Press; 1990:9–20.

6. Yutani C, Imakita M, Ishibashi-Ueda H, *et al.*: Quantitative analysis of myofiber disorganization and fibrosis in patients with idiopathic cardiomyopathy characterized by restrictive physiology. In *Cardiomyopathy Update 3. Restrictive Cardiomyopathy and Arrhythmias.* Edited by Olsen EGJ, Sekiguchi M. Tokyo: University of Tokyo Press; 1990:291–302.

7. McKenna WJ, Stewart JT, Nihoyannopoulos P, *et al.*: Hypertrophic cardiomyopathy without hypertrophy: two families with myocardial disarray in the absence of increased myocardial mass. *Br Heart J* 1990, 63:287–290.

8. Goodwin JF: Cardiomyopathies and specific heart muscle diseases: definitions, terminology, classifications and new and old approaches. *Postgrad Med J* 1992, 68(suppl 1):S3–S6.

9. Maisch B, Brilla C: Restrictive cardiomyopathy. *Curr Opin Cardiol* 1993, 8:447–453.

10. Keren A, Billingham ME, Weintraub D, *et al.*: Mildly dilated congestive cardiomyopathy. *Circulation* 1985, 72:302–309.

11. Katritsis D, Wilmshurst PT, Wendon JA, *et al.*: Primary restrictive cardiomyopathy: clinical and pathologic characteristics. *J Am Coll Cardiol* 1991, 18:1230–1235.

12. Schoenfeld MH, Supple EW, Dec GW Jr, *et al.*: Restrictive cardiomyopathy versus constrictive pericarditis: role of endomyocardial biopsy in avoiding unnecessary thoracotomy. *Circulation* 1987, 75:1012–1017.

13. Bertini E, Bosman C, Ricci E, *et al.*: Neuromyopathy and restrictive cardiomyopathy with accumulation of intermediate filaments: a clinical, morphological and biochemical study. *Acta Neuropathol* 1991, 81:632–640.

14. Hongo M, Fujii T, Hirayama J, *et al.*: Radionuclide angiographic assessment of left ventricular diastolic filling in amyloid heart disease: a study of patients with familial amyloid polyneuropathy. *J Am Coll Cardiol* 1989, 13:48–53.

15. Klein AL, Hatle LK, Burstow DJ, *et al.*: Doppler characterization of left ventricular diastolic function in cardiac amyloidosis. *J Am Coll Cardiol* 1989, 13:1017–1026.

16. Bessen M, Gardin JM: Evaluation of left ventricular diastolic function. *Cardiol Clin* 1990, 8:315–332.

17. Appleton CP, Hatle LK, Popp RL: Demonstration of restrictive ventricular physiology by Doppler echocardiography. *J Am Coll Cardiol* 1988, 11:757–768.

18. Carroll JD, Lang RM, Neumann AL, *et al.*: The differential effects of positive inotropic and vasodilator therapy on diastolic properties in patients with congestive cardiomyopathy. *Circulation* 1986, 74:815–825.

19. Masui T, Finck S, Higgins CB: Constrictive pericarditis and restrictive cardiomyopathy: evaluation with MR imaging. *Radiology* 1992, 182:369–373.

20. Lewis AB: Clinical profile and outcome of restrictive cardiomyopathy in children. *Am Heart J* 1992, 123:1589–1593.

21. Setaro JF, Soufer R, Remetz MS, *et al.*: Long-term outcome in patients with congestive heart failure and intact systolic left ventricular performance. *Am J Cardiol* 1992, 69:1212–1216.

22. Cohen AS: Amyloidosis. In *Harrison's Principles of Internal Medicine*, 12th ed. Edited by Wilson JD, Braunwald E, Isselbacher KJ, *et al*. New York: McGraw-Hill; 1991:1417–1421.

23. Nakayama Y, Kohriyama T, Yamamoto S, *et al.*: Electron microscopic and immunohistochemical studies on endomyocardial biopsies from a patient with eosinophilic endomyocardial disease. *Heart Vessel* 1985, 1(suppl 1):250–255.

24. Olsen EGJ: Morphological overview and pathogenetic mechanism in endomyocardial fibrosis associated with eosinophilia. In *Cardiomyopathy Update 3. Restrictive Cardiomyopathy and Arrhythmias*. Edited by Olsen EGJ, Sekiguchi M. Tokyo: University of Tokyo Press; 1990:1–8.

25. Andy JJ: The relationship of microfilaria and other helminthic worms to tropical endomyocardial fibrosis: a review. In *Cardiomyopathy Update 3. Restrictive Cardiomyopathy and Arrhythmias*. Edited by Olsen EGJ, Sekiguchi M. Tokyo: University of Tokyo Press; 1990:21–34.

26. Moraes CR: Early and late results of surgery for endomyocardial fibrosis. In *Cardiomyopathy Update 3. Restrictive Cardiomyopathy and Arrhythmias*. Edited by Olsen EGJ, Sekiguchi M. Tokyo: University of Tokyo Press; 1990:49–57.

CARDIAC MANIFESTATIONS OF NEUROMUSCULAR DISEASE

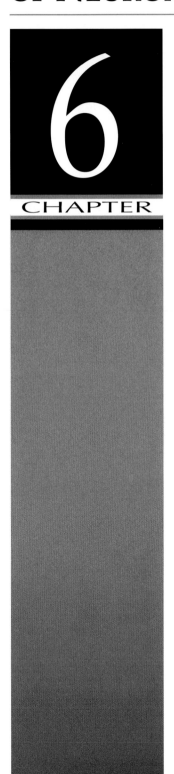

6

CHAPTER

Joseph K. Perloff

Cardiac involvement is an inherent feature of three major heredofamilial neuromyopathic diseases: the progressive muscular dystrophies, the myotonic muscular dystrophies, and Friedreich's ataxia [1]. The nonmyotonic progressive muscular dystrophies include classic, early-onset Duchenne dystrophy, late-onset Becker dystrophy, facioscapulohumeral dystrophy, and limb-girdle dystrophy. Less common nonmyotonic neuromyopathic disorders that are sometimes associated with heart disease include Charcot-Marie-Tooth disease, myotubular myopathy, Kearns-Sayre syndrome, Guillain-Barré syndrome, nemaline myopathy, myasthenia gravis, McArdle syndrome, Kugelberg-Welander disease, and periodic paralysis.

Duchenne muscular dystrophy is an X-linked recessive disorder that involves striated muscle (skeletal and cardiac), specialized cardiac tissues, smooth muscle (vasculature), and the nervous system (neurons of the central brain and cortex) [2,3]. Dystrophin, the protein product of the gene (Xp21 locus of the short arm of the X chromosome), is normally present on and limited to myogenic cells in every tissue except those of the central nervous system, and is absent or nearly so in Duchenne dystrophy [4]. There is gross, histologic, ultrastructural, and metabolic evidence that myocardial involvement initially targets the posterobasal left ventricular wall (cardiac phenotype) [2,5]. Regarding cardiac rhythm and conduction disturbances, theories of pathogenesis have focused on abnormalities presumed to originate in dystrophin-deficient specialized cardiac tissues or in small-vessel coronary arteriopathy [3].

Becker dystrophy is later in onset and slower in progression than Duchenne dystrophy [1,4], and can be diagnosed with confidence by dystrophin assays of skeletal muscle biopsies. In addition to abnormalities of the His bundle and of infranodal conduction, myocardial involvement is expressed in all four cardiac chambers.

Facioscapulohumeral dystrophy is autosomal-dominant, slowly progressive but variable in expression, and is characterized by facial and shoulder-arm weakness and atrophy [6]. The disease occasionally expresses itself in infancy and runs a rapid course. Permanent atrial paralysis, a unique electrophysiologic abnormality, is associated with a phenotypically similar but genetically different disorder—X-linked *Emery-Dreifuss dystrophy* [7]. Cardiac involvement in facioscapulohumeral dystrophy commonly takes the form of electrophysiologic abnormalities, namely, atrial fibrillation or atrial flutter, sinus node dysfunction, and less commonly as abnormalities of atrioventricular nodal or infranodal conduction [6].

Limb-girdle dystrophy refers to a heterogeneous group of muscular dystrophies [1]. Calf pseudohypertrophy sometimes occurs but is relatively late and usually mild to moderate. Because limb-girdle dystrophy is poorly defined, conclusions regarding the type and prevalence of coexisting heart disease cannot confidently be drawn. It is believed that a certain proportion of patients so diagnosed with calf pseudohypertrophy represent examples of Becker dystrophy.

Myotonic dystrophy is a relatively common autosomal-dominant multisystem neuromuscular disorder [8]. Myotonia (delayed relaxation after contraction) is provoked by voluntary, mechanical, or electrical stimulation of muscles of the hands, forearms, tongue, and jaw. The electromyogram is characteristic. Cardiac involvement, which is often the major extraskeletal muscle expression, expresses itself chiefly as abnormalities of specialized tissues including sinus node, atrioventricular node, His bundle, and bundle branches. Involvement of the myocardium is less frequent and is seldom clinically overt [8]. Abnormal ventricular function is represented chiefly by depressed contraction (systolic dysfunction), but recent

studies have identified subtle myocardial myotonia represented by slow relaxation rates in about 50% of patients.

Friedreich's ataxia is one of several types of hereditary ataxias. Cardiac involvement occurs in 90% of patients, an incidence that rises to 100% with longitudinal follow-up [9]. Phenotypically indistinguishable patients are not genetically identical because the cardiac expressions differ. Those expressions commonly take the form of hypertrophic cardiomyopathy (usually concentric, occasionally asymmetric), or less commonly global left ventricular hypokinesis that progresses to dilated heart failure [9]. Why a nonmyopathic spinocerebellar-corticospinal disorder is accompanied by two such widely divergent types of cardiac disease is unknown.

Less common neuromyopathic diseases associated with cardiac involvement include Kearns-Sayre syndrome, McArdle syndrome, periodic paralysis, and Guillain-Barré syndrome [1]. Less common neuromyopathic disorders that are sporadically or questionably associated with cardiac involvement include Kugelberg-Welander disease, myotubular myopathy, nemaline myopathy, Charcot-Marie-Tooth disease, and myasthenia gravis [1].

DUCHENNE MUSCULAR DYSTROPHY

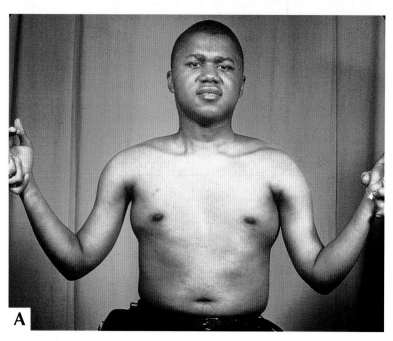
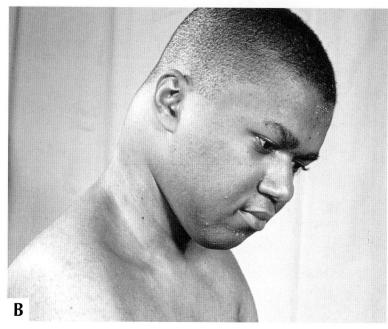

FIGURE 6-1. A 17-year-old boy with Duchenne muscular dystrophy demonstrating striking enlargement (hypertrophy-pseudohypertrophy) of the deltoid and pectoralis major muscles (**A**) and of the trapezius (**B**). There is also enlargement of the calves, which is the earliest clinical expression (phenotype) of human Duchenne dystrophy in skeletal muscle. Such calf enlargement has been called "pseudohypertrophy" because of extensive infiltration if not replacement by connective tissue and fat. However, before age 2 years, connective tissue and fat can be minimal, so calf enlargement is due to true hypertrophy rather than pseudohypertrophy. Exceptionally, regional muscle enlargement (hypertrophy-pseudo-

hypertrophy) in Duchenne dystrophy can be striking in muscle groups other than the calves, as is illustrated here. Animal models shed further light on hypertrophy, at least in striated muscle. Dystrophin-deficient mice and cats do not experience overt clinical dystrophy but instead manifest hypertrophy of striated muscle in both the early and late stages of the disease. Especially striking is the systemic striated muscle hypertrophy in dystrophin-deficient cats that have a paucity of overt muscle necrosis but remarkable hypertrophy of individual muscle fibers. The hypertrophy-pseudohypertrophy distribution shown in this patient is rare in humans with Duchenne dystrophy, but is typical of the dystrophin-deficient cat.

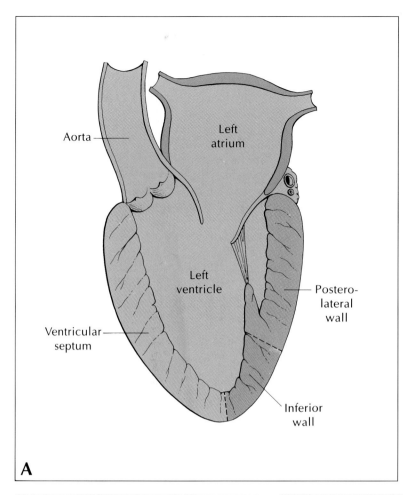

A

Aorta

Left atrium

Left ventricle

Postero-lateral wall

Ventricular septum

Inferior wall

FIGURE 6-2. A, The posterolateral (infra-atrial) involvement of the left ventricle in Duchenne dystrophy. **B,** Photomicrograph of the left atrium, mitral valve, and infra-atrial (posterolateral) wall of the left ventricle. Note extensive fibrosis of the posterobasal left ventricle with scattered foci of myocardial fibers. The small area of endocardial thickening on the posterior wall of the left atrium was due to a jet lesion from mitral regurgitation caused by dysfunction of the posterior papillary muscle. Ventricular septum (**C**) and posterobasal (**D**) portions of the left ventricular wall. In contrast to the posterobasal wall, which shows extensive connective tissue proliferation with scattered islands of myocardial fibers, no fibrous scars are present in the ventricular septum (hematoxylin and eosin, × 25). A reduction in or loss of electromotive force caused by the location of myocardial dystrophy in the posterobasal and contiguous lateral left ventricular walls is believed to be responsible for the characteristic scalar electrocardiogram, and is represented by tall right precordial R waves and deep but narrow Q waves in leads 1, aVL, and the left precordium. Duchenne dystrophy emerges as a unique form of heart disease characterized by a genetically determined predilection for specific regions of myocardium.

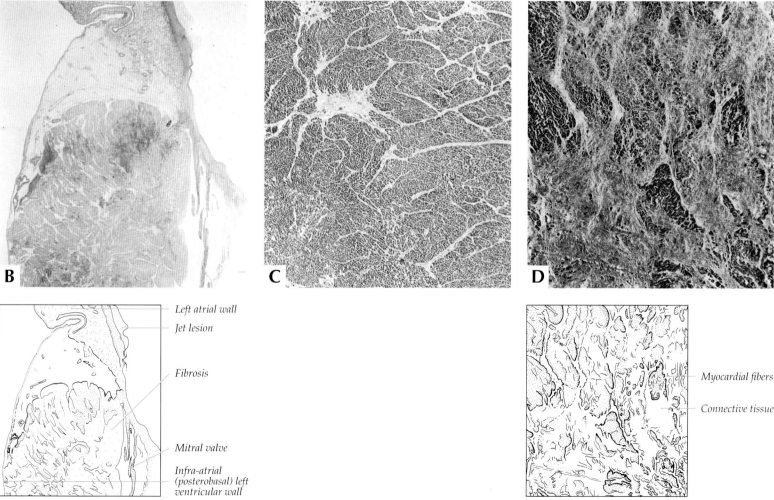

B

C

D

Left atrial wall

Jet lesion

Fibrosis

Mitral valve

Infra-atrial (posterobasal) left ventricular wall

Myocardial fibers

Connective tissue

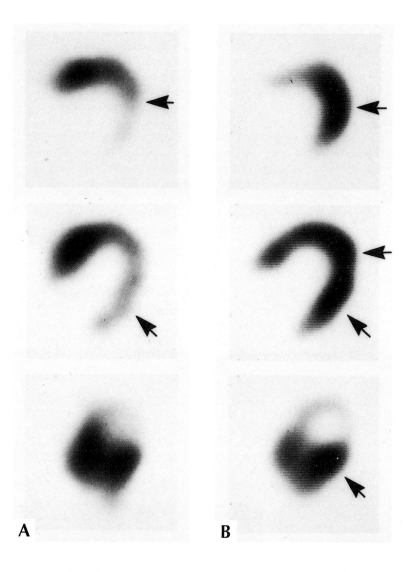

FIGURE 6-3. Regional myocardial uptake of $^{13}NH_3$ and ^{18}fluorodeoxyglucose in three contiguous positron computed tomograms of the left ventricular myocardium in a patient with Duchenne muscular dystrophy. There is a segmental decrease in $^{13}NH_3$ activity in the posterolateral left ventricle (*arrows* in **A**) with a discordant increase in ^{18}fluorodeoxyglucose concentration in the same region (*arrows* in **B**). This patient had a posterolateral thallium-201 defect, posterolateral akinesis on technetium-99m radionuclide imaging, and a left ventricular ejection fraction of 46%. Accelerated exogenous glucose utilization in the posterobasal and contiguous lateral left ventricular walls of patients with Duchenne dystrophy provide evidence of a regional myocardial metabolic abnormality. $^{13}NH_3$ activity is reduced in segments in which uptake of exogenous glucose is accelerated. These sites correspond to those of primary dystrophic replacement found at necropsy. It is believed that the regional myocardial abnormalities of ^{18}fluorodeoxyglucose and $^{13}NH_3$ activity represent secondary metabolic alterations initiated by the basic defect in the cardiac plasma cell membrane. These alterations are represented in striated muscle by the absence from the sarcolemmal membrane of dystrophin, which is the protein product of the Duchenne muscular dystrophy gene. Current ultrastructural and biochemical evidence supports the proposition that the fundamental structural and biochemical abnormalities in Duchenne dystrophy reside in the plasma cell membrane.

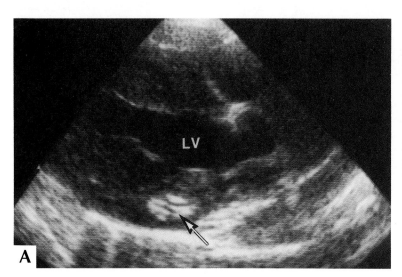

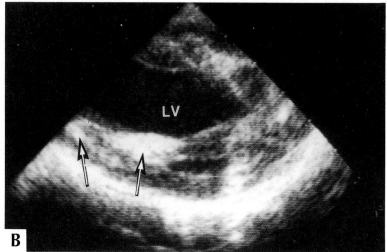

FIGURE 6-4. Two-dimensional echocardiograms from a 7-month-old female dog (**A**) and an 8-month-old male dog (**B**) with Duchenne muscular dystrophy. These X-linked dystrophin-deficient dogs have a mutation in the homologue of the Duchenne locus and exhibit histopathologic abnormalities similar to those of human Duchenne dystrophy. The phenotypic expressions of X-linked canine muscular dystrophy are closer to those in humans when compared with muscular dystrophy in the mouse or cat, and localization of myocardial involvement in the canine model is similar to that in humans with Duchenne dystrophy. These modified parasternal long-axis views of the left ventricle (LV) show hyperechoic lesions clumped in the posterior left ventricular wall at the level of the chordae tendineae (*arrow* in *A*), and in the papillary muscle and contiguous left ventricular wall (*arrows* in *B*).

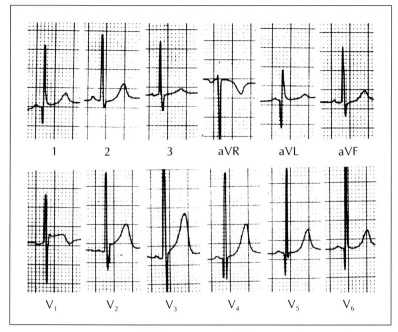

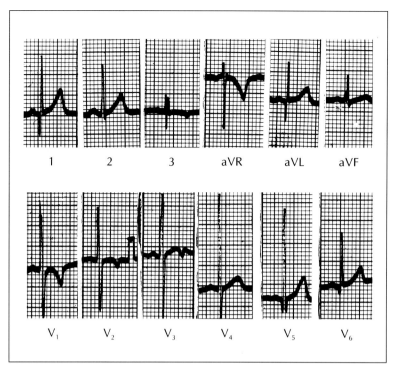

FIGURE 6-5. Typical electrocardiogram of Duchenne muscular dystrophy in a 10-year-old boy. The P-R interval is short (0.10 seconds in lead 2; *see* Fig. 6-11). The QRS complex shows an anterior shift in the right precordial leads (tall R waves) and deep but narrow Q waves in leads 1, aVL, and V_{4-6}. A reduction in or loss of electromotive force caused by myocardial dystrophy in the posterobasal and contiguous lateral left ventricular walls is believed to be responsible for the QRS pattern. The standard scalar electrocardiogram is the simplest and most reliable tool for detecting cardiac involvement in Duchenne dystrophy. Abnormal electrocardiograms are present even in early childhood. Tall right precordial R waves and increased R:S amplitude ratios, together with deep Q waves in leads 1, aVL, and V_{5-6}, are characteristic of classic, rapidly progressive X-linked Duchenne dystrophy.

FIGURE 6-6. Twelve-lead scalar electrocardiogram in an obligate female carrier of the Duchenne muscular dystrophy gene. The tracing is similar, if not identical, to the typical scalar electrocardiogram in boys who overtly express Duchenne muscular dystrophy. The tall right precordial R waves and deep but narrow Q waves in leads 1, aVL, and V_5 reflect posterobasal and lateral left ventricular extension of myocardial dystrophy in the female carrier.

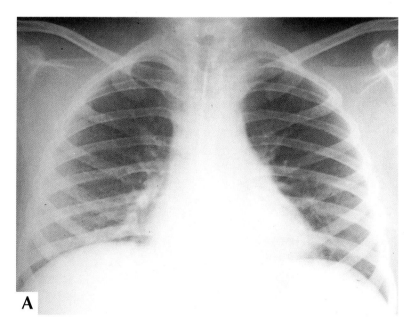

A

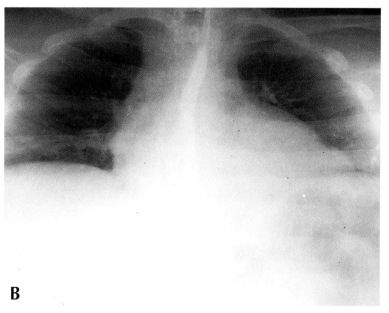

B

FIGURE 6-7. Radiographic illustration of the different degrees of diaphragmatic dystrophy in two boys aged 13 (**A**) and 16 (**B**) years with Duchenne muscular dystrophy. Note moderate elevation of the diaphragm in the 13-year-old compared with striking elevation that coincided with virtually no diaphragmatic excursions during inspiration in the 16-year-old.

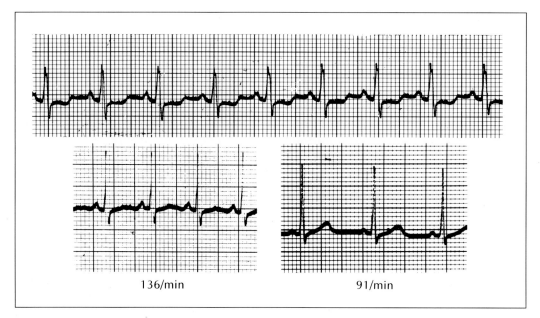

136/min   91/min

FIGURE 6-8. Two types of sinus tachycardia have been documented in Duchenne muscular dystrophy and are shown in these rhythm strips: upper, persistent sinus acceleration (minimal heart rate during a 24-hour period not less than 100 bpm in patients older than 12 years of age, or not less than 110 bpm in younger patients); and lower, labile sinus tachycardia (during waking hours or sleep), so designated when a rate acceleration, without change in P-wave morphology, is inappropriate, *ie,* unprovoked by a definable circumstantial cause. Episodes of labile sinus tachycardia are either gradual in onset (brief warm-up) or abrupt (within one beat). The upper rhythm strip illustrates persistent sinus tachycardia in a 10-year-old boy with Duchenne muscular dystrophy. Note the ST segment depression. The lower rhythm strip illustrates labile sinus tachycardia in a 6-year-old boy. The mechanism or mechanisms of these two types of sinus accelerations have not been established.

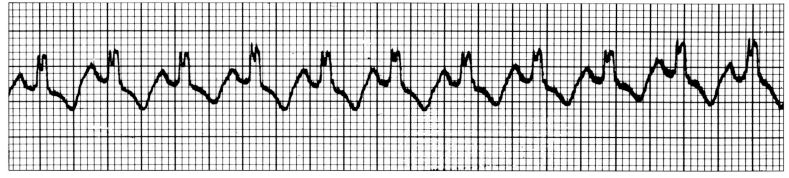

FIGURE 6-9. Rhythm strip from a 12-year-old boy with Duchenne muscular dystrophy. This tracing of lead 2 shows atrial flutter with 2:1 conduction. The most important disturbance in atrial rhythm in Duchenne dystrophy is atrial flutter, which is a rare tachyarrhythmia in children but a relatively common and often preterminal tachyarrhythmia in patients with Duchenne dystrophy. In addition, atrial premature beats, intermittent atrial ectopic rhythms, junctional rhythm, and sustained supraventricular tachycardia occur (*see* Fig. 6-11). An abnormal P-wave terminal force is evidence of prolonged intra-atrial conduction. There are focal areas of fibrosis at the cellular level and loss of thick and thin myofilaments at the subcellular level in atrial myocardium. Focal areas of fibrosis are associated with increased intercellular resistance and slowed conduction, which facilitate re-entrant arrhythmias. Slowed intra-atrial conduction is the electrophysiologic substrate associated with atrial flutter and fibrillation.

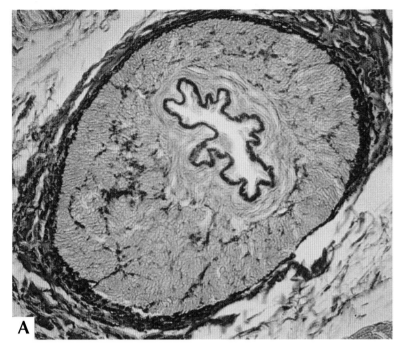

A

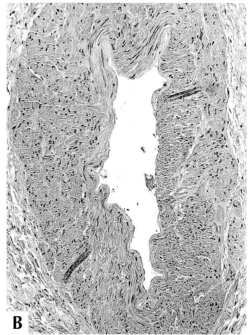

B

FIGURE 6-10. Histologic sections of small intramural coronary arteries in the left atria of two patients with Duchenne dystrophy. **A,** Striking hypertrophy of medial smooth muscle with luminal narrowing (Verhoeff-von Gieson elastic tissue stains, × 260). **B,** Medial smooth muscle hypertrophy causing a thick wall and a moderately narrowed lumen in an intramural coronary artery from the right atrium in the region of the sinus node (hematoxylin and eosin, × 25). The coronary arteriopathy is characterized principally by striking hypertrophy of the media with luminal

narrowing, and less commonly by coexisting cystic degeneration. The dystrophin content of vascular smooth muscle cells (shown here) is similar to that of striated myofibers. The smooth muscle form of dystrophin is believed to be slightly smaller than the predominant striated muscle dystrophin, implying that a smaller form might represent a vascular smooth muscle isoform. A fundamental question is why dystrophin deficiency in the vascular smooth muscle of Duchenne dystrophy (in contrast to striated muscle) expresses itself chiefly as hypertrophy rather than necrosis.

A. RHYTHM ABNORMALITIES

Sinus node
   Sinus tachycardia
      Labile (gradual or abrupt)
      Persistent
   Sinus arrythmia—marked
   Shifting atrial pacemaker
Atrial ectopic rhythms
   Flutter
   Fibrillation
   Supraventricular tachycardia
   Junctional
Ventricular ectopic rhythms
   Premature ventricular beats—
      uniform, multiform, single, couplets
   Nonsustained ventricular tachycardia

B. CONDUCTION ABNORMALITIES

Prolonged intra-atrial conduction
Atrioventricular conduction
   Accelerated (short P-R interval)
   Prolonged (long P-R interval)
Infranodal
   Right ventricular conduction delay
   Right bundle branch block
   Left anterior fascicular block
   Left posterior fascicular block
   Complete heart block

FIGURE 6-11. At least two variables are relevant in attempting to understand the rhythm (**A**) and conduction (**B**) disturbances in Duchenne dystrophy: abnormalities that might originate in specialized cardiac tissues, or abnormalities that might be consequences of the small vessel coronary arteriopathy, particularly in the atria (*see* Fig. 6-10). Relevant here is whether a relationship exists between the coronary arteriopathy (medial smooth muscle hypertrophy) and disturbances in rhythm and conduction. A sec-

ond fundamental concern centers on specialized cardiac tissues. It is not currently known whether the plasma cell membrane of specialized cardiac tissues contains dystrophin as does the cell membrane of cardiac muscle. If cell membranes of specialized cardiac tissues normally contain dystrophin, it can then be hypothesized that in Duchenne dystrophy these cell membranes may be dystrophin-deficient, and that this dystrophin deficiency may affect specialized tissue membrane viability and function.

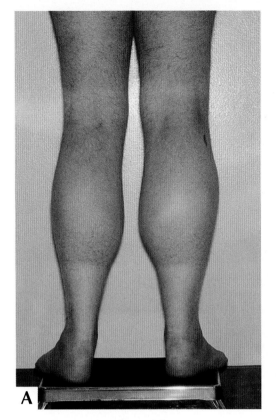
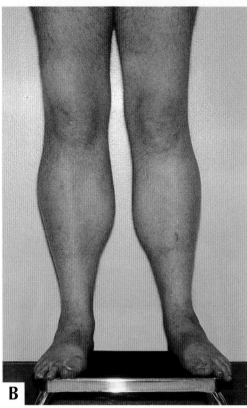

FIGURE 6-12. The calves of a 31-year-old man with late-onset, slowly progressive Becker dystrophy. **A,** The posterior aspect of the calves shows striking enlargement, with the right calf slightly larger than the left. **B,** The anterior view of the calves illustrates the disproportionate increase in size of the right compared with the left calf. Proximal leg muscle dystrophy is present more so on the left than on the right.

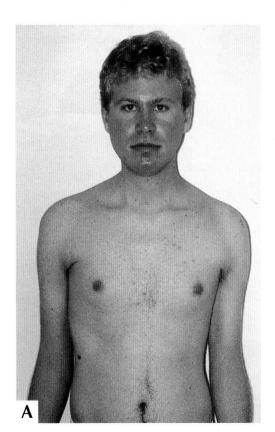
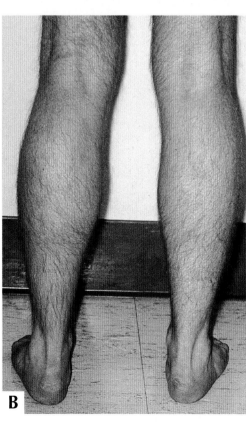

FIGURE 6-13. A 22-year-old man with late-onset, slowly progressive Becker muscular dystrophy. The 12-lead scalar electrocardiogram showed left anterior fascicular hemiblock with QRS prolongation. The two-dimensional echocardiogram disclosed a moderately enlarged, globally hypokinetic left ventricle. **A,** Dystrophy of shoulder girdle, arms, and pelvic girdle (not shown). **B,** Asymmetric calf pseudohypertrophy, greater on the left side than on the right. Dystrophy of proximal leg muscles is not shown.

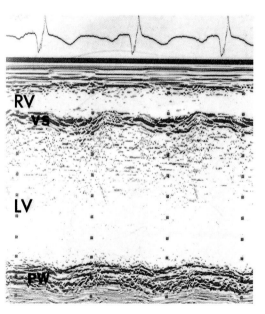

FIGURE 6-14. M-mode echocardiogram from a 20-year-old man with Becker dystrophy. The left ventricle (LV) is dilated, and the relatively thin ventricular septum (VS) and posterior wall (PW) are hypokinetic. The right ventricle (RV) is not dilated. This echocardiogram resembles that of dilated cardiomyopathy.

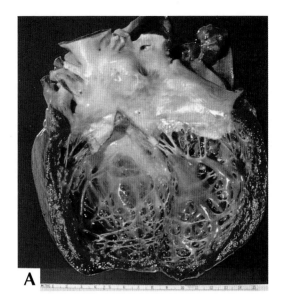

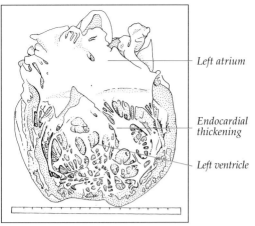

Left atrium

Endocardial thickening

Left ventricle

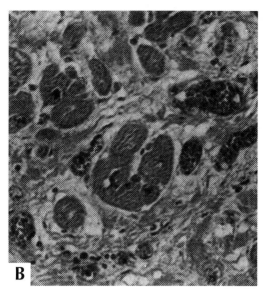

A

B

FIGURE 6-15. Gross and microscopic cardiac pathologic specimens from a 45-year-old man with late-onset, slowly progressive Becker muscular dystrophy. (For electrocardiogram, *see* Fig. 6-16.) **A,** The left ventricle was dilated and flabby with focal endocardial thickening. The left atrium was also dilated. **B,** Microscopic section from the left ventricle shows marked confluent scarring with variations in fiber size. No significant coronary artery disease was identified. In Becker dystrophy, the pro-

tein product of the gene is present but is abnormal in molecular weight, while in Duchenne dystrophy the protein product is absent or scanty but of normal molecular weight. In contrast to Duchenne dystrophy, cardiac involvement in Becker dystrophy involves all four chambers, with dilatation and failure of the ventricles in addition to abnormalities of the His bundle and infranodal conduction that express themselves as fascicular block and complete heart block as shown in Fig. 6-16.

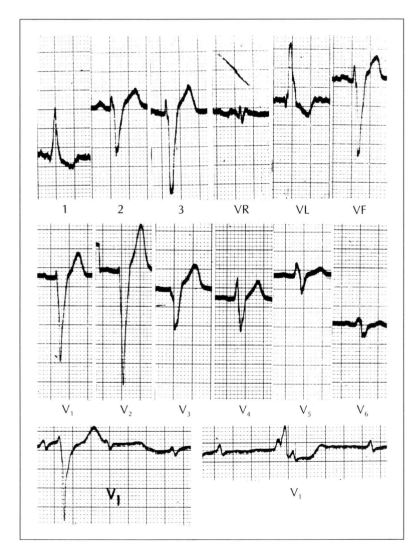

FIGURE 6-16. Twelve-lead scalar electrocardiogram from a 40-year-old man with late-onset, slowly progressive Becker dystrophy (same patient as in Fig. 6-15). There is left axis deviation, a QRS interval of 0.14 seconds, small Q waves in leads 1 and aVL, and loss of R-wave amplitude in leads V_2 and V_3. The lower tracings, taken 4 years later and 1 year before death, show complete heart block with a variable QRS configuration.

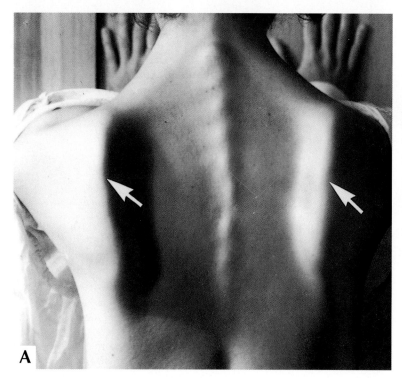

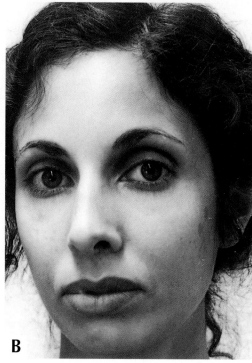

FIGURE 6-17.
Facioscapulohumeral dystrophy in a 32-year-old woman. **A,** There is typical winging of the scapulae (*arrows*) as the patient exerts pressure on the shoulder girdle by leaning against a wall with arms extended. **B,** The face is in repose (myopathic), while the corners of the mouth show the dimpling that is typical of facioscapulohumeral dystrophy and create the impression of an enigmatic smile.

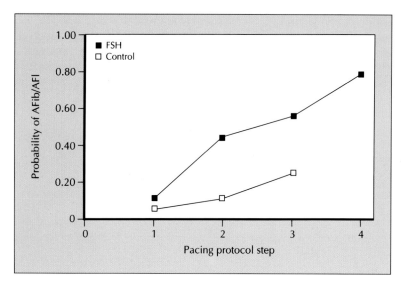

FIGURE 6-18. Cumulative incidence of initiation of atrial fibrillation (AFib) or atrial flutter (AFl) for each step in a pacing protocol designed to determine the susceptibility of patients with facioscapulohumeral (FSH) muscular dystrophy to the induction of atrial fibrillation or flutter. A quadripolar catheter was used for stimulation and mapping at multiple right atrial sites. Left atrial stimulation was achieved via the coronary sinus. Patients with facioscapulohumeral dystrophy were compared with control patients. Steps 1, 2, and 3 are high right atrial pacing at cycle lengths of 600, 500, and 400 ms, respectively. Step 4 is pacing at the same cycle lengths at additional right atrial sites. Cardiac involvement in facioscapulohumeral dystrophy takes the form of electrophysiologic derangements characterized chiefly by susceptibility to inducible atrial arrhythmias (atrial fibrillation and atrial flutter) and by sinus node dysfunction in patients devoid of clinically overt cardiac disorders apart from those that might appear on the surface electrocardiogram. P-wave abnormalities are relatively common and are unrelated to atrial size based on echocardiographic assessment. Broad bifid P waves or prolonged P-terminal components in electrocardiogram lead V_1 (left atrial), or increased amplitude of the initial component of the P wave in lead 2 (right atrial) implies abnormalities of intra-atrial conduction. Electrophysiologic abnormalities outside of the atria are less common in facioscapulohumeral dystrophy. It is believed that the genetic marker in facioscapulohumeral muscular dystrophy results in a comparatively benign form of the electrophysiologic cardiac involvement expressed in phenotypically similar Emery-Dreifuss dystrophy and its genetic variants.

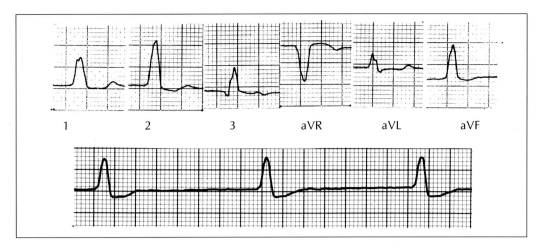

FIGURE 6-19. Limb leads and rhythm strip from a 16-year-old boy with Emery-Dreifuss muscular dystrophy. This tracing shows left bundle branch block. The rhythm strip discloses fine atrial fibrillation that is virtually indistinguishable from the absent electrical activity of atrial standstill. The ventricular response is slow. A pacemaker was inserted a month later. Emery-Dreifuss dystrophy is phenotypically similar, but not identical, to facioscapulohumeral dystrophy. Cardiac involvement in Emery-Dreifuss dystrophy and its genetic variants takes the form of permanent atrial paralysis, atrial arrhythmias, and abnormalities of atrioventricular conduction. Criteria for the diagnosis of atrial paralysis include the absence of P waves on the scalar, esophageal, and intracardiac electrocardiograms; lack of response to direct (intracardiac) electrical or mechanical stimulation of the atria; the absence of a-waves in the jugular venous and right atrial pressure pulses; and immobility of the atria on fluoroscopy or on two-dimensional echocardiography. The entire atrial myocardium ultimately becomes inexcitable.

LIMB-GIRDLE DYSTROPHY

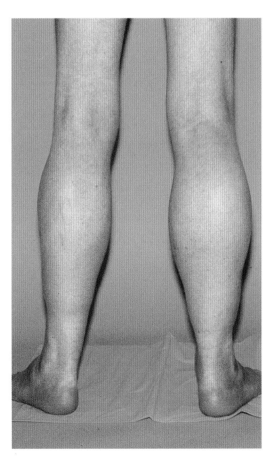

FIGURE 6-20. Calf pseudohypertrophy in a 52-year-old man believed to have limb-girdle muscular dystrophy. The distinction from Becker dystrophy was based on dystrophin assays of a skeletal muscle biopsy. This patient had no clinically detectable cardiac involvement. Disorders of cardiac muscle (cardiomyopathy) and of the cardiac conduction system have been reported in limb-girdle dystrophy, but without dystrophin assays to confirm the diagnosis. It is likely that a number of patients diagnosed as having limb-girdle dystrophy with calf pseudohypertrophy represent examples of Becker muscular dystrophy.

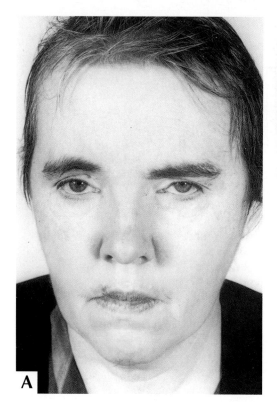

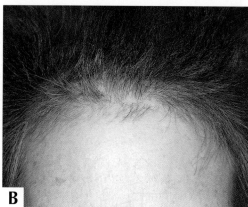

FIGURE 6-21. Patients with myotonic muscular dystrophy (Steinert's disease). **A,** The appearance of this 50-year-old woman with myotonic muscular dystrophy is characteristic: the typical expressionless facies, and thin, graying hair. This patient also had cataracts. **B,** Close-up view of another adult woman with myotonic muscular dystrophy showing the receding hairline and premature graying. Myotonic muscular dystrophy is a systemic disease with important nonmyotonic-nonmyopathic features including disorders of smooth muscle (esophagus, colon, uterus), the central nervous system (mental retardation), the endocrine system (testicular atrophy), the eyes (cataracts, retinal degeneration), and the skin (premature balding as illustrated here). Cardiac involvement, which is often the major extraskeletal muscle expression of myotonic dystrophy, manifests itself chiefly as abnormalities of specialized tissues, less frequently of myocardium.

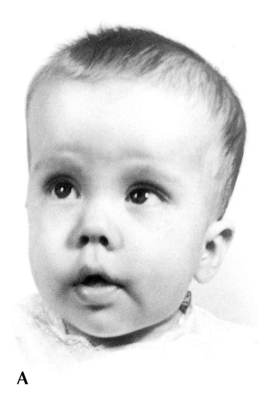

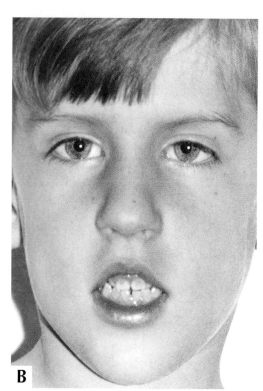

FIGURE 6-22. Facial appearance of the infantile and childhood form of myotonic dystrophy (**A** and **B**). One characteristic feature is the "cupid's bow" of the upper lip. This type of myotonic muscular dystrophy occurs in offspring of mothers with Steinert's disease. The disorder expresses itself in infants as hypotonia and facial paralysis without myotonia, at least initially. Studies on cardiac involvement are limited but have reportedly disclosed atrioventricular and intraventricular conduction defects, and less commonly, reduced left ventricular systolic function.

MYOTONIC MUSCULAR DYSTROPHY SCALAR ELECTROCARDIOGRAM

VARIABLE	PATIENTS, n
Heart rate <60 bpm	7
Normal P wave	
P-R interval ≥100 ms	10
QRS duration ≥100 ms	10
QRS axis -30° or more	8
Right bundle branch block	2
Bifascicular block	1
Abnormal Q waves	
aVL	3
1, aVL	1
V$_{1-3}$	1
One or more abnormalities	20
Normal tracings	5

FIGURE 6-23. Prevalence of scalar electrocardiographic abnormalities in myotonic muscular dystrophy (*see also* Fig. 6-26). (*Data from* Perloff and coworkers [8].)

RHYTHM ABNORMALITIES

Sinus bradycardia (30–50 bpm)
Sinus arrhythmia
Atrial arrhythmias
    Sinus pauses ≥1.5 s
    Wandering pacemaker
    Premature atrial beats
        Single
        Paired
    Supraventricular tachycardia 140–200 bpm (unsustained)
    Atrial ectopic rhythm 50–80 bpm (unsustained)
    Junctional escape rhythm
Ventricular arrhythmias
    Premature ventricular beats (occasional to frequent)
        Uniform
        Multiform
    Bigeminy-trigeminy (occasional to frequent)
    Ventricular tachycardia (frequent) up to 10 seconds

FIGURE 6-24. Rhythm abnormalities in myotonic muscular dystrophy (*see also* Figs. 6-27 and 6-28).

CONDUCTION ABNORMALITIES

	PATIENTS, n (%)
Intra-atrial conduction	
Increased atrial refractory period	0
Prolonged sinoatrial conduction time	0
Increased A-H interval	1
Abnormal atrioventricular node	
Premature Wenckebach's disease with pacing	1
Dual atrioventricular nodal pathways	5
His-Purkinje conduction	
Increased H-V interval	14
Prolonged right bundle branch effective refractory period	4
Abnormal response to atrial pacing or extrastimuli	4
Left anterior fascicular block	8
Left posterior fascicular block	0
Bifascicular block	1
Right bundle branch block	2
Left bundle branch block	0
Complete atrioventricular block	0
QRS prolongation	10
Total with His-Purkinje conduction	**20 (80%)**

FIGURE 6-25. Conduction abnormalities in myotonic muscular dystrophy (*see also* Figs. 6-27 and 6-28). (*Data from* Perloff and coworkers [8].)

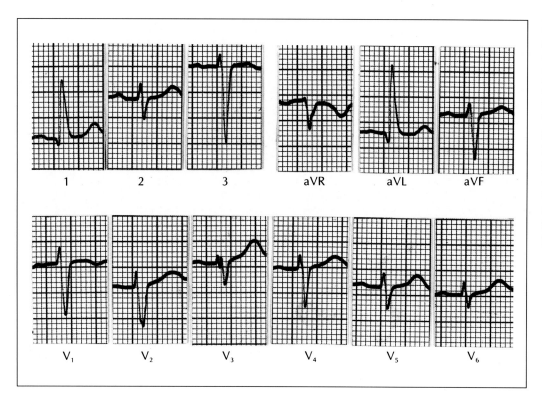

FIGURE 6-26. Typical electrocardiogram from an adult man with myotonic muscular dystrophy. There is P-R interval prolongation (0.20 seconds) and left anterior fascicular block. Cardiac involvement is relatively selective in myotonic dystrophy, primarily targeting specialized tissues, and more specifically the His-Purkinje system. The most common electrocardiographic abnormalities—prolongation of the P-R interval, left anterior fascicular block, and increased QRS duration—reflect the His-Purkinje disease that can progress rapidly, culminating in fatal Stokes-Adams episodes unless anticipated by pacemaker insertion.

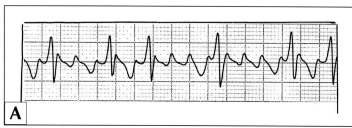

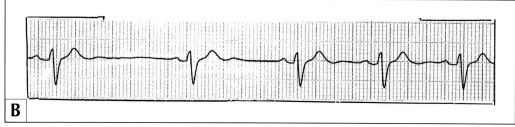

FIGURE 6-27. Rhythm strips from a 54-year-old man with myotonic muscular dystrophy. **A,** Atrial flutter with variable 2:1 and 4:1 atrioventricular conduction. **B,** After reversion to sinus rhythm there was bradycardia with marked sinus arrhythmia. Cardiac involvement in myotonic muscular dystrophy targets specialized tissues including sinus node, atrioventricular node, His bundle, and bundle branches (*see* Fig. 6-25). High-degree heart block requires pacemaker support (*see* Fig. 6-28).

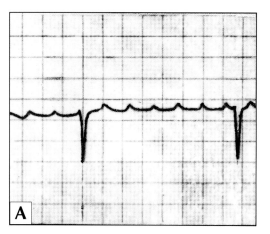 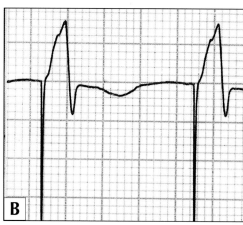

FIGURE 6-28. Rhythm strip from a 34-year-old man with myotonic muscular dystrophy. Lead V_1 (**A**) shows atrial flutter with high-degree heart block. A syncopal episode prompted insertion of a right ventricular pacemaker, shown in the tracing of lead V_6 (**B**). Myocardial dystrophy may be responsible for atrial and ventricular arrhythmias, including premature atrial beats, atrial flutter (as illustrated here), atrial fibrillation, premature ventricular beats, and ventricular tachycardia (*see* Fig. 6-24). High-degree heart block reflects preferential selection of the His-Purkinje system.

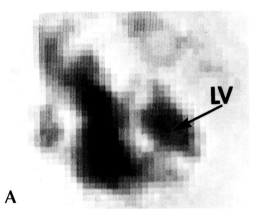 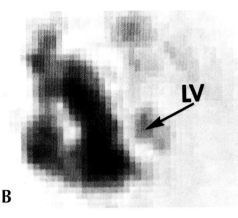

FIGURE 6-29. Technetium-99m radionuclide angiography in an adult man with myotonic muscular dystrophy. **A,** End-diastole. **B,** End-systole. Left ventricular (LV) ejection fraction was normal with the patient at rest. Occult clinical involvement of the myocardium can be assessed by radionuclide angiography during exercise. In a minority of myotonic muscular dystrophy patients who are capable of sufficient exercise to permit assessment, a less than normal increase in LV ejection fraction reflects a relatively subtle abnormality of systolic function.

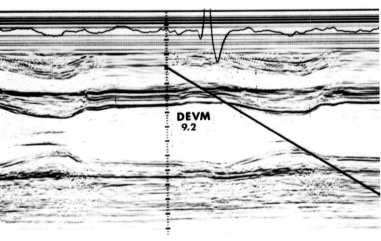

FIGURE 6-30. M-mode echocardiographic method of measuring the diastolic endocardial velocity maximum (DEVM) of the posterior left ventricular wall in a patient with myotonic muscular dystrophy. The dark diagonal line is aligned with the fastest early diastolic relaxation line of the posterior wall endocardium. The large dots on the vertical scale equal 1 cm; the horizontal distance between markers is 1 second. The DEVM in this patient is 9.2 cm/s. Normal is 18±3 cm/s. Half of the myotonic muscular dystrophy patients studied had abnormally slow echocardiographic relaxation rates of the posterior left ventricular wall.

FRIEDREICH'S ATAXIA

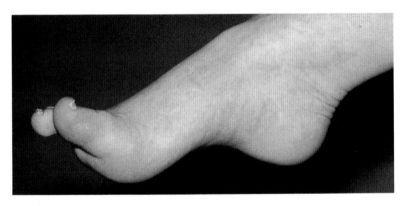

FIGURE 6-31. One of the typical phenotypic features of Friedreich's ataxia is the foot deformity characterized by pes cavas with hammer toe. The same foot deformity occurs in Charcot-Marie-Tooth disease but less frequently and usually to a lesser degree.

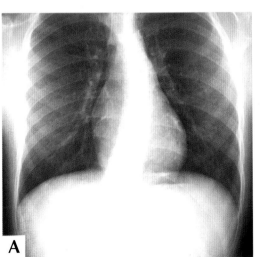 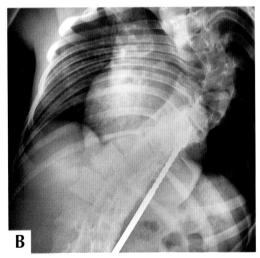

FIGURE 6-32. Radiographs from two patients with Friedreich's ataxia. **A,** This 12.5-year-old girl had moderate scoliosis to the left. **B,** This 13-year-old boy had dramatic thoracic scoliosis to the left with appreciable lumbar scoliosis to the right despite a Harrington rod. Cardiac involvement in the 13-year-old patient took the form of global left ventricular hypokinesis that progressed to dilated heart failure. Scoliosis as well as pes cavas generally develop within a few years of the clinical onset of Friedreich's ataxia. The scoliosis may progress rapidly, culminating in gross distortion, as is illustrated here.

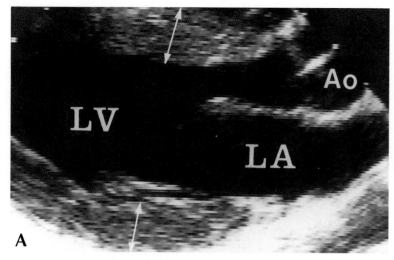
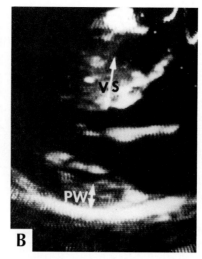

FIGURE 6-33. **A,** Two-dimensional echocardiogram (parasternal long axis diastolic frames) from a 14-year-old girl with Friedreich's ataxia and concentric hypertrophy (*arrows*) of the left ventricle (LV). **B,** Two-dimensional echocardiogram (parasternal long axis) from a 17-year-old boy with Friedreich's ataxia and hypertrophic cardiomyopathy characterized by disproportionate thickness (*arrows*) of the ventricular septum (VS) compared with the posterior wall (PW). The most common echocardiographic finding in Friedreich's ataxia is concentric (symmetric) left ventricular hypertrophy. Asymmetric septal hypertrophy occurs less frequently, and is occa-

sionally accompanied by a left ventricular to aortic systolic gradient. Septal cellular disarray, which is the histologic hallmark of genetic hypertrophic cardiomyopathy, has not been identified in necropsy studies of Friedreich's ataxia—an observation that may in part explain why the potentially malignant ventricular arrhythmias that prevail in genetic hypertrophic cardiomyopathy are essentially unknown in Friedreich's ataxia. In hypertrophic cardiomyopathy of Friedreich's ataxia, systolic ventricular function is normal, not supernormal, and diastolic function is not deranged as in genetic hypertrophic cardiomyopathy. Ao—aorta; LA—left atrium.

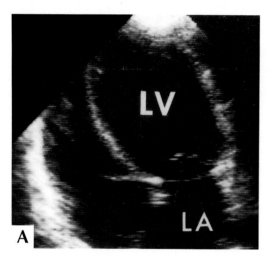
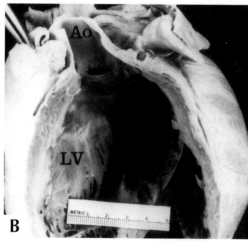
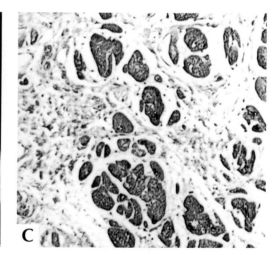

FIGURE 6-34. **A,** Two-dimensional echocardiogram from a 17-year-old boy with Friedreich's ataxia. His echocardiogram changed from normal at age 13 years to nondilated global hypokinesis shown here 3 to 4 years later. **B,** At necropsy, the gross specimen showed a left ventricle (LV) normal in size or only mildly dilated with normal thickness of flabby walls. **C,** Microscopic section from the left ventricular free wall shows marked connective tissue replacement. Small-vessel coronary artery disease was specifically sought but not identified. This patient typifies the less common form of cardiac involvement in Friedreich's ataxia that initially expresses itself as nondilated

global hypokinesis. Dilated failure of the left ventricle generally follows. In contrast to the favorable cardiac prognosis in patients with Friedreich's ataxia and hypertrophic cardiomyopathy, the outlook is poor in patients with global hypokinesis whether or not the left ventricle is dilated. The latter is a fundamentally different type of cardiac involvement designated as dystrophic, in contrast to the hypertrophic type of involvement. Atrial arrhythmias (flutter and fibrillation) and ventricular arrhythmias are features of the nonhypertrophic form of cardiomyopathy. Ao—aorta; LA—left atrium.

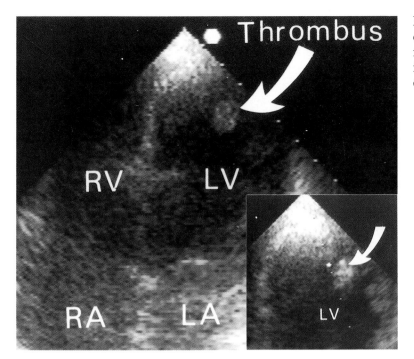

FIGURE 6-35. Two-dimensional echocardiogram from a 41-year-old woman with Friedreich's ataxia. The left ventricle (LV) was nondilated but globally hypokinetic. A thrombus (*arrow*) in the left ventricular apex (**inset**) announced itself as a cerebral embolus. LA—left atrium; RA—right atrium; RV—right ventricle.

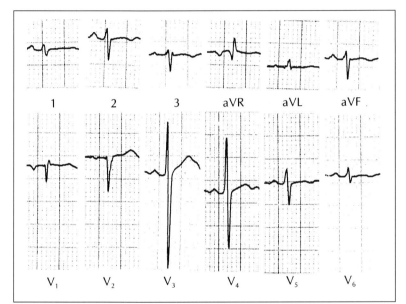

FIGURE 6-36. Twelve-lead scalar electrocardiogram from a 16-year-old boy with Friedreich's ataxia. The only overt clinical expression of cardiac involvement was the electrocardiogram shown here. The QS deformities in leads V_1 and V_2 are believed to represent regional myocardial dystrophy. There was no relationship between this type of initial force deformity and either regional wall motion abnormalities in the two-dimensional echocardiogram or the subsequent development of global left ventricular hypokinesis.

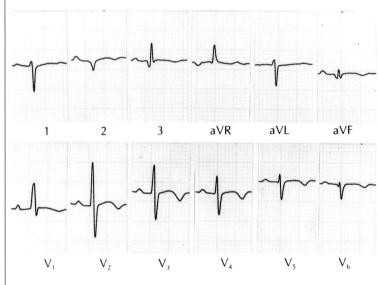

FIGURE 6-37. Electrocardiogram from a 28-year-old man with Friedreich's ataxia. Although there is right axis deviation, more important are the 40-ms Q waves in leads 2, 3, and aVF, and the prominent 60-ms R wave in lead V_1. This electrocardiographic pattern is believed to reflect the loss of inferior and posterior electrical forces, but occurred without a corresponding regional wall motion abnormality on two-dimensional echocardiography (*see* Fig. 6-36).

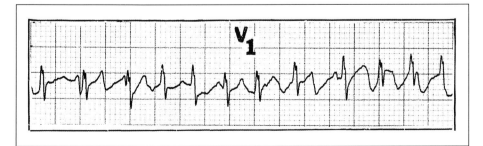

FIGURE 6-38. Rhythm strip showing coarse atrial fibrillation with a rapid ventricular response in a 39-year-old woman with Friedreich's ataxia and nondilated global left ventricular hypokinesis (*see* Figs. 6-34 and 6-35). Atrial fibrillation is an occasional and physiologically hazardous accompaniment of Friedreich's ataxia with global left ventricular hypokinesis, in contrast to stable sinus rhythm or inappropriate sinus tachycardia in patients with Friedreich's ataxia and hypertrophic cardiomyopathy (*see* Fig. 6-33).

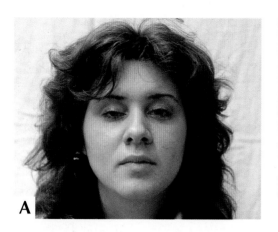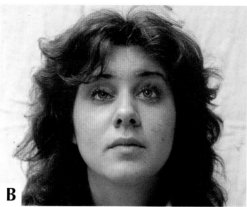

FIGURE 6-39. Kearns-Sayre syndrome is a mitochondrial myopathy expressed as external ophthalmoplegia, pigmentary retinopathy, and cardiac involvement that typically afflicts specialized conduction tissues culminating in complete heart block [10]. This 18-year-old girl with Kearns-Sayre syndrome and bilateral asymmetric ptosis had pigmentary retinopathy and an electrocardiogram that progressed from normal to bifascicular block. **A,** The asymmetric ptosis is present when the patient looks straight ahead. **B,** Ptosis of the right lid persists during upward gaze.

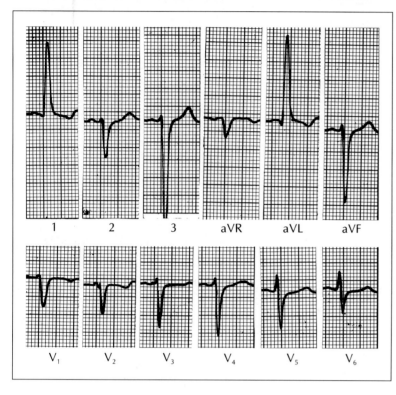

FIGURE 6-40. Twelve-lead scalar electrocardiogram from a 14-year-old girl with Kearns-Sayre syndrome. There is left anterior fascicular block and right bundle branch block (bifascicular block); 4 years earlier, the electrocardiogram showed isolated left anterior fascicular block. The patient had bilateral asymmetric ptosis that was especially apparent on upward gaze. Ophthalmologic examination disclosed pigmentary retinopathy. Skeletal muscle biopsy identified ragged red fibers in the trichrome stain. Clinically overt myocardial disease is exceptional in Kearns-Sayre syndrome, despite the fact that ultrastructural abnormalities, especially in mitochondria, are well established. Two derangements of the specialized conduction pathways generally coexist: 1) gradually progressive impairment of infranodal conduction (left anterior hemiblock, right bundle branch block, and complete heart block), and 2) enhancement of atrioventricular nodal conduction. The morphologic basis for impaired infranodal conduction lies in the extensive changes in distal portions of the His bundle extending to the origins of the bundle branches. Evidence of enhanced atrioventricular nodal conduction has been identified by His bundle electrograms.

McArdle Syndrome

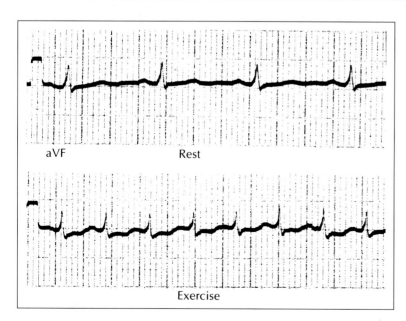

FIGURE 6-41. McArdle syndrome is a metabolic myopathy (phosphorylase deficiency) resulting in inadequate skeletal muscle glycolysis and pain in exercising muscles [1]. The most common cardiac manifestation is a striking acceleration of heart rate at the onset of exercise. These rhythm strips were taken from a 40-year-old woman with biopsy-proven McArdle syndrome. The tracings illustrate the characteristic rapid onset of sinus tachycardia in response to minimal exercise. The sinus rate at the inception of casual exercise as shown in these tracings is typical of the syndrome. McArdle syndrome (type 5 glyconeogenesis) is autosomal-recessive, rarely autosomal-dominant, and is somewhat more frequent in males than in females. The disorder is characterized initially by painful cramps in exercising muscles, often accompanied by myoglobinuria. McArdle syndrome is a myophosphorylase deficiency disease. A defect in this enzyme results in an inability to utilize glycogen as a source of energy. Minor degrees of exercise are accompanied by sudden and excessive accelerations in heart rate and by hyperventilation. These abnormalities are believed to result from abnormal vasoregulatory responses rather than from intrinsic cardiac or lung disease. McArdle syndrome usually begins before adolescence, but occurs from infancy to adulthood with a broad range of severity.

REFERENCES

1. Perloff JK: Neurological disorders and heart disease. In *Heart Disease*, 4th ed. Edited by Braunwald E. Philadelphia: WB Saunders; 1992:1810–1826.

2. Perloff JK, Henze E, Schelbert HR: Alterations in regional myocardial metabolism, perfusion and wall motion in Duchenne muscular dystrophy studied by radionuclide imaging. *Circulation* 1984, 69:33–42.

3. Perloff JK, Moise S, Stevenson WG, *et al.*: Cardiac electrophysiology in Duchenne muscular dystrophy: from basic science to clinical expression. *J Cardiovasc Electrophysiol* 1992, 3:394–409.

4. Hoffman EP, Kunkel LM: Dystrophin abnormalities in Duchenne/Becker muscular dystrophy. *Neuron* 1989, 2:1019–1029.

5. Mann O, deLeon AC, Perloff JK: Duchenne muscular dystrophy: the electrocardiogram in female relatives. *Am J Med Sci* 1968, 255:376–381.

6. Stevenson WG, Perloff JK, Weiss JN, *et al.*: Facioscapulohumeral muscular dystrophy: evidence for selective, genetic electrophysiologic cardiac involvement. *J Am Coll Cardiol* 1990, 15:292–299.

7. Emery AEH: X-linked muscular dystrophy with early contractures and cardiomyopathy (Emery-Dreifuss type). *Clin Genet* 1987, 32:360–367.

8. Perloff JK, Stevenson WG, Roberts NK: Cardiac involvement in myotonic muscular dystrophy (Steinert's disease): a prospective study of 25 patients. *Am J Cardiol* 1984, 54:1074–1081.

9. Child JS, Perloff JK, Bach PM: Cardiac involvement in Friedreich's ataxia. *J Am Coll Cardiol* 1986, 7:1370–1378.

10. Roberts NK, Perloff JK, Kark RAP: Cardiac conduction in the Kearns-Sayre syndrome (a neuromuscular disorder associated with progressive external ophthalmoplegia and pigmentary retinopathy). *Am J Cardiol* 1979, 44:1396–1400.

The Heart in Nutritional Deficiencies

7

CHAPTER

Chuichi Kawai and Yasuyuki Nakamura

Except for carnitine deficiency, most of the diseases described in this chapter are caused by deficiencies of certain nutrients, and are endemic. *Beriberi disease* is due to a deficiency of thiamine (vitamin B_1) among populations in the Orient whose staple diet consists of polished rice [1], and is characterized by a high cardiac output. *Keshan disease*, found mainly in China, is caused by selenium deficiency [2], and is characterized by heart failure and, histologically, multifocal necrosis and replacement fibrosis [2–5]. *Kwashiorkor syndrome*, found in Africa, results from a deficiency of protein relative to calories. Its characteristic features are general muscle wasting, loss of subcutaneous fat, and atrophy of most organs, including the heart [6].

Malnutrition and protein-caloric deficiency are prevalent in many underdeveloped countries. However, cardiac changes in these diseases have become a worldwide concern in recent years in cases in which similar conditions prevail, *eg*, beriberi heart disease in nonconfined urban areas in Gambia and West Africa [7]; a certain Japanese population that ingests excessive amounts of sweet carbonated drinks, instant noodles, and polished rice without thiamine supplementation [8]; Keshanlike disease in patients on long-term home parenteral nutrition in the United States [9]; or kwashiorkor syndrome in patients with anorexia nervosa [10] in many industrialized countries [11]. In the West, sporadic cases of beriberi can be seen in alcoholics, especially beer drinkers, because of the displacement of thiamine-containing food by alcohol with a high carbohydrate content [12]. Relative thiamine deficiency may also be induced by a hypermetabolic state, such as fever, thyrotoxicosis, and exercise, or by poor intake due to anorexia in those individuals who have chronic diseases including malignancy and acquired immunodeficiency syndrome [11]. Increased urinary excretion of thiamine due to prolonged use of diuretics [13,14] may also play a role.

All of these nutritional diseases are preventable if appropriate measures are taken, but not all of these diseases are curable once they develop. Theoretically, the preventive measures may appear to be easily undertaken, but practically it is difficult to begin such measures in affected areas. The problem is not merely a medical matter, but more a public health problem or sociopolitical issue. As physicians who have high standards and professional knowledge of the problem, we are expected not merely to describe diseases, but to do our part to resolve the underlying problems.

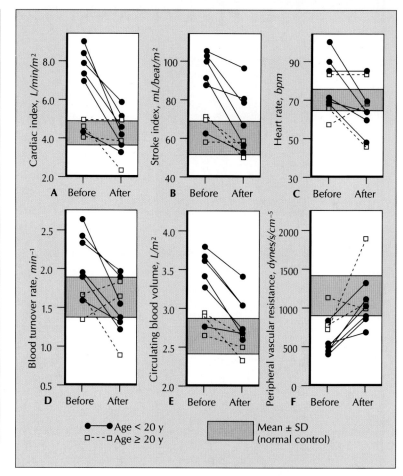

FIGURE 7-1. Structure of thiamine phosphate esters. Four different thiamine esters can be found in animal tissues, including free thiamine, thiamine monophosphate (TMP), thiamine pyrophosphate (TPP), and thiamine triphosphate. Among these thiamine phosphate esters, TPP is most abundant, comprising about 80% of the total thiamine. Five percent to 10% of thiamine is TMP and free thiamine. Vitamin B_1, as TPP, is essential in carbohydrate metabolism. TPP (cocarboxylase) is a coenzyme of dehydrogenases in the formation of acetyl–coenzyme A (CoA) from pyruvate and of succinyl-CoA from alpha-ketoglutarate in oxidative phosphorylation. This coenzyme is also tightly bound to transketolase in the pentose phosphate pathway. Therefore, carbohydrate metabolism is markedly impaired in thiamine deficiency.

FIGURE 7-2. Hemodynamic changes in beriberi heart disease before and after treatment in patients younger and older than 20 years of age. Wet beriberi disease is characterized by edema, ranging from pure peripheral edema to anasarca associated with overt heart failure. Congestive heart failure is generally of the high-output type, demonstrating increases in cardiac index (**A**), stroke index (**B**), heart rate (**C**), blood turnover rate (**D**), circulating blood volume (**E**), and decreased peripheral vascular resistance (**F**), which is prominent in patients under 20 years of age before and after treatment of beriberi heart disease. (*Adapted from* Kawai and coworkers [8]; with permission.)

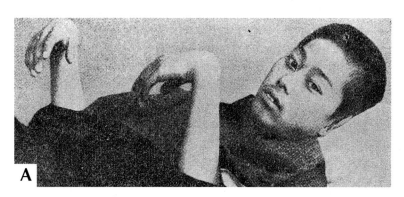

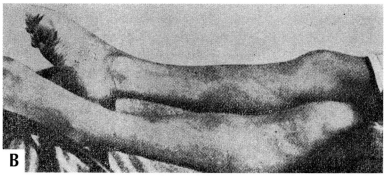

FIGURE 7-3. Paralysis of extremities in beriberi disease. Clinically, beriberi can be divided into three types: dry, wet, and "shoshin" beriberi. Dry beriberi is manifested as both motor and sensory peripheral polyneuropathy, characterized by paralysis of the extremities and decreased or absent knee and ankle jerks. In the upper extremities paralysis begins from the fingers and ascends, involving the extensors earlier and more seriously than the flexors, and eventually resulting in claw-hand (**A**). In the lower extremities, motor palsy begins from the toes, and dorsal flexion becomes difficult due to involvement of the peroneal nerve. If paralysis further involves the thigh muscles, gait becomes difficult and the foot contracts in the form of "pes equinovarus" (**B**). (*Adapted from* Inoue and Katsura [1]; with permission.)

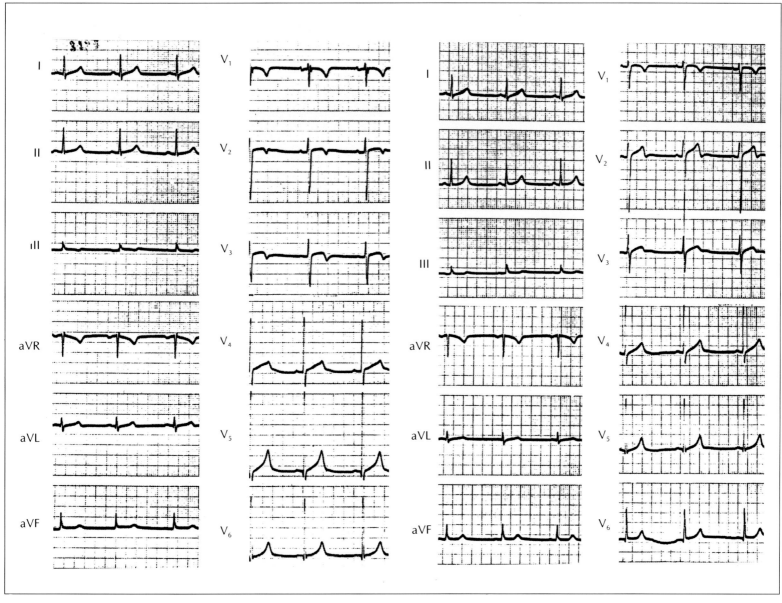

FIGURE 7-4. Electrocardiogram before (**A**) and after (**B**) treatment of beriberi heart disease. There is an increase in heart rate and prolongation of the Q-T interval. With treatment, both heart rate and Q-T interval decrease in most cases. The electrocardiogram shows inverted, diphasic, or depressed T waves. Such abnormalities of the T wave occur mainly in the right precordial leads, but in some cases also appear in the left precordial and limb leads. These T-wave abnormalities are not specific for beriberi heart disease, but could be improved with treatment. Note inverted T waves in leads V_1 through V_3 before treatment (*A*), which normalized in leads V_2 and V_3 after treatment (*B*). Not infrequently, T-wave abnormalities can be recognized retrospectively after treatment. (*Adapted from* Wakabayashi and coworkers [13]; with permission.)

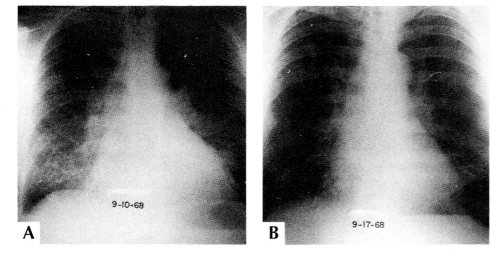

FIGURE 7-5. Chest roentgenograms in a 42-year-old patient with "shoshin" beriberi. In contrast to mild beriberi disease recently observed in Japan, "shoshin" (Japanese for "acute damage to the heart") beriberi is characterized by the sudden onset of severe biventricular failure associated with hypotension, tachycardia, lactic acidosis, and cardiovascular shock. **A,** The chest roentgenogram reveals generalized cardiomegaly and pulmonary vascular congestion with a small right pleural effusion on the day of admission. **B,** Pulmonary vascular congestion disappeared and heart size decreased 1 week after treatment, which included 100 mg of intravenous thiamine hydrochloride, nasal oxygen, digoxin, and morphine sulfate. This fulminant form of beriberi is occasionally seen in infants or pregnant women but can be found even in healthy young individuals with only minimal prodromal symptoms. Death may ensue within hours unless properly treated. Typical shoshin beriberi is now rare in developed countries. (*Adapted from* Jeffrey and Abelmann [15]; with permission.)

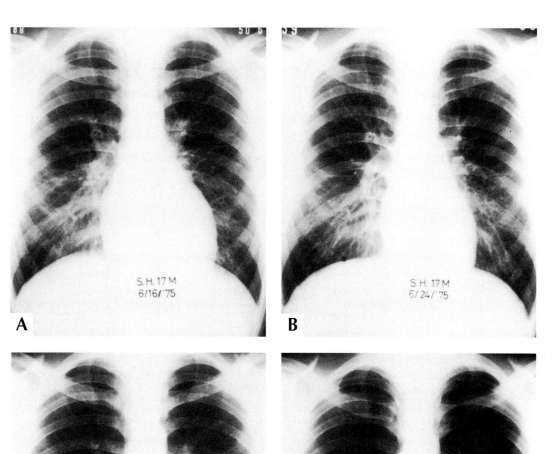

FIGURE 7-6. Chest roentgenograms in the course of treatment in beriberi heart disease usually show biventricular enlargement, pulmonary congestion, and pleural effusions. In recently reported mild cases in Japanese teenagers, the cardiac silhouette was within normal limits or was slightly enlarged before treatment (**A**). The heart size promptly began to decrease 8 days after the beginning of therapy (**B**), became still smaller after 15 days (**C**), and remained the same despite the discontinuation of treatment (**D**). Note that the cardiac silhouette appears normal at first glance, but diminishes clearly after treatment, revealing retrospectively the presence of cardiac enlargement at the onset of illness. (*Adapted from* Wakabayashi and coworkers [13]; with permission.)

DIAGNOSTIC CRITERIA FOR BERIBERI HEART DISEASE

Clinical features
  Dependent edema
  Low peripheral vascular resistance: decreased minimum blood pressure
    and increased pulse pressure
  Hyperkinetic circulatory state: midsystolic murmur and third heart sound
  Enlarged heart
  T-wave changes (inverted, diphasic, depressed) on electrocardiogram
  Peripheral neuritis
  Dietary deficiency for at least 3 months or chronic alcoholism
Presence of thiamine deficiency
  Decrease in blood thiamine concentration
  Decrease in erythrocyte transketolase activity
  Increase in TPP effect
Improvement after adequate thiamine therapy

FIGURE 7-7. Diagnostic criteria for beriberi heart disease. Laboratory diagnosis for thiamine deficiency can be made by demonstration of a decrease in the blood thiamine level, a decrease in erythrocyte transketolase activity, and an increase in thiamine pyrophosphate (TPP) effect (0% to 14% is normal; 15% to 24% represents a borderline response; and 25% or more indicates thiamine deficiency). The TPP effect is the percentage stimulation of transketolase activity above the original activity produced by adding TPP to the hemolyzed erythrocytes before assay. It reflects the proportion of the apoenzyme not saturated with coenzyme (TPP). (*Adapted from* Wakabayashi and coworkers [13]; with permission.)

TREATMENT AND PREVENTION

TREATMENT

Mild beriberi heart disease

Rest

Well-balanced diet, consisting of appropriate protein, lipids, and carbohydrate with thiamine supplementation

50 to 100 mg IV of thiamine hydrochloride or thiamine propyldisulfide, followed by 10 to 50 mg three times daily for 1 week, and then the same dose orally as maintenance therapy

"Shoshin" beriberi

Prompt 100 mg IV of thiamine hydrochloride or thiamine propylsulfide, followed by 10 to 50 mg three times daily for 1 week, and then the same dose orally as maintenance therapy

Digitalis should be given very cautiously

Diuretics if necessary

Coexistent acidosis may require therapy

PREVENTION

Ingestion of germ-retaining polished rice, undermilled rice (eg, 70% milled rice) or rice enriched with thiamine

Avoidance of excessive intake of sweet carbonated drinks and strenuous exercise during hot summer

Avoidance of long-term administration of potent diuretics; patients with congestive heart failure on long-term diuretics should be monitored carefully for a possible thiamine deficiency

Thiaminase, contained in clams, raw fish, or ferns, may sometimes cause beriberi; cooking (eg, baking or boiling) inactivates thiaminase

FIGURE 7-8. Treatment and prevention of beriberi heart disease. Dramatic improvement after thiamine administration in young patients with beriberi heart disease confirms the diagnosis. Even a sufficient supply of thiamine, however, sometimes fails to provide prompt amelioration of clinical features in elderly patients with an evident thiamine deficiency.

KESHAN DISEASE

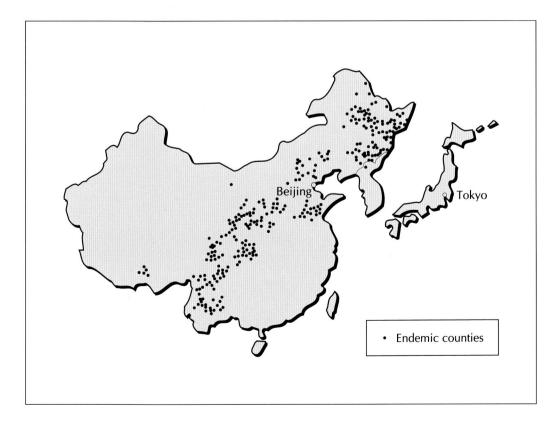

• Endemic counties

FIGURE 7-9. The characteristic distribution of Keshan disease in China is beltlike, *ie*, from northeast to southwest across the plowing area, where the elements in the soil were washed away by seasonal river floods. The affected sites are usually focally distributed in hilly land at 1000 to 3000 m above sea level. The disease is rare in high mountains or plains. (*Adapted from* Yu [3]; with permission.)

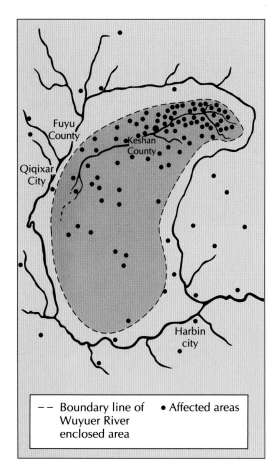

FIGURE 7-10. The distribution of Keshan disease in the Wuyuer River Basin. Keshan disease has been prevalent in China for more than 100 years. The first epidemiologic, clinical, and pathologic surveys of this disease were carried out in 1935, when there was a violent outbreak in Keshan County, Heilongjiang Province, northern China, and the disease was named after that region. The endemic areas are distributed in the higher areas of the Wuyuer River Basin. (*Adapted from* Yu [3]; with permission.)

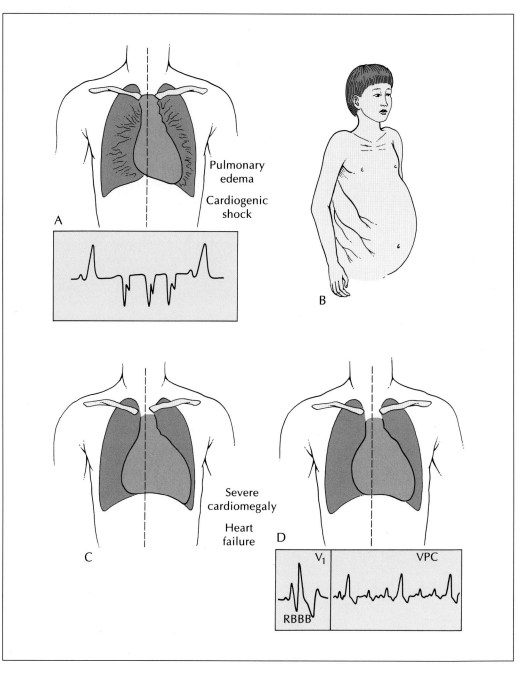

FIGURE 7-11. Types of Keshan disease. **A,** Acute Keshan disease involves sudden onset with acute heart failure such as cardiogenic shock, severe arrhythmia, and pulmonary edema. ST-T changes can be noted on electrocardiogram. **B,** Subacute Keshan disease, the most prevalent type at present, is predominant in children with generalized edema and heart failure of subacute onset. **C,** The chronic type involves moderate to severe cardiomegaly with a varying degree of heart failure. **D,** Latent disease involves mild cardiomegaly with normal heart function. Electrocardiographic changes of right bundle branch block (RBBB) and ventricular premature contractions (VPC) may also be present.

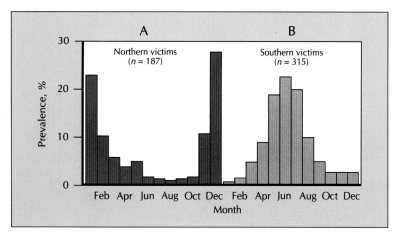

FIGURE 7-12. The monthly distribution of Keshan disease. The seasonal prevalence in northern China (**A**) differs from that in southern China (**B**). Seventy-five percent of the 187 cases observed in northern China occurred from November to February, but 72% of the 315 southern cases were observed from May to August. (*Adapted from* Ge and coworkers [4]; with permission.)

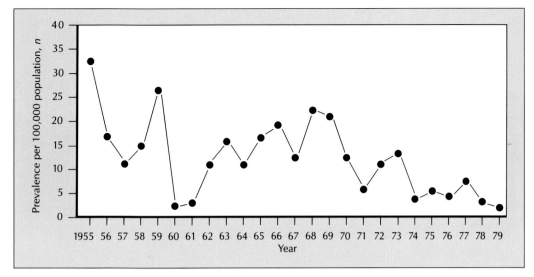

FIGURE 7-13. The incidence of Keshan disease in Heilongjiang Province from 1955 to 1979. Keshan disease was prevalent in this region in some years and in others it was rarely seen. In Heilongjiang Province in 1955 the prevalence rate was 32.7/100,000 population, but in 1961 it was only 1.9/100,000. Sometimes during a prevalent year, several counties in one province, or several communes in one county, were attacked by the disease. During large outbreaks, the prevalence rate in one county could be as high as 980/100,000, as it was in Shangzhi County of Heilongjiang Province in 1969. (*Adapted from* Yu [3]; with permission.)

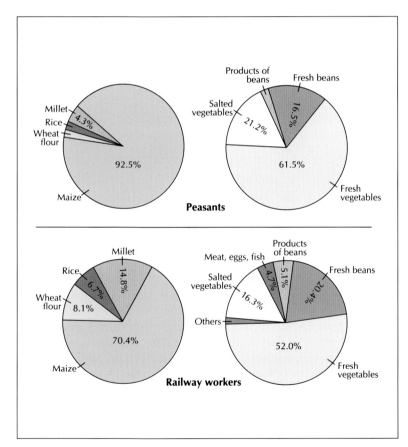

FIGURE 7-14. Mean dietary proportion of staple and subsidiary foods of peasants and railway workers in China. Coal miners, foresters, railway workers, and others living in the same endemic area as peasants, who ate commercial agricultural products rather than food produced by the peasants, did not have Keshan disease. The peasants, who ate the agricultural products (mostly maize) from their own fields, had a very simple diet compared with that of the railway workers. (*Adapted from* Yu [3]; with permission.)

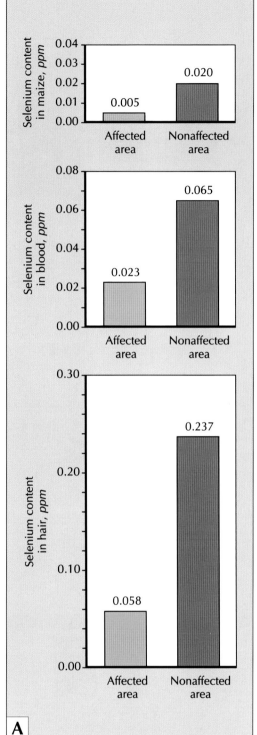

FIGURE 7-15. There is evidence in favor of and against selenium deficiency as the etiology of Keshan disease [2]. Positive evidence includes the following. **A,** There is a very low selenium content in endemic grain, and in the hair and blood of the inhabitants in endemic areas. (*continued*)

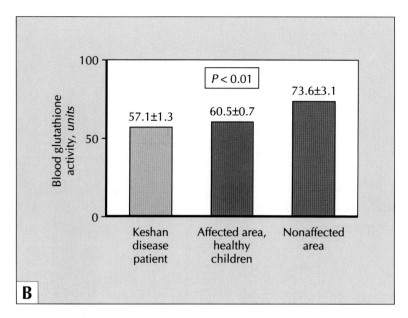

	INCIDENCE PER 1000, %	
Year	Treated children	Untreated children
1976	0.17	2
1977	0.22	1.57
1978	0.15	1.69
1979	0.47	1.34
1980	0.29	1.07
Total	0.27	1.55

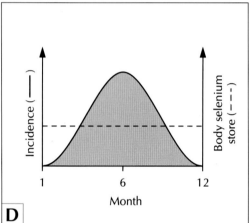

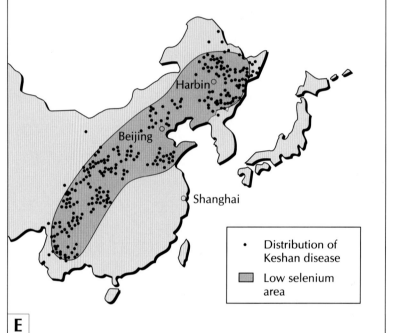

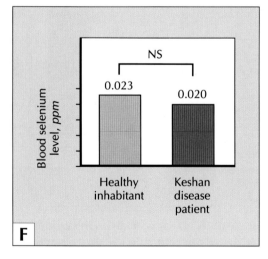

FIGURE 7-15. (*continued*) **B,** There is little glutathione peroxidase activity in the whole blood of the inhabitants. **C,** The dietary supplementation of selenium markedly diminishes the incidence. Negative evidence includes the following. **D,** The seasonal variation in the incidence of the disease (*see* Fig. 7-11) is not accompanied by changes in body selenium stores, which can remain almost constant. **E,** Not all selenium-deficient areas are necessarily endemic. **F,** There are no differences in blood selenium levels between healthy and diseased children from the same affected area. Secondary factors for Keshan disease include vitamin E deficiency, some toxins, hypoxia, and virus.

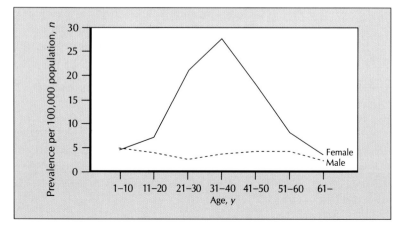

FIGURE 7-16. The incidence of acute Keshan disease in different age groups from 1955 to 1964 in Heilongjiang Province. Ninety-nine percent of the patients lived on grains from their own fields, and 80% of these were young women of child-bearing age and infants after lactation. (*Adapted from* Yu [3]; with permission.)

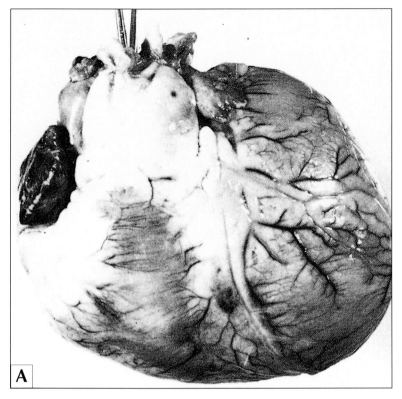

A

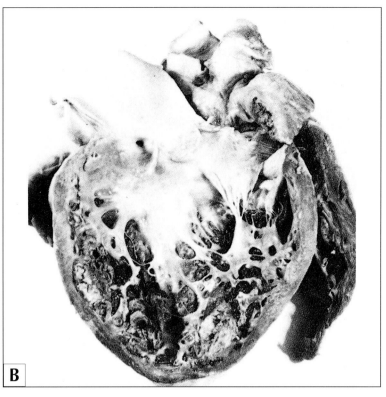

B

FIGURE 7-17. Gross pathology of Keshan disease. **A,** The heart from a 43-year-old man with chronic Keshan disease. Extreme dilatation of all cardiac chambers and the globular appearance are visible. **B,** The heart of a 21-year-old woman with chronic Keshan disease shows extreme dilation of the left ventricle and numerous mural thrombi embedded in the deepened intertrabecular spaces. The left ventricular thickness was usually within the normal range or even less than normal, especially in the apical region, but apical

aneurysm, often seen in chronic Chagas' disease, was not found. In greatly dilated hearts, the trabeculae carneae had lost their columnar shape and were thinned out and interwoven, forming netlike structures with deepened lacunae that favored the formation of mural thrombi, such as is seen in *B*. Most of the above features are indistinguishable from those of dilated cardiomyopathy. (*Adapted from* Li and coworkers [5]; with permission.)

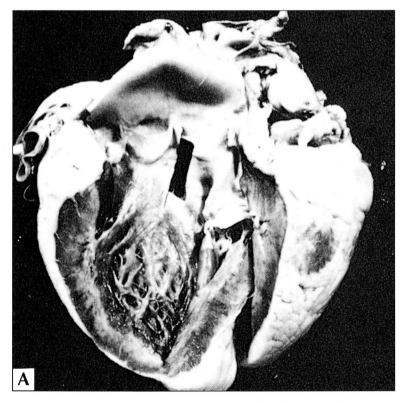

A

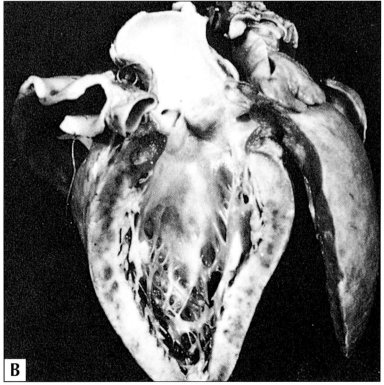

B

FIGURE 7-18. Macroscopic changes in multifocal necrotic lesions. **A,** Subendocardial yellow-gray zonal necrosis in the left ventricular wall of the heart from a 26-year-old woman with acute Keshan disease. This change reflected the severe myocardial parenchymal degeneration and early necrosis, and appeared mainly in acute cases such as this.

B, Multiple small, slightly pitted, dark red foci in the left ventricular wall of the heart from a 7-year-old girl with subacute Keshan disease. The lesion represents the dissolving and early healing phase of cardiac necrosis. Such findings are not commonly seen in dilated cardiomyopathy. (*Adapted from* Li and coworkers [5]; with permission.)

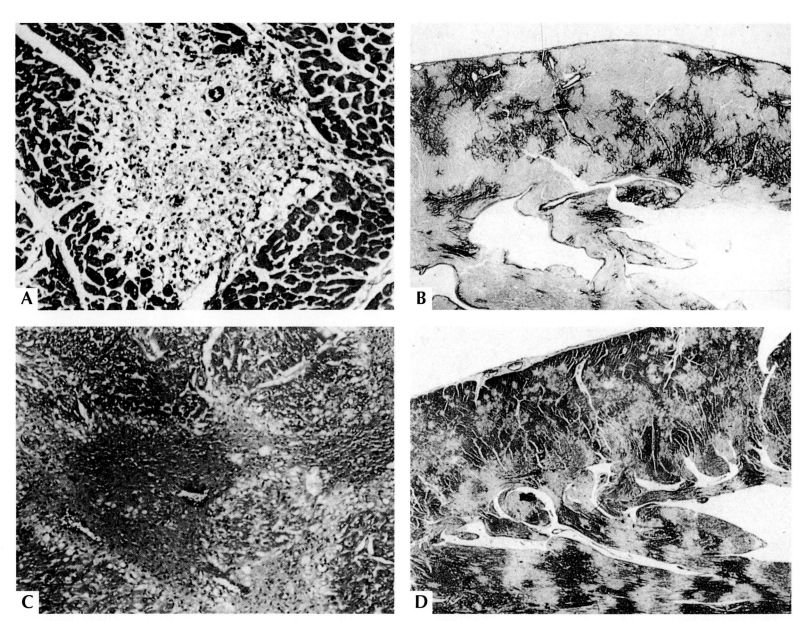

FIGURE 7-19. Microscopic changes of the Keshan diseased heart. **A,** Well-circumscribed necrotic focus in the myocardium (hematoxylin and eosin, x 120). Multifocal necrosis and replacement fibrosis of the myocardium are the characteristic features of Keshan disease. The necrotic foci varied in size and are often well circumscribed, resulting in scattered replacement fibrosis. **B,** Multiple foci of scarring in the left ventricular wall (van Gieson's stain, x 6) differentiated chronic Keshan disease from congestive cardiomyopathy and chronic myocarditis, in which interfiber and perivascular fibrosis are particularly prominent. In large, old scars dilated sinusoid or giant capillary-like blood vessels are often found. **C,** Centrally located, dense scar surrounded by a rim of myocytolysis (hematoxylin and eosin, x 50). The myocardial lesions of Keshan disease can develop repeatedly, with fresh and old lesions coexisting in the same heart. As a rule, the left ventricle is damaged prior to the right, and the inner zone of the ventricular wall prior to the outer. **D,** Miliary foci disseminated throughout the left ventricular wall, resembling clusters of grapes in the outer and middle layers, and expanding and merging in the inner layer, with a segmental distribution in the papillary muscle (phosphotungstic acid-hematoxylin stain, x 6). (*Adapted from* Li and coworkers [5]; with permission.)

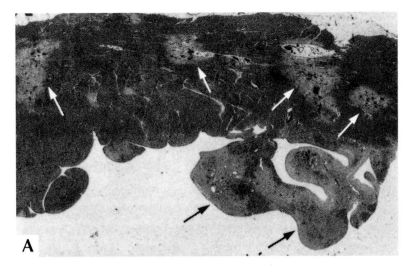

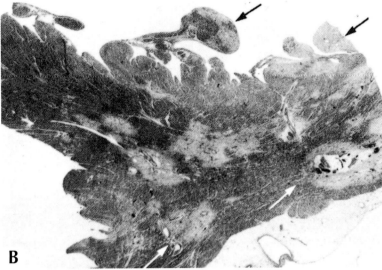

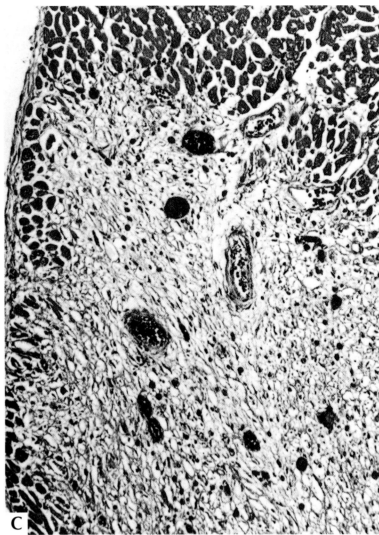

FIGURE 7-20. Keshan disease in a patient on home parenteral nutrition in the United States. This patient with chronic idiopathic intestinal pseudo-obstruction maintained on home parenteral nutrition for 6 consecutive years died from cardiomyopathy and ventricular fibrillation. Postmortem examination of the heart revealed widespread myocytolysis and replacement fibrosis similar to that seen in Keshan disease. Selenium deficiency in this patient was documented with extremely low concentrations of selenium and decreased activity of the selenoprotein, glutathione peroxidase, in blood, heart, liver, and skeletal muscle. A, and B, Low-magnification photomicrographs of full-thickness anterior (*A*) and posterior (*B*) walls of the left ventricle, showing serpiginous subendocardial (*black arrows*) and subepicardial (*white arrows*) vascular scars of the heart (hematoxylin and eosin, × 2.5). C, Higher-magnification view of a subendocardial focus of myocytolysis and replacement fibrosis with numerous small, thin-walled, engorged blood vessels (hematoxylin and eosin, × 160). (*Adapted from* Fleming and coworkers [9]; with permission.)

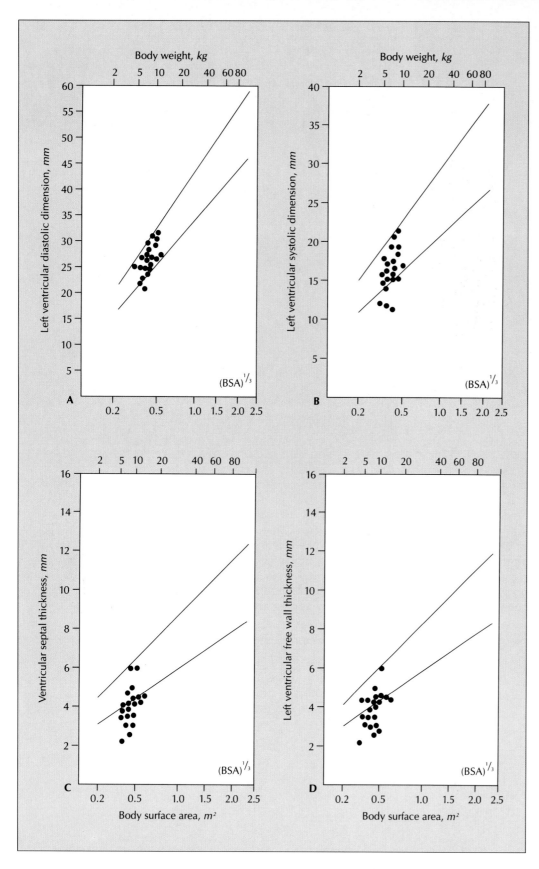

FIGURE 7-21. Heart size in kwashiorkor syndrome. Left ventricular diastolic (**A**) and systolic (**B**) dimensions according to body surface area (BSA) with 95% prediction intervals drawn for assessment. Interventricular septal thickness (**C**) and left ventricular free wall thickness (**D**) according to BSA with the 95% prediction intervals drawn for assessment. Echocardiographic assessment of left ventricular chamber size and wall thickness in 21 patients with kwashiorkor but without severe, dehydrating diarrheal disease, septicemia, or preexisting cardiac disease, revealed that the left ventricular end-diastolic and end-systolic dimensions for BSA were within the 95% predictive values in most of the patients (*A* and *B*). However, interventricular septal thickness for BSA was below the 5th percentile in 81% of the patients and left ventricular free wall thickness for BSA was below the 5th percentile in 71%. Overall, 76% of the patients had values equal to or below the 5th percentile for one or both variables. Only one of the 21 patients had a shortening fraction below the normal range. Thus, the kwashiorkor heart has reduced myocardial mass with preserved left ventricular function. (*Adapted from* Bergman and coworkers [16]; with permission.)

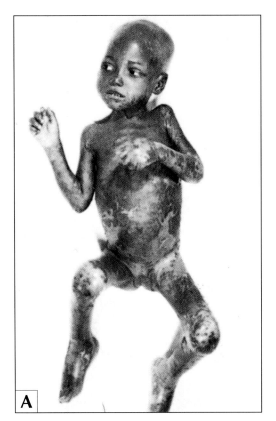

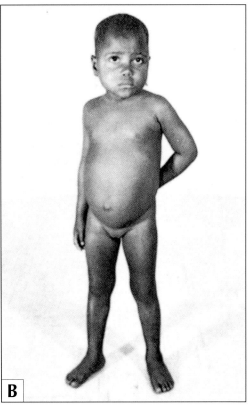

FIGURE 7-22. Kwashiorkor, which is most common in Africa, affects primarily persons on a high-carbohydrate, low-protein diet, such as those eating cassava as the staple food. **A,** A case of kwashiorkor in a 3.5-year-old Nigerian girl 48 hours after onset of therapy. Note peripheral edema, evidence of wasting in the upper arms and thorax, exfoliative dermatitis, and gray hair stubble. (The patient's head has been shaved.) **B,** Two months later, the same child had black hair and dark healthy skin, and was sturdy, ambulatory, and vigorous. In treating kwashiorkor, caution must be taken to give balanced nutrition. In many cases, there is concomitant magnesium deficiency, and therefore, usual hyperalimentation alone without adequate magnesium supplements may result in hypomagnesemia, *ie,* brief periods of apnea, electrocardiographic changes mimicking those of hypocalcemia or hypokalemia, and a wide range of neurologic manifestations. (*Adapted from* Whittemore and Caddell [6]; with permission.)

CARDIAC FUNCTION IN KWASHIORKOR

	LVEDV, mL	CO, L/min	CI, L/min/m²	EF, %	VCF, cir/s	LVM, g	LVM/KG BODY WEIGHT, g
Controls (*n*=26)	35.78±9.96	2.75±0.77	4.97±1.4	67±7.8	1.59±0.33	32.44±11.64	2.42±0.87
Patients (*n*=25)	25.12±6.07	2.03±0.45	5.95±1.95	62.4±10.7	1.52±0.34	25.75±8.09	4.44±1.45

FIGURE 7-23. Cardiac function in kwashiorkor. Echocardiographic evaluation of left ventricular function and mass was performed in children with severe protein energy malnutrition (kwashiorkor) and in normal children (controls) in India [17]. Left ventricular end-diastolic volume (LVEDV), stroke volume, and cardiac output (CO) were reduced in proportion to a decrease in body size of the patients, so that the cardiac index (CI) was not reduced but rather slightly increased in the patients. The mean left ventricular mass (LVM) in the kwashiorkor patients was lower than that in the controls; however, LVM/kg body weight was significantly increased in the kwashiorkor patients, suggesting relative cardiac sparing. Systolic function indices such as ejection fraction (EF), percentage fractional shortening, and velocity of circumferential fiber shortening (VCF) were not significantly different in the patients compared with the normal children.

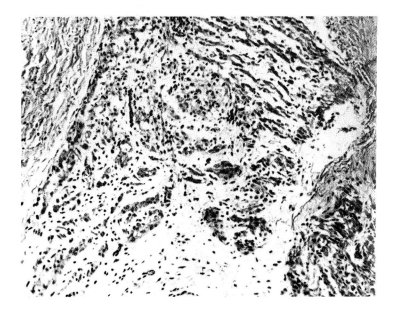

FIGURE 7-24. Conduction system of the heart in kwashiorkor. Note wasting of the conduction fibers in the atrioventricular bundle with interstitial edema of the heart in kwashiorkor. Sims [18] examined conduction tissue of the heart in seven cases of kwashiorkor, and found atrophic changes and myocytolysis in five cases. No cellular reaction or fibrous repair was found in relation to the area of myocytolysis. These findings may be associated with a disturbance of atrioventricular conduction during life, perhaps accounting for some of the unexplained sudden deaths occurring in children with kwashiorkor. (*Adapted from* Sims [18]; with permission.)

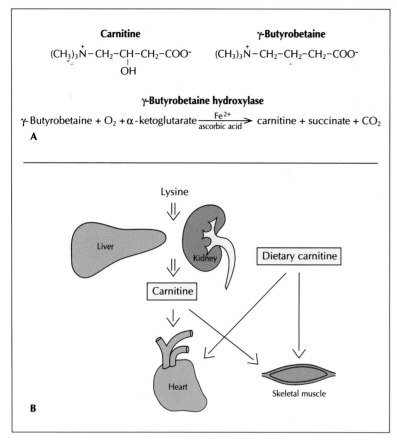

FIGURE 7-25. **A,** Biosynthesis of carnitine proceeds through successive methylations, using methyl groups derived from S-adenosylmethionine, of either free or protein-bound lysine to give ε-N-trimethyllysine, which is then metabolized by a series of reactions with the loss of carbons to yield Y-butyrobetaine. The latter is then hydroxylated to form carnitine in a reaction catalyzed by Y-butyrobetaine hydroxylase. **B,** The process takes place in the liver and kidney. Both skeletal and cardiac muscles use lipid in addition to carbohydrate as the main energy source. The heart is unable to synthesize carnitine and therefore its concentration depends on intake from diet or release from the liver and kidney, or both.

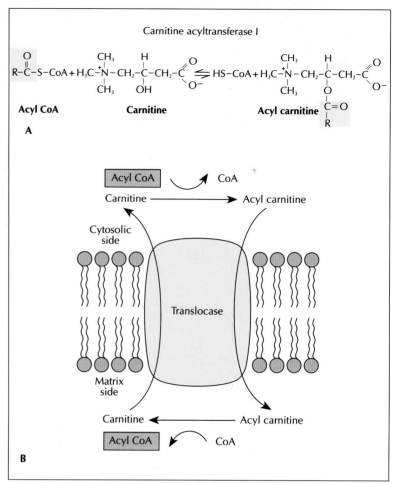

FIGURE 7-26. Metabolic roles of carnitine. **A,** Long-chain acyl coenzyme A (CoA) molecules, the activated form of long-chain fatty acids on the outer mitochondrial membrane, do not readily transverse the inner mitochondrial membrane into the mitochondrial matrix, where they are to be oxidized. Therefore, a special transport mechanism is needed. Carnitine carries activated long-chain fatty acids across the inner mitochondrial membrane. The acyl group is transferred from the sulfur atom of CoA to the hydroxyl group of carnitine to form acyl carnitine. This reaction is catalyzed by carnitine acyltransferase I, which is located on the cytosolic face of the inner mitochondrial membrane. **B,** Acyl carnitine is then transported across the inner mitochondrial membrane by translocase. The acyl group is transferred back to CoA on the matrix side of the membrane. This reaction, which is catalyzed by carnitine acyltransferase II, is thermodynamically feasible because the O-acyl link in carnitine has a high group-transfer potential. Finally, carnitine is returned to the cytosolic side by the translocase in exchange for incoming acyl carnitine. Both skeletal and cardiac muscles use lipid in addition to carbohydrate as the main energy source. Carnitine depletion results in depressed mitochondrial oxidation of fatty acids and in cytoplasmic accumulation of lipids. (*Adapted from* Stryer [19]; with permission.)

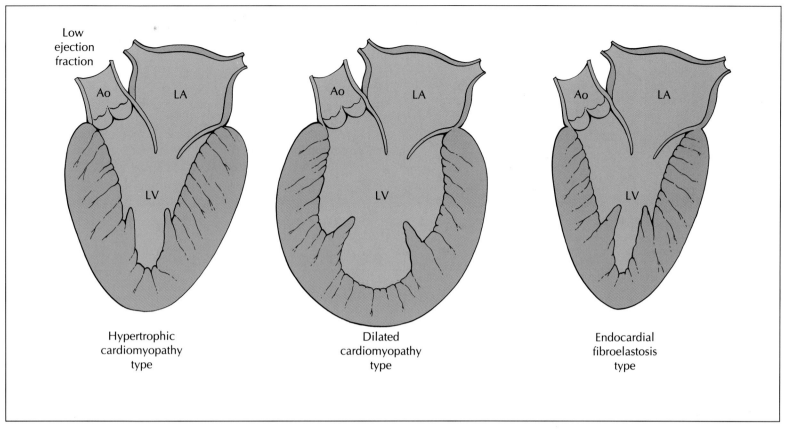

FIGURE 7-27. Cardiac manifestations in carnitine deficiency. Carnitine deficiency in humans is classified as myopathic or systemic according to the clinical presentation. Myopathic forms are characterized by normal plasma concentrations but low skeletal-muscle carnitine concentrations, with progressive muscle weakness. Systemic forms are characterized by low plasma and tissue carnitine concentrations with multisystem involvement.

Cardiac involvement has been described in patients with both forms of carnitine deficiency. Cardiac manifestations in carnitine deficiency are variable and many types have been reported: a hypertrophic cardiomyopathy type with a decreased ejection fraction, a type that resembles dilated cardiomyopathy, and an endocardial fibroelastosis type have been reported.

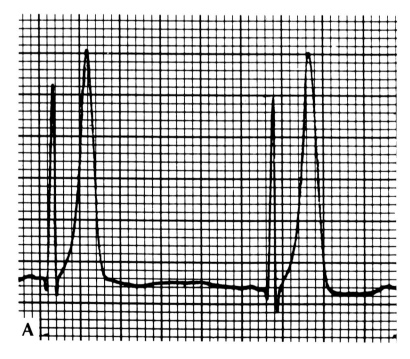

FIGURE 7-28. Electrocardiograms in carnitine deficiency are also variable. **A,** An electrocardiogram from a school-age girl with systemic carnitine deficiency who presented with familial endocardial fibroelastosis. Bizarre T-wave enlargement similar to that seen in extensive posterior-wall ischemia and in hyperkalemia can be seen. In a series of 11 children with cardiac involvement associated with abnormal carnitine metabolism, the most frequent electrocardiographic abnormality was tachycardia. T-wave abnormalities with inversion in leads V_4 to V_6 were seen in four patients and diffusely low voltage was seen in three patients. Signs of left and right ventricular hypertrophy were common. (*continued*)

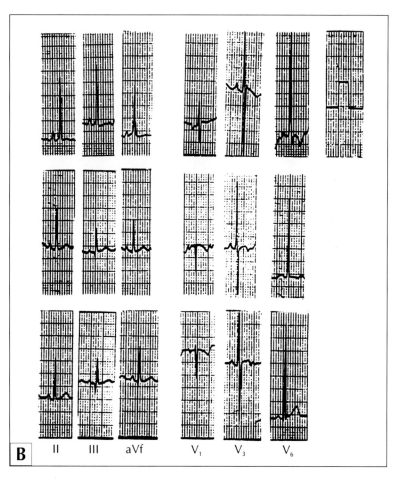

FIGURE 7-28. (*continued*) **B,** Serial changes in the electrocardiogram in a patient with carnitine deficiency before and after oral L-carnitine therapy. *Top,* Pretreatment electrocardiogram showing ST segment depression in the precordial leads and T-wave inversion in lead V_6, as well as evidence of bilateral atrial enlargement and left ventricular hypertrophy. *Middle,* After 3 months of therapy, there are increased T-wave amplitudes in leads II, III, and aVF and less inversion in lead V_6. *Bottom,* After 14 months of therapy the T wave in lead V_6 was normal. High voltage QRS is still present in leads V_3 and V_6. (*Adapted from* Tripp and coworkers [20] and Ino and coworkers [21]; with permission.)

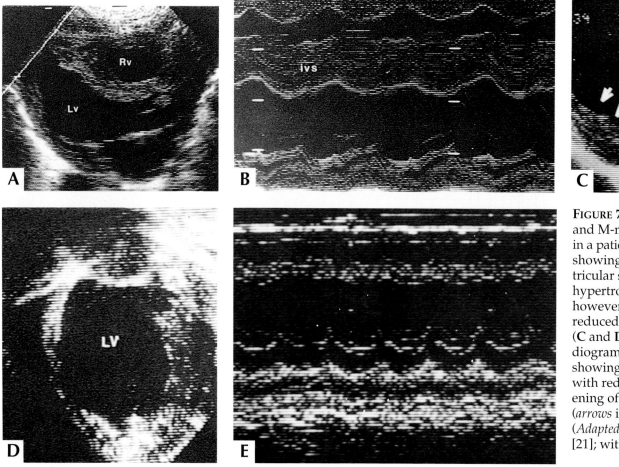

FIGURE 7-29. Two-dimensional (**A**) and M-mode (**B**) echocardiograms in a patient with carnitine deficiency showing a hypertrophied interventricular septum (ivs). Unlike typical hypertrophic cardiomyopathies, however, the ejection fraction was reduced (25%). Two-dimensional (**C** and **D**) and M-mode (**E**) echocardiograms of a 7-month-old patient showing a dilated left ventricle (LV) with reduced function and thickening of the LV posterior wall (*arrows* in **C**). RV—right ventricle. (*Adapted from* Ino and coworkers [21]; with permission.)

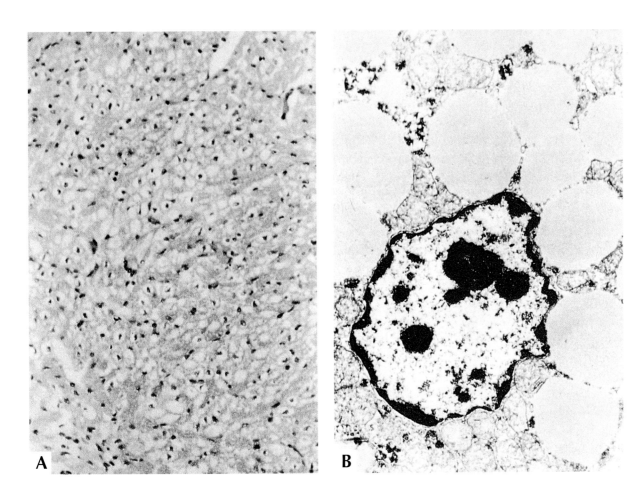

FIGURE 7-30. Histopathologic changes in carnitine deficiency. **A,** Light microscopic section of the left ventricular myocardium showing myocyte vacuolization due to fatty change. **B,** Electron microscopic section showing cytoplasmic lipid deposits adjacent to the nucleus and mitochondria. (*Adapted from* Ino and coworkers [21]; with permission.)

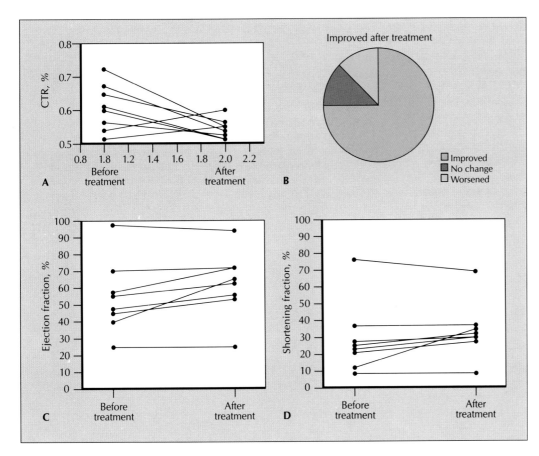

FIGURE 7-31. **A** through **D,** Chest radiographic, electrocardiographic, and echocardiographic findings before and after L-carnitine treatment in eight patients. Six of eight patients on carnitine supplementation improved clinically during the 3 months to 2 years of follow-up [20]. The cardiothoracic ratio (CTR) decreased significantly after treatment in five patients. In four, the electrocardiogram showed improvement in ST-T waves but mild left ventricular hypertrophy persisted. Echocardiographic improvement in ejection and shortening fractions and ventricular chamber size occurred in five patients without significant reduction in posterior wall thickness.

ETIOLOGY AND TREATMENT OF NUTRITIONAL HEART DISEASES

DISEASE	ETIOLOGY	TREATMENT
Keshan disease	Selenium deficiency	Selenium supplements
Kwashiorkor	Protein deficiency	Protein and magnesium supplements
Carnitine deficiency	Inborn error of metabolism	Carnitine supplements

FIGURE 7-32. Etiologies and treatment of nutritional heart diseases.

REFERENCES

1. Inoue K, Katsura E: Clinical signs and metabolism of beriberi patients. In Beriberi and Thiamine. Edited by Shimazono N, Katsura E. Kyoto/Tokyo: Vitamin B Research Committee of Japan/Igaku Shoin Ltd; 1965:29–63.

2. Yang G, Chen J, Wen Z, *et al.*: The role of selenium in Keshan disease. *Adv Nutr Res* 1984, 6:203–231.

3. Yu W-H: A study of nutritional and biogeochemical factors in the occurrence and development of Keshan disease. *Jpn Circ J* 1982, 46:1201–1207.

4. Ge K, Xue A, Bai J, *et al.*: Review of Keshan disease: an endemic cardiomyopathy in China. *Virchows Arch A Pathol Anat Histopathol* 1983, 401:1–15.

5. Li G, Wang F, Kang D, *et al.*: Keshan disease: an endemic cardiomyopathy in China. *Hum Pathol* 1985, 16:602–609.

6. Whittemore R, Caddell JL. Metabolic and nutritional diseases. In *Heart Disease in Infants, Children, and Adolescents*, ed. 2. Edited by Moss AJ, Adams FH. Baltimore. Williams & Wilkins; 1983:579–602.

7. Rolfe M, Walker RW, Samba KN, *et al.*: Urban beri-beri in The Gambia, West Africa. *Trans R Soc Trop Med Hyg* 1993, 87:114–115.

8. Kawai C, Wakabayashi A, Matsumura T, *et al.*: Reappearance of beriberi heart disease in Japan: a study of 23 cases. *Am J Med* 1980, 69:383–386.

9. Fleming CR, Lie JT, McCall JT, *et al.*: Selenium deficiency and fatal cardiomyopathy in a patient on home parenteral nutrition. *Gastroenterology* 1982, 83:689–693.

10. Schocken DD, Holloway JD, Powers PS: Weight loss and the heart: effects of anorexia nervosa and starvation. *Arch Intern Med* 1989, 149:877–881.

11. Butterworth RF, Gaudrhau C, Vincelettr, *et al.*: Thiamine deficiency in AIDS. *Lancet* 1991, 338:1086.

12. Braunwald E, Grossman W: Clinical aspects of heart failure: beriberi heart disease. In *Heart Disease*, ed 4. Edited by Braunwald E. Philadelphia: WB Saunders; 1992:461–462.

13. Wakabayashi A, Yui Y, Kawai C: A clinical study on thiamine deficiency. *Jpn Circ J* 1979, 43:995–999.

14. Yui Y, Itokawa Y, Kawai C: Furosemide-induced thiamine deficiency. *Cardiovasc Res* 1980, 14:537–540.

15. Jeffrey FE, Abelmann WH: Recovery from proved shoshin beriberi. *Am J Med* 1971, 50:123–128.

16. Bergman JW, Human DG, De Moor MMA, *et al.*: Effect of kwashiorkor on the cardiovascular system. *Arch Dis Child* 1988, 63:1359–1362.

17. Kothari SS, Patel TM, Shetalwad AN, *et al.*: Left ventricular mass and function in children with severe protein energy malnutrition. *Int J Cardiol* 1992, 35:19–25.

18. Sims BA: Conduction tissue of the heart in kwashiorkor. *Br Heart J* 1972, 34:828–829.

19. Stryer L: *Biochemistry*, ed 3. New York; WH Freeman; 1988.

20. Tripp ML, Katcher ML, Peters HA, *et al.*: Systemic carnitine deficiency presenting as familial endocardial fibroelastosis: a treatable cardiomyopathy. *N Engl J Med* 1981, 305:385–390.

21. Ino T, Sherwood G, Benson LN, *et al.*: Cardiac manifestations in disorders of fat and carnitine metabolism in infancy. *J Am Coll Cardiol* 1988, 11:1301–1308.

CHAGAS' DISEASE

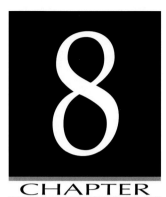

8

CHAPTER

Harry Acquatella

In 1909, the Brazilian physician Carlos Chagas described a disease, which is caused by the protozoan *Trypanosoma cruzi*. Confined within ecologic units composed of infected sylvatic or peridomestic mammals and sylvatic triatomid vectors, it exists only in the Americas. Human infection occurs by penetration of these ecotopes. In Latin America it is estimated that about 16 million people are infected and another 90 million are at risk of acquiring the parasite. The initial infection occurs largely unnoticed in childhood only to become clinically manifest in adulthood. Chagas' disease mainly affects people of the lowest socioeconomic level.

In recent decades substantial migration of infected rural dwellers to urban communities has occurred. After living several decades in nonendemic areas, subjects with chronic Chagas' disease may be misdiagnosed as having ischemic heart disease or idiopathic dilated cardiomyopathy. Exposed to urban risk factors, these individuals may also present in combination with other cardiac disorders. A positive epidemiology and serology thus does not necessarily mean that cardiac symptoms are of chagasic origin in a particular patient. The diagnosis must also rely on a combination of clinical findings known as the *chagasic syndrome*. Peculiar to chagasic myocarditis is the frequently focal nature of the scarring lesions at the left ventricular apex.

Transmission of Chagas' disease via blood transfusion is a real threat even in nonendemic countries. Since at present neither a cure nor eradication is possible, prophylactic measures are of the utmost importance. Programs to control Chagas' disease are based on good epidemiologic data, housing improvement, elimination of the vectors, and community education. Only a few countries have implemented these preventive measures on a large scale.

PARASITE CYCLE

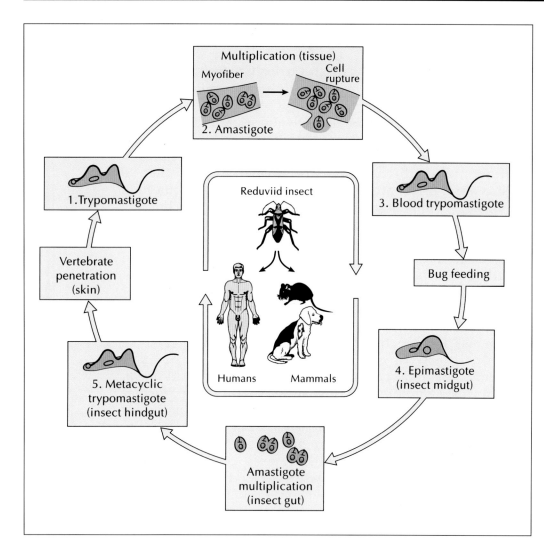

FIGURE 8-1. Chagas' disease is caused by *Trypanosoma cruzi*, a protozoan present in sylvatic mammals of the Americas such as armadillos, rodents, and opossums, as well as in domestic animals. It has vertebrate and invertebrate cycles. Transmission to humans is by reduviid bugs while feeding, by fecal contamination rather than inoculation. After initial trypomastigote (flagellate form) parasitemia [1], the parasites penetrate cardiac muscle and other tissue cells where they transform into amastigotes (aflagellate form) [2]. Intracellular parasite multiplication may lead to cell rupture with passage into the circulation or parasitism of other tissues including various ganglionic plexuses and segments of the alimentary tract. The cycle is completed when feeding bugs pick up blood trypomastigotes [3]. The trypanosomes become epimastigotes in the insect midgut [4], and then multiply and migrate to the hindgut where they become metacyclic trypomastigotes [5], the infective form in humans. Continuous transmission is independent of human infection.

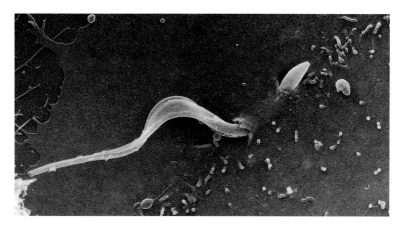

FIGURE 8-2. Scanning electron micrograph of *Trypanosoma cruzi* trypomastigotes actively entering mammalian cells. Immediately after invasion, the parasites can be found inside endocytic vacuoles in macrophages, fibroblasts, epithelial and endothelial cells, muscle, and nerve cells. Attachment of the parasite is an active process that requires energy, which can be inhibited by drugs affecting *T. cruzi* energy conservation. (*Adapted from* Schenkman and coworkers [3]; with permission.)

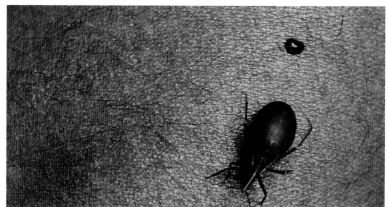

FIGURE 8-3. *Rhodnius prolixus* (nymph stage) after having a meal. The abdomen is greatly swollen from sucked blood even after defecation (dark bright spot behind the insect). The infection is acquired through the skin or mucosa by penetration of infecting forms of *Trypanosoma cruzi* present in the insect feces. (*Adapted from* The Pan American Health Organization [2]; with permission.)

GEOGRAPHIC DISTRIBUTION AND PREVALENCE

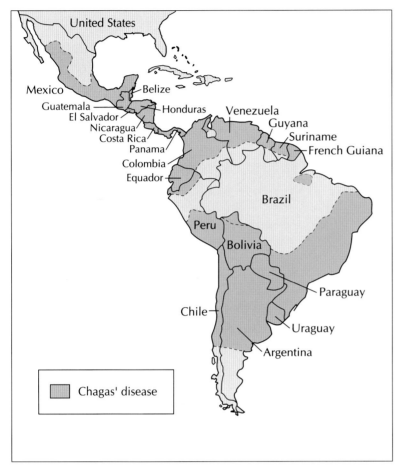

FIGURE 8-4. Distribution of Chagas' disease in the Americas. The extent of Chagas' disease depends on the geographic distribution of the triatomid vectors of *Trypanosoma cruzi* (shaded areas). There are significant differences among insect species of ecotope habitats: *Triatoma infestans* (southern South America) and *Rhodnius prolixus* (northern South America) are well adapted to human dwellings, while *T. protracta* (North America) is sylvatic. *T. dimidiata, T. sordida, T. brasiliensis,* and *Panstrongylus megistus* are in the process of adapting to the human habitat while preserving an extensive sylvatic ecotope [4]. These differences have implications for both human infection and control programs. In geographic areas where domiciliary vectors predominate, high rates of human infection exist, but insect eradication programs are more prone to be effective. Areas harboring vectors living in mixed ecotopes are the most challenging to control. Human infection is rare in areas having exclusively sylvatic (woodland) vectors. (*Adapted from Epidemiol Bull PAHO* [5]; with permission.)

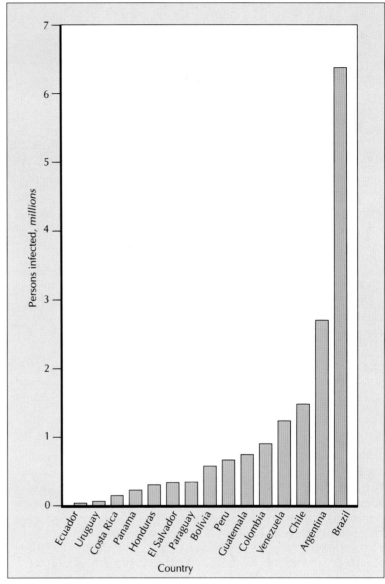

FIGURE 8-5. Prevalence of human *Trypanosoma cruzi* infection in Latin America from 1980 to 1986 [6]. The countries with the four highest rates have established prophylactic control programs. Although the prevalence in the United States is not known [7], emigration of about 5 million people from Latin America in the last three decades allows for an estimate that 50,000 to 100,000 immigrants have *T. cruzi* infection in the United States [8].

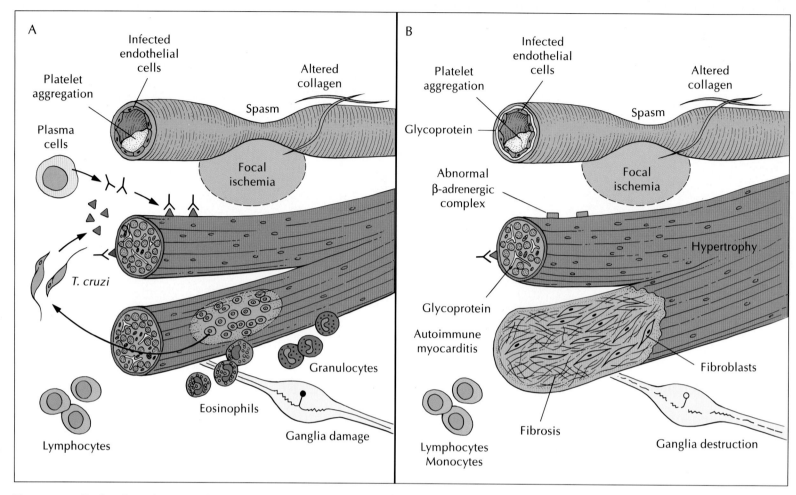

FIGURE 8-6. Pathophysiologic mechanisms proposed to explain the cardiac damage induced by *Trypanosoma cruzi*. **A,** Acute Chagas' disease. The penetration of the parasite into the cardiocyte exerts direct mechanical damage and may lead to myofibrillar rupture. Intense inflammation of the endomysium is denoted by infiltration composed of granulocytes, eosinophils, lymphocytes, histiocytes, and macrophages. Cytotoxic T lymphocytes are sensitized by *T. cruzi* antigens (*triangles*). Antibodies (*inverted Y's*) are produced by plasma cells, which might cross-react with tissue. T lymphocytes release lymphokines attracting and activating macrophages and platelet activator factor, which may promote platelet aggregation and thromboxane A$_2$ release. Intense vasculitis and abnormalities in the coronary microcirculation may lead to microvascular hyper-activity (spasm). These microvascular changes may lead to focal ischemia. Infected endothelial cells have an increased platelet-binding and enhanced endothelium-platelet interaction. Intra-cardiac lesions of the autonomic nervous system (ganglia damage) include periganglionitis, perineuritis, neuronal cell depletion, and Schwann cell damage. **B,** Chronic Chagas' disease. Destruction of cardiocytes and fibrotic replacement are accompanied by hypertrophy of the remaining myocardiac cells. Myocyte

hypertrophy and fibrosis interplay in a ventricular remodeling process that may take years. Myocyte ultrastructural abnormalities include mitochondrial atrophy, edema, and severe contractile system lysis. Deposition of a glycoprotein-like substance may appear in the tubular T system, and in the basement membrane of cardiac myocytes and of the endothelium. A mononuclear and lymphocytic infiltrate predominates. The absence of parasites has stimulated the concept of an autoimmune myocarditis, by virtue of cross-reactivity with mammalian tissue antigens. *T. cruzi* epimastigote forms may share antigenic determinants with mammalian striated and cardiac muscle sarcoplasmic reticulum. Extensive vagal aganglionosis and intracardiac autonomic damage may induce autonomic dysfunction (slow heart rate response to exercise, postural hypotension). Alteration of the β-adrenergic receptor complex in acute and chronic Chagas' disease may occur. Extracellular matrix abnormalities (altered collagen) have been observed in chronic murine chagasic myocarditis and *in vitro T. cruzi*–infected endothelial cells. This could allow cardiac muscle fiber slippage, fiber realignment, and wall thinning, leading to ventricular remodeling. (*Adapted from* Weber and coworkers [53]; with permission.)

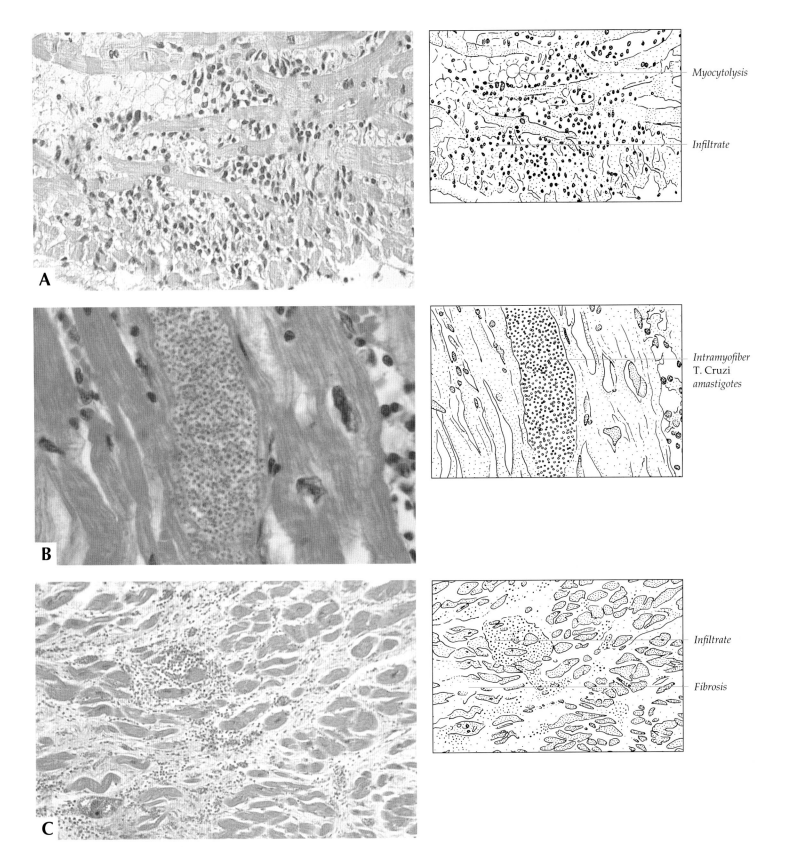

FIGURE 8-7. A, Endomyocardial biopsy section obtained from a patient with a 1-month clinical history of acute chagasic infection. Extensive myocardial fiber necrosis (myocytolisis) is accompanied by an inflammatory lymphocytic infiltrate. **B,** Autopsy section from a patient with chronic chagasic myocarditis shows an intramyofiber *Trypanosoma cruzi* amastigote nest. Parasites are rarely detected histologically in chronic cases. **C,** The chronic form may have diffuse or focal inflammatory infiltrates, predominantly of mononuclear cells (lymphocytes, monocytes, and plasma cells). Degeneration, fragmentation, and destruction of myocardial fibers are present along with interstitial fibrosis. (Courtesy of J.A. Suarez.)

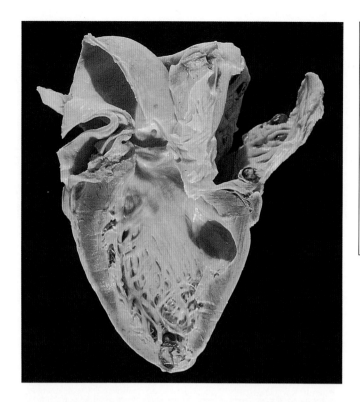

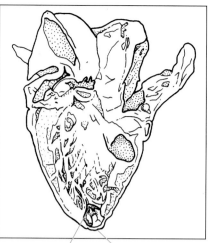

Thrombus   Apical aneurysm

FIGURE 8-8. The heart from a patient who died suddenly shows a narrow-neck typical chagasic left ventricular apical aneurysm that is partially thrombosed. Approximately half of all patients with chronic Chagas' disease have an apical lesion. Various pathophysiologic mechanisms have been suggested to explain its origin, such as a dysautonomic imbalance with increased sympathetic drive, increased wall stress on the apex, microvascular lesions, and herniation through the apical myocardial spiral bundles. Right ventricular apical aneurysms are found at autopsy in about 10% to 20% of patients.

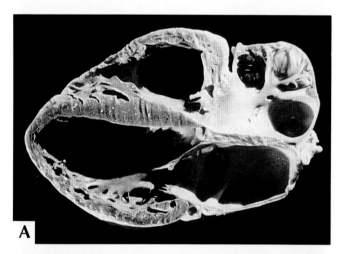

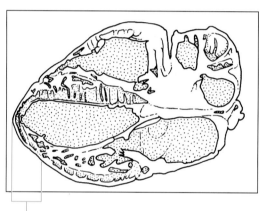

Apicoposterior scarring

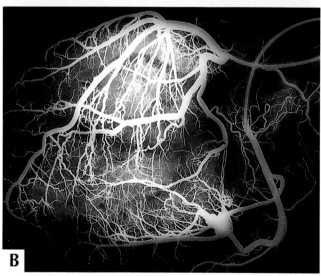

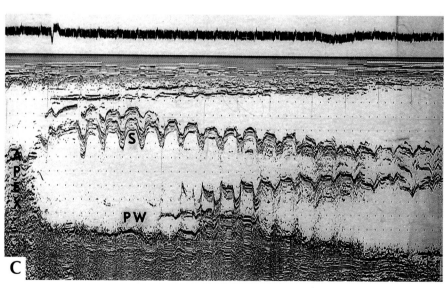

FIGURE 8-9. Fibrosis of the left ventricular apicoposterior wall from a patient dying in congestive heart failure. **A,** Left ventricular long-axis slice displays the apicoposterior scarring. Septal thickness is normal. **B,** Postmortem barium filling of the coronary arteries shows absence of obstruction. **C,** Slow-sweep M-mode echocardiogram scan of the long axis of the left ventricle shows preserved inward systolic thickening of the septum (S) in contrast to the noncontracting thin fibrotic posterior wall (PW). Approximately 20% of chagasic patients in heart failure may have free wall left or right ventricular localized areas of fibrosis. (*Parts A and C adapted from* Acquatella and coworkers [10]; with permission.)

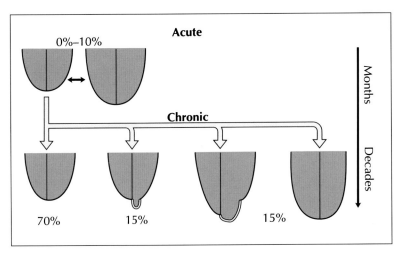

FIGURE 8-10. Scheme of the natural history of Chagas' heart disease represented by relative ventricular size. Primary infection occurs mostly unrecognized. Clinically apparent acute chagasic myocarditis may appear in up to 10% of persons (usually children) living in endemic areas. Chronic Chagas' disease takes years to develop into three clinical groups. A latent asymptomatic phase (indifferentiate form) develops in about 70% of seropositive persons. The rest become symptomatic with mild to moderate to severe heart damage. The main symptoms arise from arrhythmias, embolism, or heart failure. The yellow border represents the left ventricular apical aneurysm.

DIAGNOSIS OF ACUTE AND CHRONIC CHAGAS' DISEASE

	ACUTE	CHRONIC
Epidemiology		
Infection acquisition		
Natural	Endemic area	Endemic area
Through blood transfusion, pregnancy, or accident	Yes	Yes
Parasite		
Blood (Giemsa stain)	Possible	Extremely rare
Culture	Possible	Extremely rare
Xenodiagnosis	More than 50%	About 20%–30%
Polymerase chain reaction	Under investigation	Under investigation
Serology		
Immunoglobulins	IgM-IgG after 2–3 wk	IgG
Serology		Highly sensitive and specific in 97%, titers
Complement fixation		1:32 or more, false-positive found in
Immunofluorescence		leishmaniasis, schistosomiasis,
Hemagglutination		and immunologic disorders
Clinical findings		
Acute symptoms	Fever, malaise, nodes, generalized swelling, Romaña's sign (highly suspicious)	None
Heart size	Normal or enlarged	Normal or enlarged
Presentation	Acute myocarditis or chronic changing due to acute immune depression by AIDS, transplant, or cancer chemotherapy	Asymptomatic, arrhythmias, embolism, heart failure
Apical lesion	Possible	Aneurysm in about 50%
Electrocardiogram	Tachycardia, nonspecific ST-T changes	Right bundle branch block, left anterior hemiblock, ventricular extrasystoles, abnormal Q, AV block

FIGURE 8-11. The clinical diagnosis of Chagas' disease is based on the triad of positive epidemiology, positive serology, and a combination of clinical findings (eg, suggestive electrocardiographic abnormalities, apical aneurysm). Xenodiagnosis involves noninfested reduviid bugs that are fed with blood from presumed infected humans (or animals). After several weeks *Trypanosoma cruzi* may be demonstrated in the bugs. Polymerase chain reaction laboratory technique allows amplification of a specific DNA genome sequence of the parasite present in tissue or other material [11]. AIDS—acquired immunodeficiency syndrome.

ACUTE DISEASE

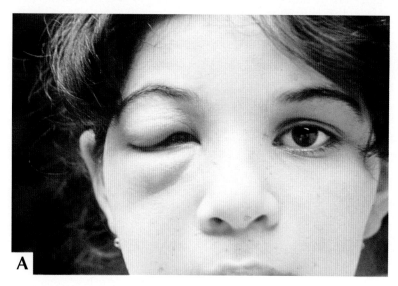

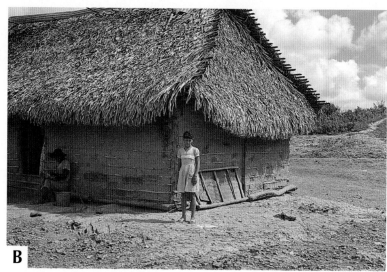

FIGURE 8-12. A, Romaña's sign is indicative of *Trypanosoma cruzi* conjunctival penetration seen during acute Chagas' disease. It consists of unilateral bipalpebral edema of abrupt onset, pink-violescent color, conjunctival congestion, and swelling of satellite nodes. It is a most useful clinical sign. Auto-inoculation by eye scratching with contaminated hands is possible. It has been reproduced experimentally in monkeys. **B,** Primitive housing, made of mud-plastered walls and a ceiling of dried palm tree leaves, is ideal for harboring reduviid insects. Infective bug droppings that fall from the ceiling may also contaminate the eye. Natural acute Chagas' infection almost always occurs in persons living in these ranchos or favelas. (Part A *adapted from* The Pan American Health Organization [2]; with permission.]

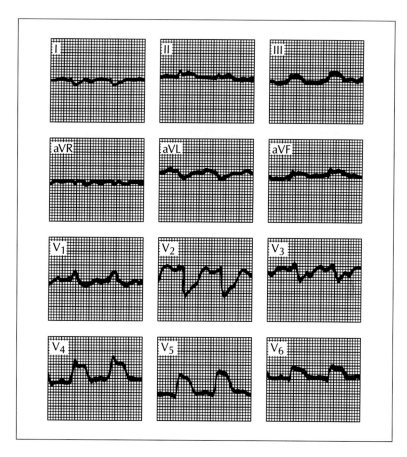

FIGURE 8-13. Electrocardiogram from a 25-year-old physician accidentally infected in the laboratory with *Trypanosoma cruzi* cultures who died after 5 weeks of heart failure from acute chagasic myocarditis. Right bundle branch block and monophasic extreme ST segment shift suggestive of a recent acute myocardial infarction are present. At autopsy, acute necrotizing panmyocarditis was more intense in the anterolateral and posterior walls of the left ventricle. Intramyocardial *T. cruzi* amastigote nests were seen. The majority of patients with acute disease do not present with this extremely aggressive form. (*Adapted from* Rosenbaum [12]; with permission.)

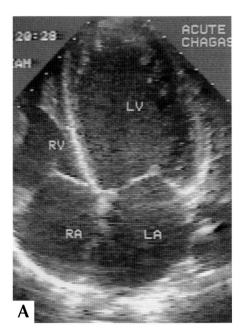 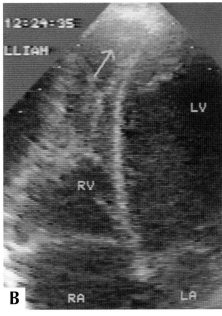

FIGURE 8-14. Two-dimensional echocardiographic four-chamber apical view from an 11-year-old boy with a 1-month history of acute chagasic myocarditis. **A,** The left ventricle (LV) was moderately dilated and diffusely hypokinetic, with intracavitary echoes. Moderate mitral regurgitation was present on Doppler studies. **B,** The right ventricular (RV) apex had a systolic bulge (*arrow*), suggesting that apical abnormalities may appear early in the disease. Both atria were dilated. The echocardiographic examination has also proved to be of great diagnostic help in chronic cases. LA—left atrium; RA—right atrium.

CHRONIC DISEASE

CLINICAL CLASSIFICATION AND FINDINGS IN CHRONIC CHAGAS' DISEASE			
	ASYMPTOMATIC	SYMPTOMATIC	
Group	A or I	B or I	C or III
Clinical history	Unremarkable, referral by positive serology	Palpitations, dizziness, syncope, fatigue, asthenia, shortness of breath, embolism	
NYHA classification	—	I–II	III–IV
Physical examination	Unremarkable	Regurgitant murmurs, S₃, venous and liver congestion, edema, pulmonary rales	
Electrocardiogram	N-A	N-A	A
Heart size (by radiography)	N	N/increased	Increased
Echocardiography and ventricular angiography			
Apical lesion	Akinesis/dyskinesis	Akinesis or aneurysm in approximately 50%	
Other focal scarring	No	Posterior wall in approximately 10%–20%	
Chamber size	N	N/increased	Increased
Ejection fraction	N	N/decreased	Decreased
Apical thrombus	Rare	10%–30%	
Diastolic function	N-A	Abnormal relaxation and filling	
Endomyocardial biopsy			
Light microscopy	N/chronic myocarditis	Chronic myocarditis, progression of changes, glycoprotein-like deposits, contractile system lysis	
Ultrastructure	N/T-tubules incipient dilatation, mitochondrial and nuclear changes		

FIGURE 8-15. Classification into three groups (A, B, C or I, II, III) is most useful because each group has a different clinical course (*see* Fig. 8-28). Epidemiologic surveys show that about three quarters of seropositive people are asymptomatic (indeterminate form). Approximately half of asymptomatic people have normal electrocardiograms, but cardiac damage may be demonstrated by other methods such as echocardiography, left ventriculography, or myocardial biopsy. The presence of other cardiac disorders (hypertension, ischemic heart disease) may pose clinical difficulties in ascertaining the contribution of Chagas' disease to the heart damage of a particular patient. A—abnormal; N—normal; NYHA—New York Heart Association.

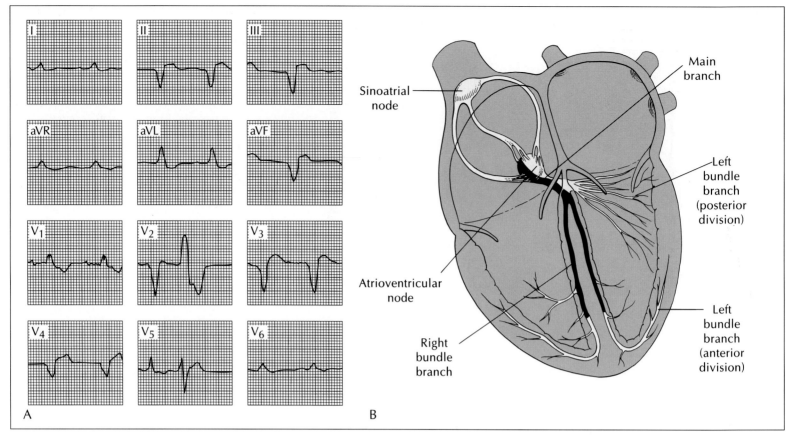

FIGURE 8-16. A, Electrocardiogram typical of chronic Chagas' disease shows right bundle branch block, left anterior hemiblock, poor precordial R-wave progression, ST segment elevation on precordial leads, and ventricular extrasystoles. **B,** Diagram of the conduction system. Autopsy of the same patient revealed scattered lymphocytes, mild diffuse and distal fibrosis of the inferior portion of the atrioventricular node, and selective involvement of the right portion of the His bundle, right bundle, and of the anterior portion of the left bundle were seen. A good correlation existed between the electrocardiographic and histopathologic findings (*Adapted from* Andrade and coworkers [13]; with permission.)

ELECTROCARDIOGRAPHIC FINDINGS IN ENDEMIC AREAS

ECG abnormality		ABNORMAL		RBBB		LAHB		VPC	
Serology		+	-	+	-	+	-	+	-
Study	**Persons studied, n**								
Diaz et al. [14]	280	32.7	3.4	13.5	0	—	—	15.4	1.1
Rosenbaum and Cerisola [15]	1354	27.7	10.9	9.7	0.9	—	—	7.3	2
Pifano et al. [16]	7000	22.9	6.1	7.1	2.2	—	—	4.2	0.6
Maguire et al. [17]	644	20.2	6	10.7	0.3	3.2	2.7	7.5	5.4
Baruffa et al. [18]	1332	30.2	9.9	4.7	0.1	8.9	1.8	5.7	0.6
Acquatella et al. [19]	1698	30.2	2.4	16.8	1.3	16.5	3.9	18.2	4.3
Estimated risk ratio		2.8	—	13	—	3.3	—	4	—

FIGURE 8-17. Electrocardiographic (ECG) surveys performed in Brazil, Argentina, and Venezuela before (1949 to 1985) and after (1987) the introduction of Chagas' control measures. The ECG combination of right bundle branch block (RBBB), left anterior hemiblock (LAHB), first- or second-degree atrioventricular block (not shown), and ventricular premature contraction (VPC) is highly suggestive of chagasic origin. ECG has become the epidemiologic method of choice for screening heart damage in rural areas because it is inexpensive, transportable, and easy to read. Comparison of the age-related rates of ECG abnormalities before and after Chagas' control programs were introduced did not differ significantly [19].

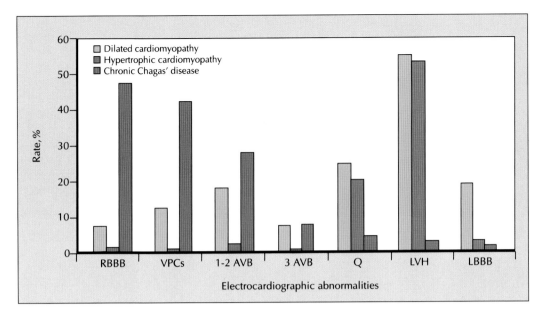

FIGURE 8-18. Differences in the rates of some electrocardiographic abnormalities found in patients with dilated cardiomyopathy, hypertrophic cardiomyopathy [20], and chronic Chagas' disease [21]. LBBB—left bundle branch block; LVH—left ventricular hypertrophy; Q—pathologic Q wave; RBBB—right bundle branch block; VPCs—ventricular premature contractions; 1-2 AVB—first and second degree atrioventricular block; 3 AVB—third degree atrioventricular block.

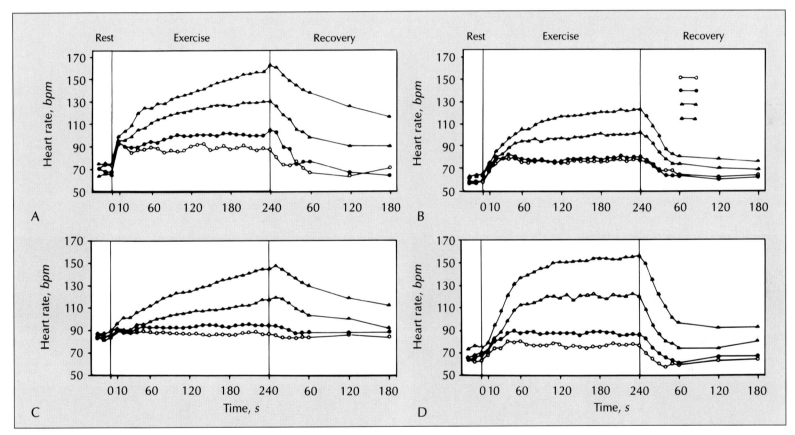

FIGURE 8-19. Changes in heart rate response during bicycle exercise. **A,** Normal control patient. **B,** Asymptomatic chagasic patient without cardiac disease. **C** and **D,** Chagasic patients with typical electrocardiograms but normal echocardiograms. Chagasic patients had a significantly abnormal lower heart rate increase in the first 10 seconds of cycle exercise at different workloads. Heart rate responses at 1 to 4 minutes of exercise were unaltered in all patients. The abnormal initial heart rate response was attributed to depression of parasympathetic efferent action on the sinus node, while the preserved late heart response indicated an unimpaired adrenergic sympathetic stimulation of the sinus node. Power spectral analysis of heart rate variability had also showed an abnormal response to the upright position [22]. Interestingly, experiments suggest that chagasic IgG binding may desensitize or down-regulate cardiac muscarinic cholinergic receptors [23]. It seems that abnormal parasympathetic function before the clinical appearance of significant myocardial dysfunction seems to be a unique aspect of the disease. (*Adapted from* Gallo and coworkers [24]; with permission.)

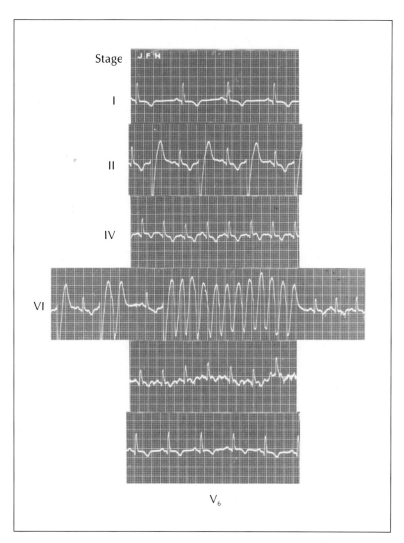

FIGURE 8-20. Electrocardiographic lead V_6 tracings obtained during a treadmill stress test (Naughton protocol) from a 37-year-old patient with chronic Chagas' disease. Upper strip shows T-wave inversion at rest. Ventricular bigeminy appears at stage II. The fourth strip, obtained at peak exercise, shows a couplet preceding a run of nonsustained rapid ventricular tachycardia, which prompted the interruption of the test. The fifth strip, taken immediately after exercise, shows an atrial flutter with a 4:1 conduction ratio. Normal sinus rhythm reappeared in the last strip. The patient hardly complained of symptoms. Contrary to coronary heart disease, Chagas' patients seldom develop ischemic ST-segment elevation or depression during electrocardiographic stress tests, which are useful for arrhythmia detection.

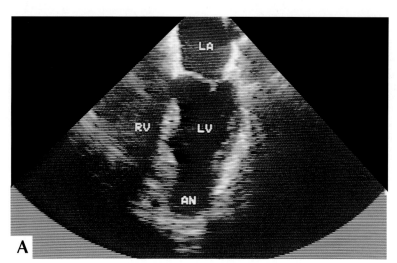

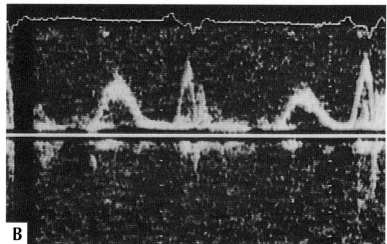

FIGURE 8-21. Two-dimensional echocardiography is helpful in characterizing ventricular function and morphology, especially of the apical lesions [10]. **A,** Transesophageal echocardiogram (transverse plane) of the long axis of the heart of a patient with a chagasic apical aneurysm (AN) of the left ventricle (LV) who had sustained multiple cerebral embolisms despite oral anticoagulation. Notice the relative shape preservation of the superior two thirds of the ventricle and the systolic bulging of the apex. No cavitary thrombus was found at the time of the examination. **B,** Pulsed Doppler examination at the tip of the mitral valve is useful in analyzing the left ventricular inflow filling characteristics. This tracing obtained from a young adult shows a lower peak velocity at early diastole than at late diastole, suggesting abnormal early filling (relaxation). The reverse occurs when left atrial pressure is increased in heart failure, whereas in early diastole peak velocity inflow is high and deceleration time is short. LA—left atrium; RV—right ventricle.

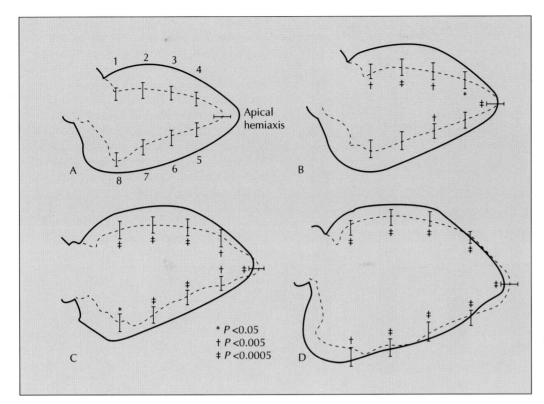

FIGURE 8-22. Cineventriculographic left ventricular outline analysis of segmental myocardial shortening of 126 chronic chagasic patients divided into groups of increasing damage. Continuous and interrupted lines denote end-diastolic and end-systolic frames, respectively. Enumeration corresponds to hemiaxes according to the Leighton method. **A,** and **B,** Asymptomatic subjects with normal electrocardiograms and chest radiographs; few had atypical chest pain. In *A*, all 30 had normal segmental shortening and volumes. In *B*, among 21 subjects, 95% had asynergy at the apex, combined or not, with significant hypokinesis of the anterior and inferomedial segments. **C** and **D,** Patients with and without heart failure, respectively. Extensive asynergy, ventricular dilatation, decreased distensibility, and depressed contractility of increased severity were found. Large apical aneurysms were found in 40%, with thrombosis in 20%. *T-bars* represent the mean percent segmented shortening ±1 SD. (*Adapted from* Carrasco and coworkers [25]; with permission.)

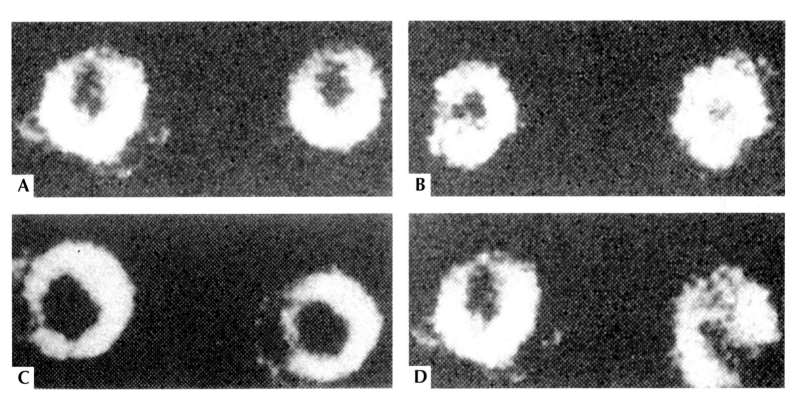

FIGURE 8-23. Examples of normal (**A**) thallium-201 effort-redistribution uptake and each type of perfusion defect found in a group of patients with Chagas' disease complaining of atypical chest pain. Reversible (**B**) and fixed (**C**) septal defects. A paradox defect (**D**) in the posterolateral region. The left and right frames represent scintigraphic left anterior oblique views for effort and redistribution, respectively, in all panels. (*Adapted from* Marin-Neto and coworkers [26]; with permission.)

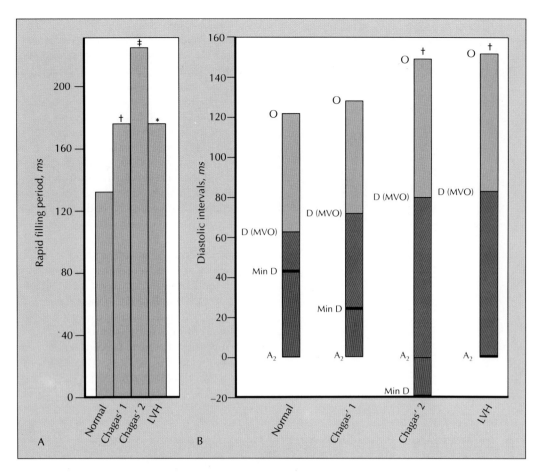

FIGURE 8-24. Abnormalities in early isovolumic relaxation assessed by left ventricular diastolic time intervals were shown by digitized simultaneous M-mode echocardiograms, phonocardiograms, and apexcardiograms in Chagas' 1 (asymptomatic) subjects, Chagas' 2 (with arrhythmias) subjects, and non-Chagas' subjects with left ventricular hypertrophy (LVH), and were compared with a normal control group. **A,** Significantly prolonged rapid filling time. **B,** Delayed closure of the aortic valve (A_2), delayed mitral valve opening (MVO), and prolonged isovolumic relaxation were observed by prolonged A_2-MVO and A_2-O-apexcardiographic O point intervals. An abnormal increase in dimensions before MVO may reflect an outward wall motion during relaxation. It appears that diastolic abnormalities may precede systolic dysfunction. Min D—M-mode electrocardiographic minimal left ventricular dimension. (*Adapted from* Combellas and coworkers [27]; with permission.)

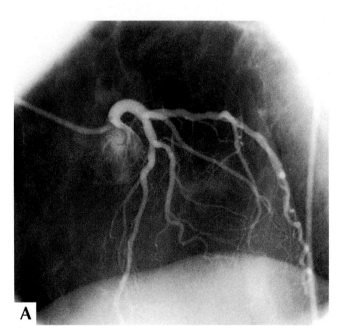

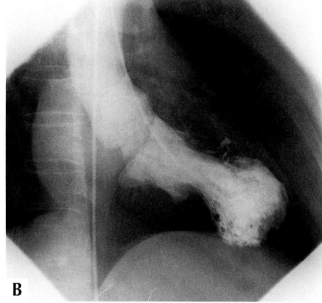

FIGURE 8-25. Chronic Chagas' disease simulating ischemic heart disease in a 55-year-old woman who complained of atypical chest pain. The electrocardiogram had QS in several precordial leads suggestive of anteroseptal myocardial infarction. **A,** Angiogram of a normal left anterior coronary artery. **B,** Right anterior view angiogram of the left ventricle shows a large apical aneurysm. This and similar patients may pose difficulties in the differential diagnosis [28]. Coronary vasospasm secondary to autonomic imbalance [26,29–31], coronary embolism with recanalization, and abnormalities in the coronary microcirculation have been suggested to explain these findings [30–32].

THERAPEUTIC MODALITIES

Parasiticide drugs	Nifurtimox (15 mg/kg for 120 d) Benznidazole (5 mg/kg for 60 d) High rate of secondary effects with both drugs [33] Indications: acute Chagas' disease, accidental contamination Uncertain benefit in chronic cases
Arrhythmias	Amiodarone: ventricular extrasystoles or tachycardia, efficacious in over 50% of treated patients [34,35] Mexiletine [36] Quinidine, disopyramide, and other class I antiarrhythmic drugs have induced a high incidence of *torsades de pointes* [34,36] Aneurysmectomy in selected cases [37] Chemical ablation in selected patients [38] Implantable defibrillator in evaluation
Complete atrioventricular block	Survival improvement in the absence of heart failure [39] Atrioventricular sequential pacing in heart failure
Heart failure	Traditional treatment: low salt, diuretics, digitalis ACE inhibitors seem to improve survival [40] Oral anticoagulants Cardiomyoplasty successful in initial small series [41] Heart transplant [42]
Dysautonomic symptoms	Gangliosides appear to ameliorate dysautonomic symptoms in selected patients [43]
Disease reactivation	Immunosuppression and transplantation may require use of benznidazole or nifurtimox in cancer chemotherapy [44], AIDS immune depression [45–47], and organ transplant chemotherapy [7,42]

FIGURE 8-26. Therapeutic modalities in Chagas' disease. Heart transplant for chronic Chagas' heart disease is associated with a high rate of *Trypanosoma cruzi* infection of the graft despite preoperative parasiticidal treatment. ACE—angiotensin-converting enzyme; AIDS—acquired immunodeficiency syndrome.

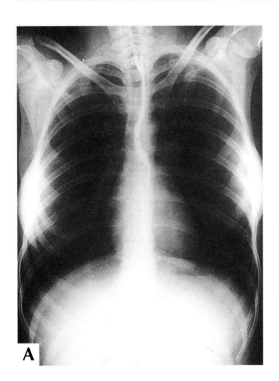

A

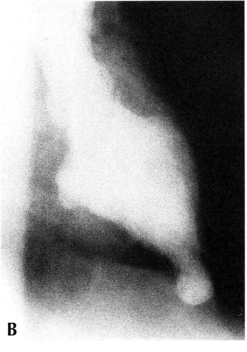

B

FIGURE 8-27. Seventeen-year follow-up of a woman who required various therapeutic procedures. **A,** Heart size was normal at age 25 when she initially consulted because of palpitations. This normal radiographic aspect is misleading because two-dimensional echocardiography showed an apical aneurysm. **B,** Angiography demonstrated a narrow-neck left ventricular apical aneurysm, normal basal and midventricular wall contractility, and normal ejection fraction. (*continued*)

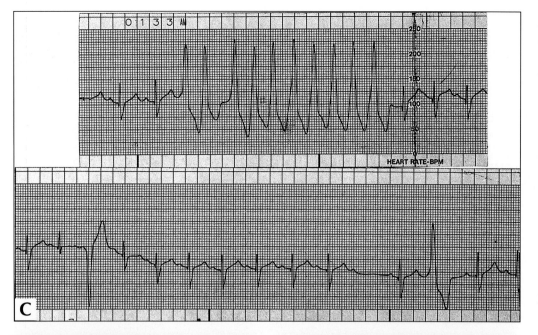

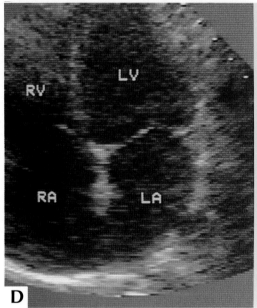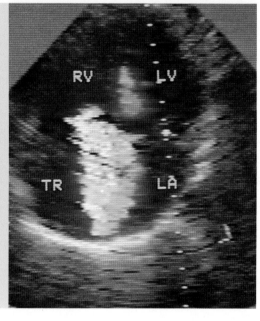

FIGURE 8-27. (*continued*) C, At age 27 she developed severely symptomatic runs of sustained and nonsustained ventricular tachycardia resistant to antiarrhythmic therapy. Results of an electrophysiologic study led to an aneurysmectomy with subsequent disappearance of the malignant arrhythmias. Two years later the patient needed a pacemaker because of multiple syncopal attacks secondary to intermittent atrioventricular block. D, At age 37, two-dimensional echocardiography disclosed an increase in ventricular size, moderately depressed ejection fraction, greatly enlarged atria (*left panel*), and severe tricuspid regurgitation on color Doppler (*right panel*). Notice the postaneurysmectomy rounded apex. E, At age 42 the patient had drug-resistant incessant atrial tachyarrhythmias with intermittent rapid ventricular response and congestive heart failure. His bundle electrogram obtained after radiofrequency ablation of the conduction system below the atrioventricular node shows a decrease in the ventricular response. CS—coronary sinus; HRA—high right atria; LA—left atrium; LV—left ventricle; PVB—premature ventricular beat; RA—right atrium; RV—right ventricle; RVA—RV apex; S—pacemaker spikes; TR—tricuspid regurgitation. (Part B *adapted from* Acquatella and coworkers [10]; with permission; part D courtesy of Victor Medina.)

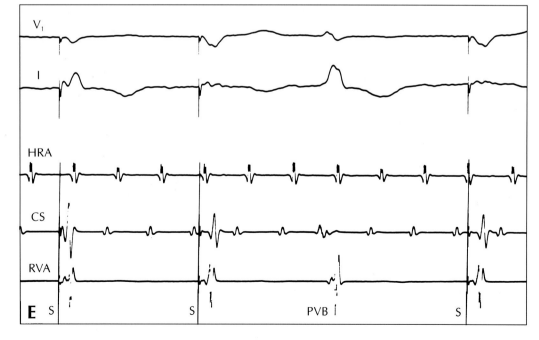

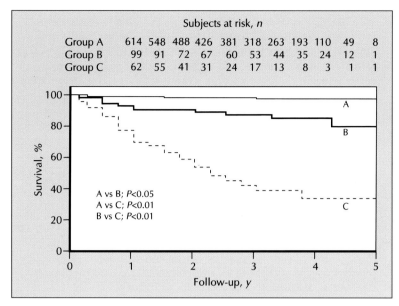

FIGURE 8-28. Survival of 775 Chagas' seropositive subjects according to clinical group classification. A denotes asymptomatic, B, moderately symptomatic, and C, severely symptomatic patients, respectively. Survival rates among the three groups were significantly different at 3 and 5 years ($P<0.01$). The 95% confidence limits at 5-year follow-up were 97% to 98.7% for group A, 72.3% to 86.2% for group B, and 14.2% to 48.8% for group C. Mortality predictors (Cox regression model) in a series of chagasic patients with abnormal electrocardiograms [48] included systolic blood pressure of less than 120 mm Hg, atrial fibrillation, cardiothoracic index greater than 55%, and an angiographic left ventricular end-diastolic volume of greater than 110 mL/m^2 ($P=0.0228$). (*Adapted from* Acquatella and coworkers [19]; with permission.)

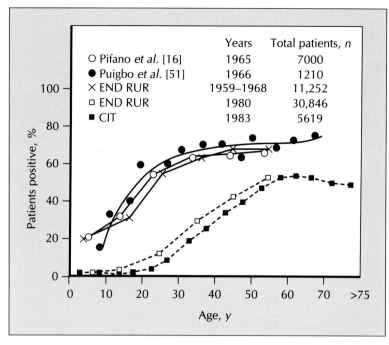

FIGURE 8-29. Decrease in the percentage of Chagas' seropositivity before and after a control program carried out in endemic communities of Venezuela between 1959 and 1983. Results of serologic surveys performed at the beginning (upper three series) and after 20 years (lower two series) show a decrease in the proportion of seropositive subjects at each age cohort, especially in subjects born during the program. Prophylactic control programs rely on housing improvement, elimination of domestic triatomid bugs, and community education [19,49–51]. CIT—Centro Investigaciones Torrealba (unpublished serology survey); END RUR—Endemias rurales (unpublished serology surveys).

REFERENCES

1. Brener Z: O parasito: relacoes hospedeiro-parasito. In *Trypanosoma cruzi e Doenca de Chagas*. Edited by Brener Z, Andrade A: Rio de Janeiro (Brazil): Editora Guanabara Koogan S.A.; 1979: 1–41.

2. Pan American Health Organization: La Historia Natural, la Epidemiologia y el Control de la Enfermedad de Chagas (curso de niveles multiples) [slides series 92]. Washington, DC: Pan American Health Organization.

3. Schenkman S, Robbins ES, Nussenzweig Y: Attachment of *Trypanosoma cruzi* to mammalian cells requires parasite energy, and invasion can be independent of the target cell cytoskeleton. *Infect Immun* 1991; 59:645–654.

4. Sherlock IA: Vetores. In *Trypanosoma cruzi e Doenca de Chagas*. Edited by Brener Z, Andrade Z. Rio de Janeiro: Editora Guanabara Kogan SA; 1979:42–88.

5. Status of Chagas' disease in the region of the Americas. *Epidemiol Bull PAHO* 1984, 5:5–9.

6. Moncayo A: Chagas' disease: epidemiology and prospects for interruption of transmission in the Americas. *World Health Stat Q* 1992, 45:276–279.

7. Kirchhoff LV: American trypanosomiasis (Chagas' disease): a tropical disease now in the United States. *N Engl J Med* 1993, 329:639–644.

8. Milei J, Mautner B, Storino R, *et al.*: Does Chagas' disease exist as an undiagnosed form of cardiomyopathy in the United States? *Am Heart J* 1992, 123:1732–1735.

9. Acquatella H, Piras R: Chagas' disease. *Curr Opin Cardiol* 1993, 8:463–472.

10. Acquatella H, Schiller NB, Puigbo JJ, *et al.*: M-mode and two-dimensional echocardiography in chronic Chagas' heart disease. *Circulation* 1980, 62:787–799.

11. Jones EM, Colley DG, Tostes S, *et al.*: Amplification of a *Trypanosoma cruzi* DNA sequence from inflammatory lesions in human chagasic cardiomyopathy. *Am J Trop Med Hyg* 1993, 48:348–357.

12. Rosenbaum MB: Chagasic myocardiopathy. *Prog Cardiovasc Dis* 1964, 7:199–225.

13. Andrade ZA, Andrade SG, Oliveira GB, Alonso DR: Histopathology of the conducting tissue of the heart in Chagas' myocarditis. *Am Heart J* 1978, 93:316–324.

14. Diaz E, Laranja FS, Pellegrino J: Primera reunion Panamericana sobre enfermedad de Chagas, Tucuman (Argentina). Tucuman; 1949:I:33–34.

15. Rosenbaum MB, Cerisola JA: Epidemiologia de la enfermedad de Chagas en la Republica Argentina. *O Hospital* 1961, 60:55–99.

16. Pifano F, Anselmi A, Makekelt GA, *et al.*: Estudios sobre la miocardiopatia chagasica en el medio rural venezolano. *Arch Ven Med Trop Parasitol Med* 1965, 5:3–67.

17. Maguire JH, Mott KE, Lehman JS, *et al.*: Relationship of electrocardiographic abnormalities and seropositivity to *Trypanosoma cruzi* within a rural community in Northeast Brazil. *Am Heart J* 1983, 105:287–294.

18. Baruffa G, Alcantara-Filho A, de Aquino-Neto JO: Estudo pareado da cardiopatia chagasica no Rio Grande do Sul, Brasil. *Mem Inst Oswaldo Cruz* 1985, 80:457–463.

19. Acquatella H, Catalioti F, Gomez-Mancebo JR, *et al.*: Long-term control of Chagas' disease in Venezuela: effects on serologic findings, electrocardiographic abnormalities, and clinical outcome. *Circulation* 1987, 76:556–562.

20. Flowers NC, Horan LG: Electrocardiographic and vectorcardiographic features of myocardial diseases. In *Myocardial Diseases*. Edited by Fowler NO. New York: Grune & Stratton; 1973:181–211.

21. Laranja FS, Dias E, Nobrega G, *et al.*: Chagas' disease: a clinical, epidemiologic, and pathologic study. *Circulation* 1956, 14:1035–1060.

22. Guzzetti S, Iosa D, Pecis M, *et al.*: Impaired heart rate variability in patients with chronic Chagas' disease. *Am Heart J* 1991, 121:1727–1734.

23. Sterin-Borda L, Gorelik G, Borda ES: Chagasic IgG binding with cardiac muscarinic cholinergic receptors modifies cholinergic-mediated cellular transmembrane signals. *Clin Immunol Immunopathol* 1991, 61:387–397.

24. Gallo Jr L, Morel-Filho J, Maciel BC, *et al.*: Functional evaluation of sympathetic and parasympathetic system in Chagas' disease using dynamic exercise. *Cardiovasc Res* 1987, 21:922–927.

25. Carrasco HA, Barboza JS, Inglessis G, *et al.*: Left ventricular cineangiography in Chagas' disease: detection of early myocardial damage. *Am Heart J* 1982, 104:595–602.

26. Marin-Neto JA, Marzullo P, Marcassa C, *et al.*: Myocardial perfusion abnormalities in chronic Chagas' disease as detected by thallium-201 scintigraphy. *Am J Cardiol* 1992, 69:780–784.

27. Combellas I, Puigbo JJ, Acquatella H, *et al.*: Echocardiographic features of impaired left ventricular diastolic function in Chagas' heart disease. *Br Heart J* 1985, 53:298–309.

28. Hagar JM, Rahimtoola SH: Chagas' heart disease in the United States. *N Engl J Med* 1991, 325:763–768.

29. Oliveira JSM, dos Santos M, Mucillo G, *et al.*: Increased capacity of the coronary arteries in chronic Chagas' disease: further support for the neurogenic pathogenesis concept. *Am Heart J* 1985, 109:304–308.

30. Bestetti RB, Ariolli MT, do Carmo JL, *et al.*: Clinical characteristics of acute myocardial infarction in patients with Chagas' disease. *Int J Cardiol* 1992, 35:371–376.

31. Morris SA, Tanowitz HB, Wittner M, *et al.*: Pathophysiological insights into the cardiomyopathy of Chagas' disease. *Circulation* 1990, 82:1900–1909.

32. Torres FW, Acquatella H, Condado J, *et al.*: Endothelium dependent coronary vasomotion is abnormal in patients with Chagas' heart disease [abstract]. *J Am Coll Cardiol* 1993, 21(suppl A):197A.

33. Ferreira H de O: Treatment of the undetermined form of Chagas' disease with nifurtimox and benzonidazole. *Rev Soc Bras Med Trop* 1990, 23:209–211.

34. Chiale PA, Halpern S, Nau GJ, *et al.*: Efficacy of amiodarone during long-term treatment of malignant ventricular arrhythmias in patients with chronic chagasic myocarditis. *Am Heart J* 1984, 107:656–665.

35. Giniger AG, Retyk EO, Laino RA, *et al.*: Ventricular tachycardia in Chagas' disease. *Am J Cardiol* 1992, 70:459–462.

36. Mendoza I, Camardo J, Moleiro F, *et al.*: Sustained ventricular tachycardia in chronic chagasic myocarditis: electrophysiologic and pharmacologic characteristics. *Am J Cardiol* 1986, 57:423–427.

37. Milei J, Pesce R, Valero E, *et al.*: Electrophysiological-structural correlations in chagasic aneurysms causing malignant arrhythmias. *Int J Cardiol* 1991, 32:65–73.

38. dePaola AAV, Gomes JA, Miyamoto MH, *et al.*: Transcoronary chemical ablation of ventricular tachycardia in chronic chagasic myocarditis. *J Am Coll Cardiol* 1992, 20:480–482.

39. Chuster M: Implante de marcapasso nas bradiarritmias chagásicas. In *Cardiopatia Chagásica*. Edited by Cancado JR, Chuster M. Imprensa oficial do estado de minas gerais: Belo Horizonte: Fundaçao Carlos Chagas, Brazil; 1985:289–297.

40. Roberti RR, Martinez EE, Andrade JL, *et al.*: Chagas cardiomyopathy and captopril. *Eur Heart J* 1992, 13:966–970.

41. Bocchi EA, Mareira LF, Bellatti G, *et al.*: Hemodynamic study during upright isotonic exercise before and six months after dynamic cardiomyoplasty for idiopathic dilated cardiomyopathy or Chagas' disease. *Am J Cardiol* 1991, 67:213–214.

42. Bocchi EA, Bellotti G, Uip D, *et al.*: Long-term follow-up after heart transplantation in Chagas' disease. *Transplant Proc* 1993, 25:1329–1330.

43. Iosa D, Massari DC, Dorsey FC: Chagas' cardioneuropathy: effect of ganglioside treatment in chronic dysautonomic patients: a randomized, double blind, parallel, placebo-controlled study. *Am Heart J* 1991, 122:775–785.

44. Villalba R, Fornées G, Alvarez MA, *et al.*: Acute Chagas' disease in a recipient of a bone marrow transplant in Spain: case report. *Clin Infect Dis* 1992, 14:594–595.

45. Rosemberg S, Chaves CJ, Higuchi ML, *et al.*: Fatal meningoencephalitis caused by reactivation of *Trypanosoma cruzi* infection in a patient with AIDS. *Neurology* 1992, 42:640–642.

46. Gluckstein D, Ciferri F, Ruskin J: Chagas' disease: another cause of cerebral mass in the acquired immunodeficiency syndrome. *Am J Med* 1992, 92:429–432.

47. Oddo D, Casanova M, Acuna G, *et al.*: Acute Chagas' disease (Trypanosomiasis americana) in acquired immunodeficiency syndrome: report of two cases. *Hum Pathol* 1992, 23:41–44.

48. Espinosa RA, Pericchi LR, Carrasco HA, *et al.*: Prognostic indicators of chronic chagasic cardiopathy. *Int J Cardiol* 1991, 30:195–202.

49. Mota EA, Guimaraes AC, Santana OO, *et al.*: A nine year prospective study of Chagas' disease in a defined rural population in northeast Brazil. *Am J Trop Med Hyg* 1990, 42:429–440.

50. Chuit R, Paulone I, Wisnivesky-Colli C, *et al.*: Result of a first step toward community-based surveillance of transmission of Chagas' disease with appropriate technology in rural areas. *Am J Trop Med Hyg* 1992, 46:444–450.

51. Control of Chagas' disease: report of a WHO expert committee. *World Health Organ Tech Rep Ser* 1991, 811:1–95.

52. Puigbo JJ, Nava-Rhode JR, Garcia-Barrios H, *et al.*: Clinical and epidemiologic study of chronic heart involvement in Chagas' disease. *Bull WHO* 1966, 34: 655.

53. Weber KT, Brilla CG, Janicki JS: Myocardial remodeling and pathologic hypertrophy. *Hosp Pract* 1991, 26: 73–80.

MYOCARDITIS

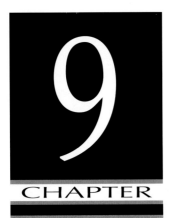

9

CHAPTER

Ahvie Herskowitz and Aftab A. Ansari

When the term *myocarditis* is used today it refers to a spectrum of nonischemic inflammatory diseases of the myocardium. A standardized histologic terminology for the morphologic classification of myocarditis has been accepted, and nucleic acid hybridization molecular techniques have affirmed that cardiotropic viruses play a role in the pathogenesis of a subgroup of patients with myocarditis and cardiomyopathy. Nevertheless, myocarditis is one of the daunting challenges in the field of cardiology today. Diagnosis of the disorder is problematic because of the lack of a distinct clinical syndrome, the lack of a universally accepted noninvasive method of diagnosis, and the focal histologic abnormalities characteristic of the disease with the inherent difficulty in the interpretation of endomyocardial biopsy findings. These barriers have prevented an accurate assessment of the true incidence and prevalence of myocarditis and have therefore blunted the analysis of its potential significance to public health.

Clinical-histologic correlations have been difficult to define in myocarditis, and no clear relationships between the extent of microscopic evidence of myocardial damage and the level of contractile dysfunction have been found. These observations have led many investigators to suspect that other immunopathogenic mechanisms may be involved. The clinical and pathologic consequences of the presence of viral genes or gene products within the myocardium in myocarditis continue to be debated intensely. Studies of the molecular basis by which putative viruses or viral sequences remain intracellular for prolonged periods of time, possibly altering the metabolic pathways of host myocytes, are in progress. The precise delineation of the role of the host immune–effector system directed at viral or cardiac peptides in the context of induced self-histocompatibility molecules expressed by myocardial cells, including monocytes, is also currently under investigation.

Increasing quantities of virologic and immunologic data suggest that subgroups of patients with myocarditis and idiopathic dilated cardiomyopathy are part of a spectrum of immune-mediated cardiac disease; therefore, a deeper understanding of the mechanisms of cardiac injury in myocarditis is fundamental for both the diagnosis of myocarditis and the development of future novel therapies. The purpose of this chapter is to review the diagnosis, causes, and immunopathogenesis of human myocarditis while weighing the evidence for and against the concept that myocarditis is an immunopathologic consequence of an initiating viral infection.

DEFINITION AND PATHOLOGY

HISTOPATHOLOGY AND IMMUNOHISTOLOGY

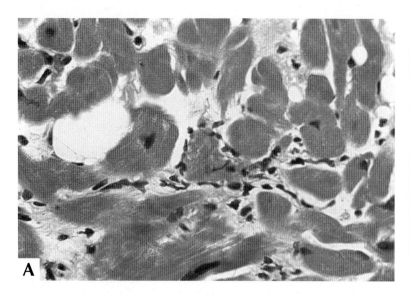

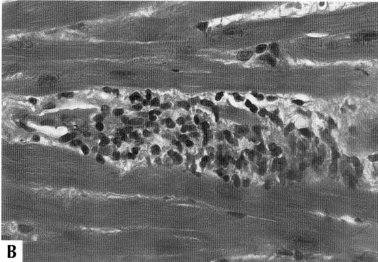

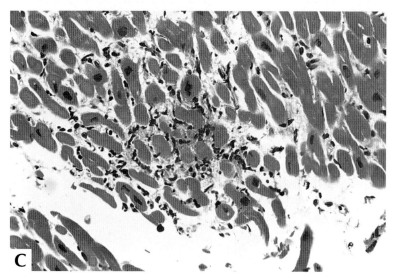

FIGURE 9-1. Histopathologic features of endomyocardial biopsy samples from patients with myocarditis (*see also* Chapter 12.) **A,** High-power photomicrograph of an endomyocardial biopsy sample stained with hematoxylin and eosin, highlighting one isolated necrotic myocyte surrounded by a mixed inflammatory infiltrate. **B,** A small cluster of longitudinally oriented myocytes engulfed in a dense inflammatory infiltrate composed primarily of mononuclear cells. Typically, outside the focus of active myocarditis, the adjacent myocardium appears relatively preserved. **C,** Cross-section of a cluster of myocytes undergoing necrosis. Interstitial inflammatory cells surround the myocytes, which no longer have crisp cellular outlines. The interstitial space between affected myocytes contains granular basophilic material that contains fibrin and fibrinogen, a likely consequence of microvascular injury. The inflammatory cells extend from the central core of necrotic myocytes into the adjacent myocardium. In 1986 and 1987 Aretz *et al.* [1,2], in an attempt to establish a uniform histologic classification for the diagnosis of myocarditis on endomyocardial biopsy, published a classification proposed by eight cardiac pathologists (the Dallas panel). Two separate classifications were described, one for the first biopsy and one for subsequent biopsies. On the first biopsy, *active myocarditis* was defined as a process characterized by an inflammatory infiltrate of the myocardium with necrosis or degeneration of adjacent myocytes not typical of the ischemic damage associated with coronary artery disease. The diagnosis of active myocarditis therefore requires the presence of myocardial inflammation as well as adjacent myocyte damage.

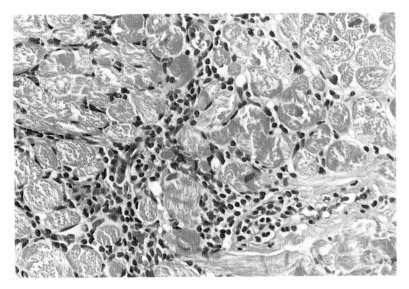

FIGURE 9-2. Some features of subtle *myocyte degenerative changes* that reflect irreversible myocyte damage. In addition to frank myocyte necrosis (*see also* Fig. 9-1), this figure demonstrates a focus of interstitial inflammatory cells surrounding individual myocytes and small myocyte clusters. Myocytes with inflammatory cells immediately adjacent to their plasma membrane contain membrane vacuoles and irregular surface outlines. These morphologic changes are similar to those noted in experimental postviral murine myocarditis during the early phases of myocyte injury.

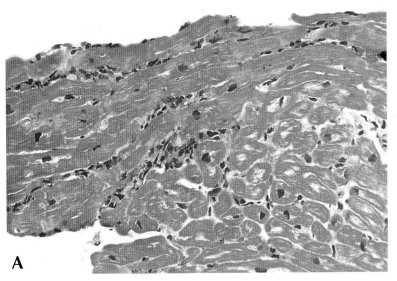

A

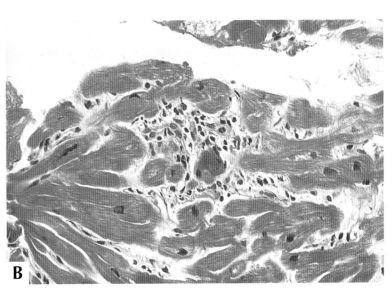

B

FIGURE 9-3. **A** and **B,** The morphologic features of *borderline myocarditis*. Borderline myocarditis is diagnosed when an unequivocal diagnosis of myocarditis cannot be made either because the inflammatory infiltrate it too sparse or because the damage to myocytes is not clearly demonstrated. Because the hearts of patients with advanced idiopathic dilated cardio-

myopathy frequently contain scattered collections of interstitial infiltrates not associated with myocyte necrosis, care must be used not to misdiagnose borderline myocarditis in cases where cardio-myopathic changes, such as extensive interstitial fibrosis and myocyte hypertrophy, are found.

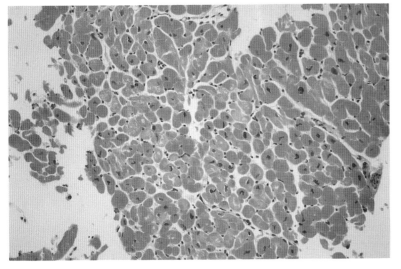

FIGURE 9-4. The histopathologic features of *no myocarditis*, which is diagnosed when the myocardium is either entirely normal or shows nonspecific changes, such as mild myocyte hypertrophy and mild interstitial fibrosis. When an endomyocardial biopsy shows no evidence of inflammation but does show more advanced features of idiopathic dilated cardiomyopathy, such as extensive interstitial fibrosis and myocyte hypertrophy, the diagnosis of "findings consistent with dilated cardiomyopathy" is commonly made. The terminology used for subsequent biopsies is *ongoing, resolving,* and *resolved* myocarditis and is reserved only for patients with previous biopsies. *Ongoing* or *persistent myocarditis* describes persistent myocardial inflammation associated with myocyte damage. Myocarditis that is resolving or healing can be morphologically identical to borderline myocarditis, although reparative interstitial fibrosis may accompany the interstitial infiltrates. Resolved or healed myocarditis is diagnosed when no remnants of an inflammatory infiltrate are found.

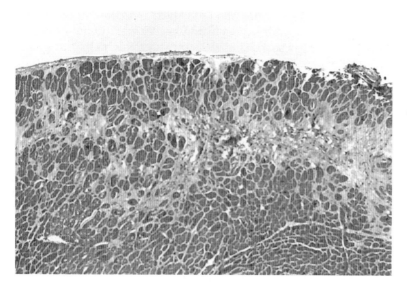

FIGURE 9-5. One of the typical histologic patterns of injury seen in endomyocardial biopsies from patients with occult ischemic heart disease. The zones of myocytolysis and replacement fibrosis are located entirely within the subendocardium. It is important to note that the definition of myocarditis specifically mentions the presence of myocyte necrosis *not typical of the ischemic damage associated with coronary artery disease.*

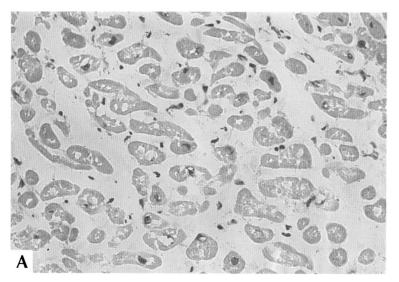

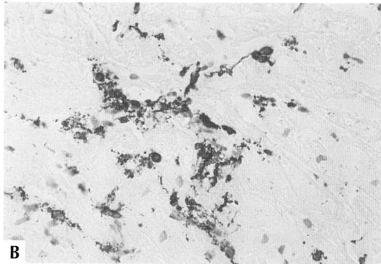

FIGURE 9-6. A, Immunoperoxidase staining with a monoclonal antibody to the common leukocyte antigen (CLA) in a paraffin-embedded endomyocardial biopsy sample that showed no myocarditis on histology. Note the lack of staining of any of the interstitial cells. **B,** A similar immunoperoxidase stain for CLA in a biopsy sample from a patient with borderline myocarditis. In contrast to *A,* a dense, focal collection of interstitial cells stain positively for the presence of CLA, identifying them clearly as leukocytes. While the Dallas criteria provide a standard, reliable histologic terminology, many centers are currently also using immunohistochemical techniques to specifically identify inflammatory cells. This strategy has gained prominence partially because of the difficulty in distinguishing myocardial lymphocytes from interstitial endothelial cells, fibroblasts, pericytes, and mast cells [3]. Standardized criteria for the immunohistologic diagnosis of myocarditis, however, have not yet been defined.

A. ETIOLOGIES OF HUMAN MYOCARDITIS: INFECTIOUS

Viral
  Coxsackievirus (A and B)
  Echovirus
  Influenza
  Cytomegalovirus
  Hepatitis
  Mumps
  Herpes simplex
  Rabies
  EBV
  HIV
Rickettsial
  Q fever
  Rocky mountain spotted fever
  Scrub typhus
Fungal
  Cryptococcus
  Candidiasis
  Histoplasmosis
  Aspergillus

Protozoal and metazoal
  Trypanosomiasis
  Toxoplasmosis
  Malaria
  Schistosomiasis
  Trichinosis
Bacterial
  Diphtheria
  Tuberculosis
  Legionella
  Brucella
  Clostridium
  Salmonella/shigella
  Meningococcus
  Yersinia
Spirochetal
  Borrelia (Lyme)

B. ETIOLOGIES OF HUMAN MYOCARDITIS: NONINFECTIOUS

Cardiotoxic drugs
  Catecholamines
  Doxorubicin
  ? Nucleoside analogues
  ? Cocaine
Systemic illness
  SLE
  Other collagen vascular
    diseases
  Sarcoidosis
  Kawasaki disease

Hypersensitivity drug reactions
  Antibiotics
    Amphotericin B
    Ampicillin
    Chloramphenicol
    Penicillin
    Tetracycline
    Streptomycin
    Sulfisoxazole
  Diuretics
    Chlorthalidone
    Acetazolamide
    Hydrochlorothiazide
    Spironolactone
  Others
    Isoniazid
    Lithium
    Methyldopa
    Tetanus toxoid
    Indomethacin

FIGURE 9-7. Infectious (**A**) and noninfectious (**B**) causes of myocarditis. Strictly speaking, the Dallas criteria are confined to cases of idiopathic myocarditis rather than cases secondary to specific infectious or noninfectious causes. The presence of cardiotropic viruses is rarely confirmed, however, and the clinical significance of such viruses is still debated. Thus, most cases of myocarditis are clinically idiopathic and likely represent the largest subgroup of cases of human myocarditis. EBV—Epstein-Barr virus; HIV—human immunodeficiency virus; SLE—systemic lupus erythematosus.

EPIDEMIOLOGIC CONSIDERATIONS

Male predisposition
Virus isolation in myocardium is rare
Fulminant presentations more common in young infants and neonates
Subacute presentations more common in adolescents and adults
Duration from initial infection to cardiac symptoms in adults may be years
5% incidence of "carditis" during viral epidemics
1%–4% incidence in autopsy series
15%–20% incidence in young subjects with sudden death

FIGURE 9-8. Epidemiologic characteristics of human myocarditis. While the true prevalence and incidence of viral myocarditis in the general population is unknown, evidence indicates that approximately 5% of a virus-infected population may experience some form of cardiac involvement associated with the acute illness. Studies of cardiac tissues from two series of unselected autopsies involving 40,000 [4] and 12,474 [5] patients showed a prevalence of myocarditis of 3.5% and 1.1%, respectively (the latter using the currently accepted Dallas criteria). In victims of unexpected sudden death and children who died violent deaths, the overall prevalence of myocarditis is also less than 5%. In cases of sudden death not associated with accidents or violence, however, the prevalence is higher, ranging from 17% to 21% [6,7]. There is also evidence that, during epidemics of coxsackievirus B, poliomyelitis, and influenza, approximately 5% to 10% [6] of affected individuals experience cardiac symptoms. Unlike adults, lethal myocarditis may occur in up to 50% of infants infected with coxsackievirus B. Coxsackievirus B, poliomyelitis, and influenza are known to produce a high prevalence of myocarditis in infected babies in the first year of life, particularly during the neonatal period. These cases of myocarditis are characterized by a fulminant course with short incubation times (frequently less than 1 week). Myocarditis becomes less common in early childhood but increases again in adolescence and adulthood. In contrast to the often fatal disease that occurs in the neonatal period, viral myocarditis in adolescents and adults usually has a delayed onset (1 to 4 weeks) and is rarely fatal.

ENTEROVIRAL INFECTIONS WITH DIAGNOSES OF CARDIOVASCULAR AND MUSCLE-JOINT DISEASES

	INFECTIONS REPORTED		CLINICAL DIAGNOSIS	
VIRUS GROUP	PATIENTS REPORTED, *n*		CARDIOVASCULAR, *n*(%)	MUSCLE-JOINT, *n*(%)
Coxsackievirus A	5781		57(0.98)	35(0.61)
Coxsackievirus B	14,934		596(3.99)	302(2.02)
Echovirus, all types	38,191		266(0.7)	223(0.58)
Enterovirus 68–71	217		0(0)	0(0)
Poliovirus 1–3	43		1(2.33)	0(0)

FIGURE 9-9. The reports of enterovirus infections made to the World Health Organization from 1975 to 1983 in relation to diagnoses of both cardiovascular and muscle joint disease. The increased prevalence of cardiovascular symptoms associated with coxsackievirus B as compared with coxsackievirus A and other enteroviruses during this period are demonstrated. The RNA viruses appear to predominate, with picornaviruses being the most commonly identified agents. Coxsackieviruses are members of the *Enterovirus* genus within the picornavirus family and are most prevalent in warm climates and in the warm season of temperate countries. Reinfection can occur, and the types of enteroviruses prevalent in any particular community as well as the cardiotropic nature of enteroviral stains are likely to vary from year to year. The association of a particular viral infection and heart disease has most often been based either on serologic studies or on the isolation or identification of the virus in tissues or fluids outside the heart. The rarity of a positive-virus isolation from myocarditis tissue probably reflects the very brief period (probably less than 1 to 2 weeks in duration) of myocardial virus replication. The identification of virus gene expression using nucleic acid hybridization techniques from the hearts of infected patients, however, probably represents nonreplicating virus (nonpermissive or latent infection). Although the initial cytopathic event in most cases of idiopathic myocarditis appears to be viral infection and replication within monocytes, the development of chronic cardiac dysfunction is probably not attributable directly to the virus. (*Adapted from* Grist [8]; with permission.)

PATHOGENESIS AND PATHOPHYSIOLOGY

ANIMAL STUDIES OF ACUTE POSTVIRAL MYOCARDITIS

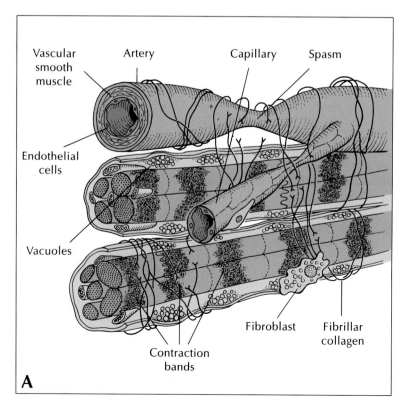

A

FIGURE 9-10. A, The early myocardial changes seen during the acute phase of experimental postviral myocarditis. These changes are complex and as yet poorly understood. The earliest light microscopic changes within the myocardium after cardiotropic viral infection are contraction band necrosis of small clusters of myocytes as well as myocyte vacuolization, both of which appear before any significant inflammatory cell response [9,10]. These abnormalities therefore likely represent either a direct cytopathic effect of myocyte viral infection or possibly concurrent viral infection of other myocardial cells, such as those that make up the microvasculature. Islands of injured myocytes appear to lose their distinct cell contours and myofilament architecture and contain characteristic eosinophilic bands or contraction bands and vacuoles. It is interesting to note that contraction band necrosis is also characteristically seen in reperfusion injury and catecholamine-induced injury. Such necrosis reflects calcium overload of myocardial cells. (*continued*)

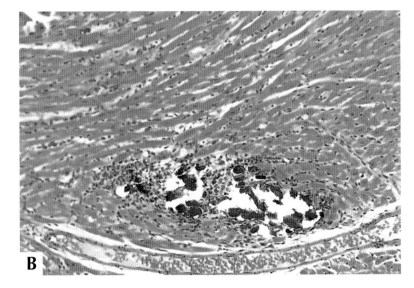

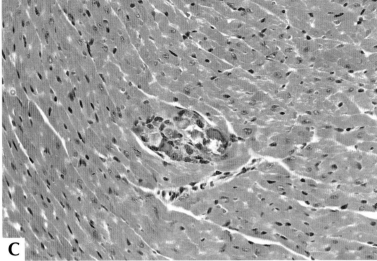

B

C

FIGURE 9-10. (*continued*) Some investigators have hypothesized that microvascular spasm with reperfusion plays a role in early post-coxsackievirus B3 (CVB3) myocardial injury [11] induced either by direct viral infection of arteriolar endothelium or smooth muscle cells or secondary effects modulated by local cytokine or nitric oxide production. Regardless of the precise mechanism of injury, therapy of acute viral myocarditis in mice with calcium channel blockers appears to ameliorate the severity of myocardial lesions. In addition, a dramatic degradation of the interstitial collagen matrix is seen, a pattern of injury similar to that of ischemia-induced myocardial stunning. Much of our understanding of the immunopathogenetic mechanisms of viral myocarditis in humans is derived from experimental studies in mice. Two human cardiotropic viruses have been well characterized in murine models: CVB3 [12,13] and cytomegalovirus (CMV) [14]. Both viruses show remarkable likenesses in their patterns of acute and chronic injury, suggesting that a number of viruses are likely to have a similar impact on human myocarditis. **B,** The histologic features of early post-CVB3 myocarditis in the mouse model. Once inflammatory cells are recruited, typically between 5 and 7 days after viral inoculation, focal zones of myocyte necrosis (frequently with superimposed calcification) are characteristically seen. Immunohistologic studies reveal that such lesions typically contain a mixed population of mononuclear cells, including natural killer cells, T lymphocytes, and macrophages. **C,** The histologic features of healed myocarditis typically found in mouse strains genetically predisposed to mild, self-remitting myocarditis. Focal sites of myocyte necrosis undergo organization and appear as discrete foci of replacement fibrosis. The adjacent myocardium is normal, with no evidence of residual myocyte hypertrophy or interstitial fibrosis.

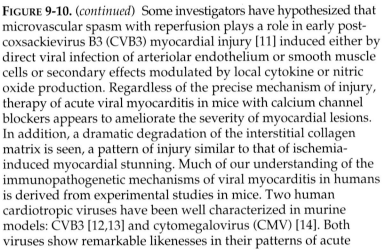

FACTORS CONTRIBUTING TO INCREASED SUSCEPTIBILITY

Hypoxia

Pregnancy

Nutritional deficiencies

Prolonged ingestion of ethanol

Forced exercise and increased afterload

Corticosteroids

Nonsteroidal anti-inflammatory agents

Radiation

Tachycardia

Myocarditic nature of the virus strain

Genetic background of the host

Therapy with proinflammatory cytokines

FIGURE 9-11. The enhancing factors that may potentiate postviral myocarditis. Immunosuppression of mice with cortisone leads to increased mortality and severe myocarditis and is associated with a 100- to 10,000-fold rise in organ viral titers. Chow *et al.* [15] recently showed that mice with severe combined immunodeficiency also develop severe and predominantly virus-mediated myocyte lysis. Using a model of severe myocarditis induced by encephalomyocarditis virus, Kishimoto *et al.* [16] showed that the maximal reduction in postinfection left ventricular ejection fraction correlated with the severity of myocardial necrosis. These findings suggest that in murine postviral myocarditis in the setting of unrestricted viral proliferation, direct viral mechanisms can be responsible for severe myocyte injury and associated myocardial dysfunction.

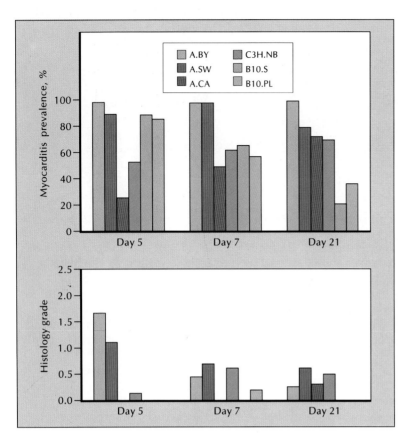

FIGURE 9-12. The prevalence and severity of myocarditis in different inbred strains of mice inoculated with coxsackievirus B3 (CVB3). The A.BY/SnJ (H-2^b), A.SW/SnJ (H-2^s), A.CA/SnJ (H-2^f), B10.SgSf (H-2^s), B10.PL/SgSf (H-2^u), and C3H.NB/SnJ (H-2^p) strains differ in prevalence, severity, and duration of myocardial disease. The influence of the major histocompatibility complex (MHC) on disease production can be demonstrated by comparing the three A strain H-2 congenic lines and the two B10 strain H-2 congenic lines. The A.BY/SnJ and A.SW/SnJ strains display the greatest susceptibility to CVB3–induced myocarditis, as demonstrated by the high incidence and severity of disease. Other studies have shown that these strains experience high mortality rates resulting from elevated peak viremia levels and a delayed neutralizing antibody response. In comparison, the A.CA/SnJ mice have a moderate incidence and severity of myocarditis. This strain typically does not experience significant mortality, has low levels of viremia, and a neutralizing antibody response appears early. This difference in postviral response can be attributed to the H-2 haplotype, which suggests that the MHC controls clearance of CVB3 particles as well as the incidence of myocarditis. Significant differences between prevalence and severity of disease in the A.SW/SnJ (H-2^s) and B10.S/SgSf (H-2^s) strains, which share the same H-2 haplotype, show that these parameters are also controlled by background genes.

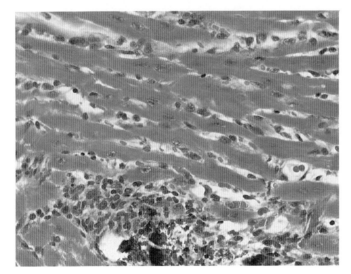

FIGURE 9-13. Medium-power photomicrograph of the left ventricular myocardium from a susceptible mouse strain 21 days after viral inoculation. A focal, cellular necrotic lesion characterized by myocyte dropout with replacement by loose fibrous connective tissue, mononuclear cells, and calcification can be seen (*bottom*). The area immediately adjacent to the necrotic lesion contains increased numbers of interstitial mononuclear cells (*upper half*). This histologic pattern of mononuclear cell infiltrates found within widened interstitial spaces, separating relatively normal appearing myocytes, is characteristic of chronic postviral murine myocarditis. Immunohistologic studies have shown that the inflammatory cell population at this stage is composed primarily of T cells, macrophages, and B cells. Cardiotropic virus cannot be cultured from heart samples after the ninth day following viral inoculation. Therefore, mouse strains that are genetically susceptible to chronic forms of myocarditis have ongoing myocardial inflammation after viral replication ceases. In addition to direct viral injury, other mechanisms contribute to the development of chronic myocyte injury in myocarditis and probably play a more significant role than direct viral injury.

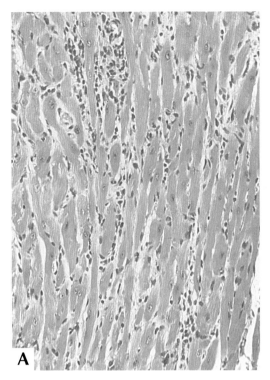

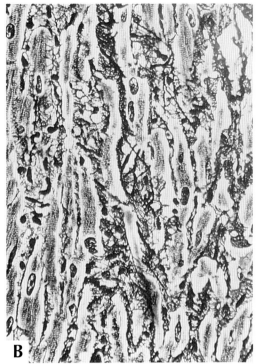

A

B

FIGURE 9-14. The association between myocardial interstitial inflammation and changes in the extracellular matrix. **A,** A portion of left ventricular myocardium with extensive interstitial mononuclear cell infiltration. **B,** A silver stain that highlights reticulin collagen fibers, demonstrating extensive reduplication of the interstitial collagen that is characteristic of chronic myocarditis. The excessive deposition of interstitial collagen in sites of mononuclear cell infiltration suggests an interaction between activated inflammatory cells and fibroblasts [17]. The development of interstitial fibrosis in the postcoxsackievirus B3 model of myocarditis is consistent with a cardiomyopathic change and is similar to the diffuse interstitial fibrosis seen in human dilated cardiomyopathy.

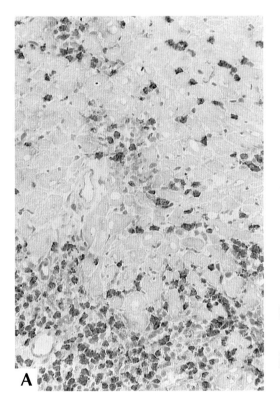

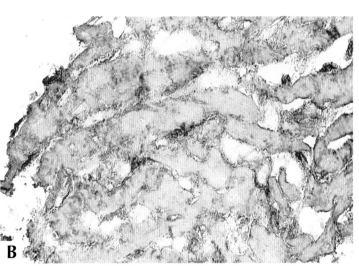

A

B

FIGURE 9-15. **A,** An immunoperoxidase stain of the inflammatory infiltrate seen in Fig. 9-13 using a monoclonal antibody to murine cytotoxic and suppressor T cells. Cytotoxic T cells are found within the focal necrotic lesion as well as within the diffuse interstitial inflammatory cells. **B,** An immunoperoxidase stain using a monoclonal antibody to the murine equivalent of major histocompatibility complex (MHC) class I. Note the diffuse expression of human leukocyte antigen ABC throughout the myocardium; such expression is not limited to zones of myocyte necrosis. From an immunopathologic perspective, ongoing myocardial inflammation can be initiated and sustained by the response of cytotoxic T cells to altered myocytes expressing endogenous viral or intracellular peptides in association with MHC class I antigens. This mechanism may result in the lysis of targeted myocytes, leading to myocarditis. In addition to such lysis, induced autoreactive T cells secondary to presentation of autoantigen peptides by myocytes in association with major histocompatibility antigens may also produce an autoimmune response that would target both virally altered and normal myocytes, resulting in myocarditis.

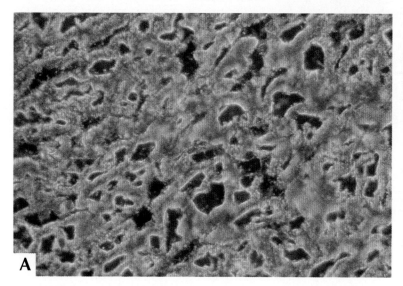

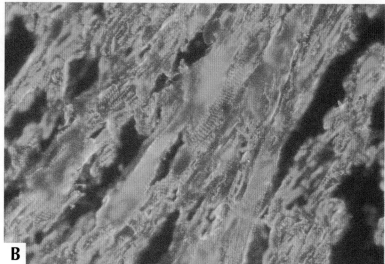

FIGURE 9-16. Representative immunofluorescence staining of normal rat heart tissue incubated with serum from infected mice susceptible to chronic myocarditis. As noted in Fig. 9-8, four strains displayed chronic myocarditis (A.BY/SnJ, A.SW/SnJ, A.CA/SnJ, and C3H.NB/SnJ). These strains produce heart-specific autoantibodies, whereas the two strains without ongoing injury (B10.S/SgSf and B10.PL/SgSf) do not. These findings suggest that postviral autoimmunity plays a role in the pathogenesis of chronic myocarditis [18]. **A,** Cross-section of myocytes with intense surface membrane fluorescence, known as antisarcolemmal antibody (ASA) pattern. **B,** Longitudinally oriented myocytes highlighting both an ASA pattern and an antifibrillary antibody (AFA) pattern of fluorescence. The AFA pattern is characterized by linear thick bands of fluorescence within the cytoplasm, perpendicular to the long axis of the myocytes. Enzyme-linked immunosorbent assay studies have shown that this pattern of immunofluorescence reactivity is associated with circulating antibodies to the cardiac myosin heavy chain. The ability of cardiac myosin to act as an autoantigen in myocarditis has been confirmed by numerous investigators, who immunized susceptible strain mice with cardiac myosin along with adjuvant. Chronic myocarditis, along with the production of myosin autoantibodies, ensues [19].

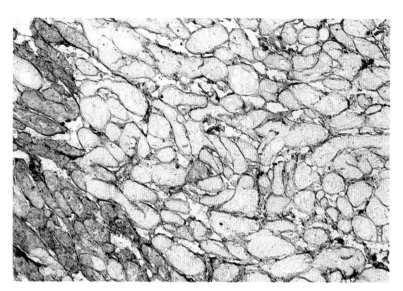

FIGURE 9-17. Myocardial IgG deposition 14 days postcoxsackie-virus B3 infection. The diffuse reactivity on myocyte sarcolemmal membranes suggests that in the setting of induced expression of major histocompatibility complex (MHC) antigens (either by primary viral infection or by secondary release of cytokines by cardiac-infiltrating cells), antibodies bind to self-peptides on the myocyte cell surface. Investigative studies have shown that in addition to myosin, other intracellular proteins (such as the two mitochondrial proteins known to be autoantigens in human myocarditis: the adenine nucleotide translocator [ANT] and the branched-chain ketoacid dehydrogenase [BCKD] complex) are transported to the myocyte cell surface during the course of chronic myocarditis. These proteins are thus presented to the immune system in the context of MHC [20]. Studies by Huber and Moraska [21] have raised the possibility that nonviral insults that produce myocarditis may similarly induce cardiac-specific autoimmunity. Adriamycin-treated mice developed myocarditis and cytolytic T lymphocytes as well as antibodies specifically reactive to only drug-treated myocytes. Thus, the antigenicity of a myocyte may change sufficiently to induce immune reactivity to new antigenic epitopes regardless of the type of toxic insult. Whether these autoantibodies are directly involved in the pathogenesis of cardiac injury or whether they represent an epiphenomenon of ongoing myocardial injury is still the subject of debate. In addition, whether autoantibodies recognize intra-cellular proteins (such as myosin, ANT, and BCKD) transported to the surface of myocytes and expressed as peptides that have been part of the MHC or normal membrane constituents, which cross-react with antigenic epitopes of these intracellular proteins, is not known.

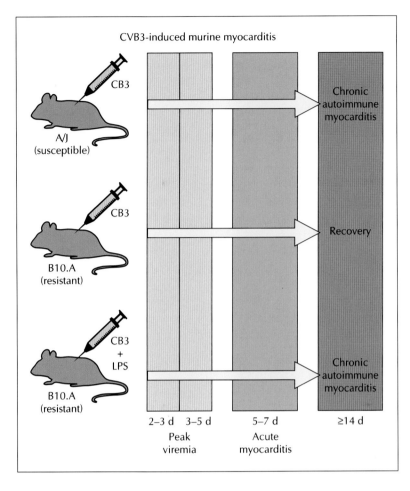

CVB3-induced murine myocarditis

FIGURE 9-18. Mouse strains genetically resistant to coxsackievirus B3 (CVB3) myocarditis develop myocarditis when treated with lipopolysaccharide (LPS). Recent studies by Lane *et al.* [22,23] demonstrated similar results when resistant mice were treated with either tumor necrosis factor-α or interleukin-1β along with the viral inoculum.

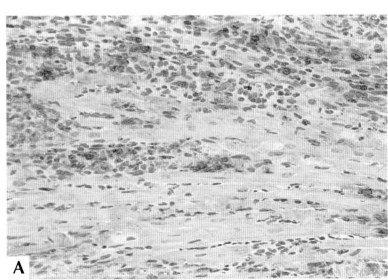

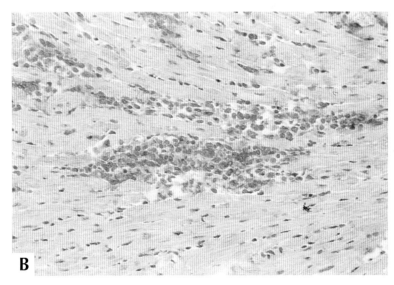

A

B

FIGURE 9-19. A and **B,** Immunoperoxidase stains of myocardium of a B.10A strain mouse, which is genetically resistant to coxsackievirus B infection. The mouse was treated with interleukin-1β at the time of viral inoculum and was sacrificed 14 days later. Intense myocardial inflammation has occurred, suggesting an enhanced role for cytokines in the development of severe myocarditis. Intense staining of a large proportion of infiltrating mononuclear cells with monoclonal antibodies to human tumor necrosis factor-α (*A*) and interleukin-1β (*B*) suggests that local cytokine production may play a direct role in myocyte injury.

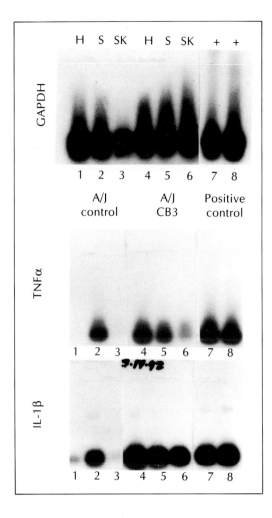

FIGURE 9-20. Autoradiogram showing bands of relative intensity for cytokine mRNA expression in samples of heart (H), spleen (S), and skeletal muscle (SK) in A/J mice 14 days after viral inoculation with coxsackievirus B3. Total cellular RNA was extracted from each tissue section and subjected to the polymerase chain reaction–amplification technique. Serial dilutions of a positive control for interleukin-1β (IL-1β), tumor necrosis factor-α (TNFα), and glyceraldehyde-3-phosphate dehydrogenase (GAPDH) were used: GAPDH internal control (*top*), TNFα (*middle*), and IL-1β (*bottom*). *Plus signs* indicate positive control. Note that control, noninfected A/J mice have no appreciable myocardial or skeletal muscle cytokine mRNA for TNFα and only small amounts of constitutive IL-1β. In contrast, the myocardium of infected mice shows significant cytokine mRNA expression for both IL-1β and TNFα, and cytokine mRNA is demonstrated also within skeletal muscle, although to a lesser extent. The immunoperoxidase findings shown in Fig. 9-13 and these data demonstrate both cytokine gene expression and cytokine protein within the myocardium during chronic myocarditis. A possible direct effect of cytokines on cardiac contractility was studied by Finkel *et al.* [24]. This study demonstrated that TNFα, IL-6, and IL-2 inhibited contractility of isolated papillary muscles of hamsters in a concentration-dependent, reversible manner. The nitric oxide synthase inhibitor Ng-monomethyl-arginine was shown to block these negative inotropic effects, thereby suggesting that the direct negative inotropic effect of cytokines is mediated through nitric oxide synthase.

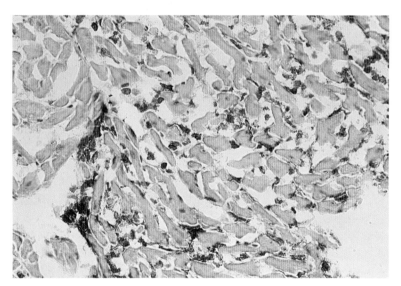

FIGURE 9-21. Immunoperoxidase stain using a monoclonal antibody to the inducible isoform of nitric oxide synthase (termed *i-NOS* or *m-NOS*). Numerous mononuclear cells stain positively for NOS within the myocarditic focus of an animal 14 days after inoculation with coxsackievirus B3. Exactly which myocardial components are potentially affected by cytokines and NOS at this point is unclear. Recent studies have hypothesized, however, that induction of cytokines and NOS within the myocardium play a role in the negative inotropism associated with endotoxemia as well as in the impaired myocardial function associated with myocarditis. Gulick *et al.* [25] demonstrated interleukin-1β and tumor necrosis factor-α inhibited β-adrenergic agonist–mediated increases in cultured cardiac myocyte contractility and intracellular cAMP accumulation. Conversely, other studies demonstrated that endotoxin impairs endothelium-dependent vasodilation in coronary arterioles [26]. These findings suggest that intrinsic control of the coronary arteriolar bed may be altered as a result of increased circulating cytokine levels. Other studies have shown the induction of myocyte cell adhesion proteins by cytokines [27]. Further study is clearly needed to elucidate which cytokines are locally produced in myocarditis to determine the effects of such cytokines on individual components of the myocardium. Understanding the functions of cytokines during the inflammatory response in myocarditis may allow the development of rational therapies to limit myocardial damage.

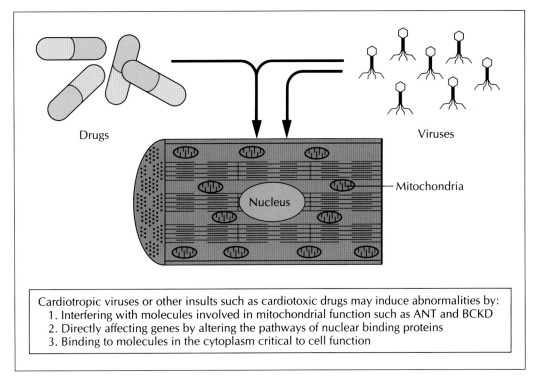

FIGURE 9-22. Direct cytopathologic effects of cardiotropic viruses and cardiotoxic drugs, such as the anthracyclines, have long been suspected to cause injury to cardiac myocytes, although the precise cytopathologic mechanisms have not been defined. In human myocarditis, clues to which cardiac proteins may be dysregulated are derived from precise characterization of circulating autoantibodies found in patients; the peptides that these autoantibodies recognize represent the growing list of putative autoantigens. The best characterized antigens are the mitochondrial proteins (*ie*, the adenine nucleotide translocator (ANT) protein and the branched-chain α-ketoacid dehydrogenase (BCKD) protein), a variety of contractile proteins, and the β-adrenergic receptor. A working hypothesis holds that viruses, either replicating or latent, and other potential toxins interfere with the synthesis, transport, or function of intracellular and cytoplasmic proteins. Other mechanisms include 1) the interference of these agents with the myriad intracellular second messenger pathways that affect the binding of nuclear binding proteins, which results in deregulation of gene transcription or 2) binding of these agents to cytoplasmic proteins that are critical for myocyte function.

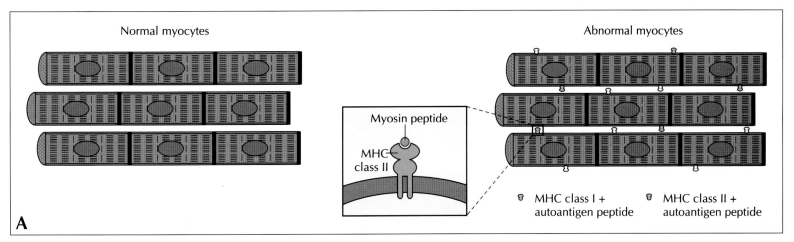

FIGURE 9-23. **A,** Normal human cardiac myocytes do not express major histocompatibility complex (MHC) class I or class II antigens. During myocarditis, however, there is a marked increase in the frequency of myocytes (abnormal myocytes) that express not only MHC class I antigens but also lower (but significant) levels of MHC class II antigens [28]. Both types of MHC molecules appear relatively stable, suggesting that they contain peptides in their peptide-binding clefts (lack of peptides leads to the expression of unstable major histocompatibility molecules). Thus, infiltrating T cells can potentially recognize myosin or other myocardial protein peptides complexed to MHC class II molecules, initiating an autoimmune response. (*continued*)

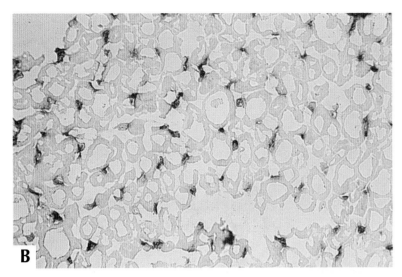

FIGURE 9-23. (*continued*) **B,** Immunoperoxidase stain of an endo-myocardial biopsy from a patient without myocarditis using a monoclonal antibody to MHC class II. Faint staining is limited to the microvasculature. **C,** A similarly stained sample from a patient with active myocarditis contrasts with *B*. In addition to increased staining within the microvasculature, intense sarcolemmal staining of individual myocytes is seen.

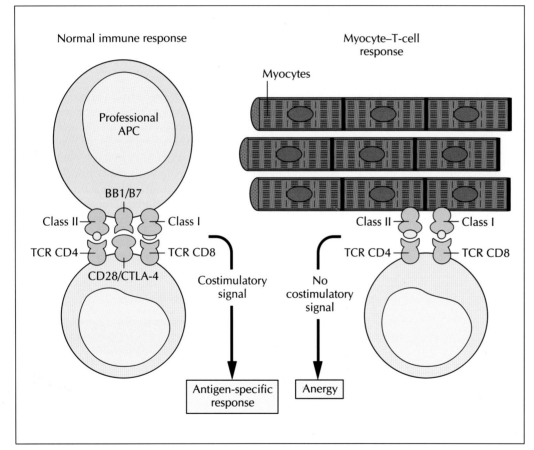

FIGURE 9-24. Normal physiologic immune responses involve recognition of the foreign peptide (in the case of autoimmune disease, a self-peptide) associated with either major histocompatibility complex (MHC) class I or class II molecules on the surface of antigen-presenting cells (APCs) by T cells via clonally rearranged T-cell surface receptors (TCRs). CD4+ T cells predominantly recognize peptides (processed from exogenously presenting antigens) complexed with MHC class II molecules, whereas CD8+ T cells predominantly recognize peptides (processed from endogenous proteins) complexed with MHC class I molecules. For the interaction to lead to a productive antigen-specific response, besides T-cell surface receptors and MHC-peptide engagement, there appears to be a requirement for interaction between other receptor-ligands termed *costimulatory signal-inducing molecules*, such as CD28/CTLA-4 on T cells and BB1/B7 on APCs. In contrast to this physiologic response between T cells and APCs, the interaction between T cells and MHC class I– and II–expressing cardiac myocytes does not appear to lead to a productive T-cell response because myocytes do not express BB1/B7 (the costimulatory molecule). This interaction leads to possible anergy [29].

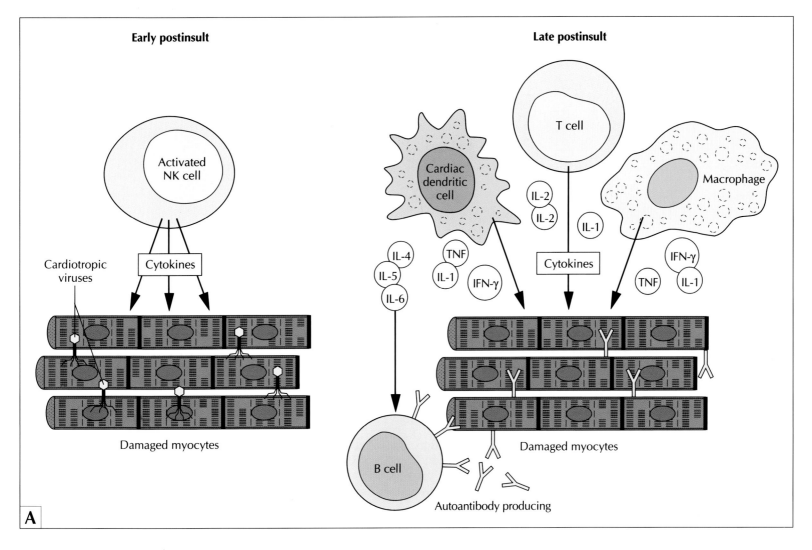

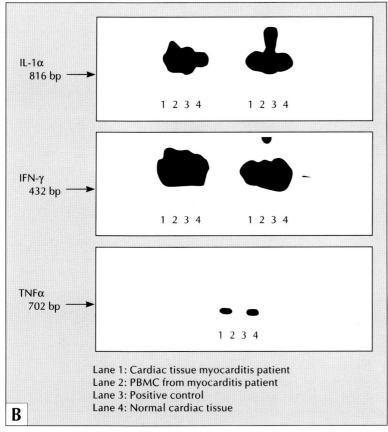

Lane 1: Cardiac tissue myocarditis patient
Lane 2: PBMC from myocarditis patient
Lane 3: Positive control
Lane 4: Normal cardiac tissue

FIGURE 9-25. A, A growing body of evidence suggests that immune-mediated cardiac myocyte injury is more likely from indirect means than from direct T cell– or natural killer (NK) cell–mediated lysis [30]. Data suggest that during the acute phase of myocarditis (early postinsult), there is a predominant infiltration of the natural killer cell lineage. It is known that natural killer cells, when activated, secrete several cytokines, some of which may be toxic to cardiac myocytes. During the chronic stage of myocarditis (late postinsult), it is envisaged that cardiac dendritic cells and infiltrating macrophages may process cardiac tissue proteins (from dying or dead myocytes in small focal areas of the myocardium) and present them to T cells. The combination of these components may become activated and secrete cytokines, such as tumor necrosis factor α (TNFα), interleukin-1β (IL-1β), and IL-2 (TH1-type CD4+ T cells). These cytokines may be toxic to cardiac monocytes and secrete helper factors and cytokines, such as IL-4, IL-5, IL-6 (TH2-type CD4+ ZT cells), which induce B cells to secrete antibodies against cardiac tissues. These antibodies may then bind to cardiac tissue surface membrane proteins and dysregulate myocyte function. **B,** An autoradiogram generated by the reverse transcriptase polymerase chain reaction amplification technique of peripheral blood mononuclear cells (PBMCs) and biopsy tissue. The patient was a child who presented with myocarditis. Increased cytokine mRNA for IL-1β and interferon-γ (IFN-γ) and, to a lesser extent, TNFα was found, indicating the presence of activated TH-1 type CD4+ T cells within the circulation and myocardium.

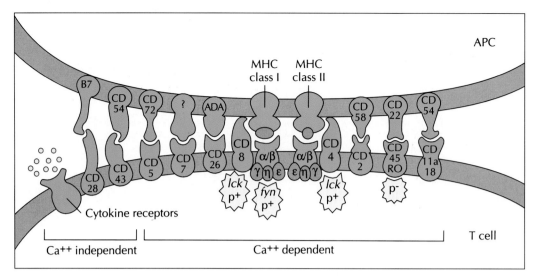

FIGURE 9-26. To define immune-mediated cardiac tissue injury, it is important to understand the nature of immune system–cardiac myocyte interaction. Within this context, it is important first to understand the nature of the receptors and ligands that are involved in physiologic responses of T cells with antigen-presenting cells (APCs). T cells express clonally rearranged T-cell receptors composed of a heterodimer of α and β chains. These receptors recognize peptides bound to major histocompatibility complex (MHC) molecules on APCs. The T-cell receptor is associated with the trimeric CD3 complex (γ δ ε chain) in the cytoplasm responsible for intracellular signalling. Besides T-cell receptor and MHC peptide engagement, there are sets of cognate receptors and ligands, some of which have been shown to promote cell adhesion and others that provide accessory or costimulatory signals. Absence of the costimulatory signals appears to lead to nonproductive T-cell activation and anergy. The cell adhesion molecules (CAM) receptor/ligands include CD43/CD54, CD5/CD72, CD26/ adenosine deaminase (ADA), CD8/MHC class I, CD4/MHC class II, CD45/RO/CD22, and CD11a/18/CD54. Those that provide costimulatory function include CD28, CTLA-4/BB1-B7, and CD2/CD58 (CD58—LFA-3; CD18—LFA-1b; CD11a—LFA-1a; CD54—ICAM-1). After effective receptor/ligand binding, enzymatic pathways of intracellular signaling (lck and fyn) are initiated; some of these pathways are Ca^{++} dependent and some are not. This mechanism leads to T-cell activation, proliferation, and release of cytokines.

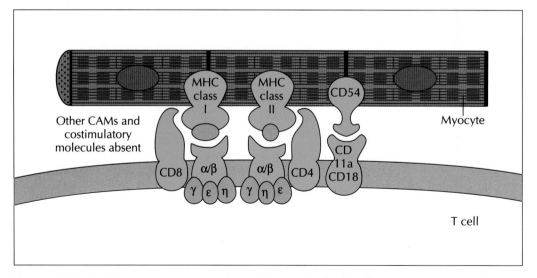

FIGURE 9-27. It is important to note that of the myriad cell adhesion proteins and costimulatory molecules, human cardiac myocytes constitutively express only CD54 (ICAM-1). Studies involving numerous cell activation agents at various concentrations for different periods have shown that the only inducible molecules on myocytes appear to be major histocompatibility complex (MHC) class I and, to a lesser extent, MHC class II. There also appears to be an increase in CD54 expression. Most other cell adhesion molecules and the costimulatory molecules cannot be constitutively expressed, and expression is not inducible. These data indicate that direct immune-mediated dialogue between T cells and cardiac myocytes may not exist [31]. CAM—cell adhesion molecules.

DIAGNOSIS

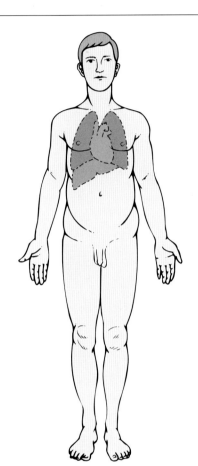

Clinical history
Preceding symptoms of: Fever and chills Upper respiratory infection Gastrointestinal symptoms Chest pain Unexplained tachycardia Short duration of cardiovascular symptoms: CHF Syncope or presyncope No previous history of heart disease

Signs
S_3 gallop Pericardial friction rub Left- or right-sided congestive heart failure Cardiogenic shock

Laboratory findings
Increase in: CPK Liver enzymes ESR Leukocyte count Serologic evidence of active viral infection EKG abnormalities: AV block and repolarization abnormalities ST-T changes including   pseudoinfarction pattern Low voltage LVH Intraventricular conduction delay or LBBB Sinus tachycardia Atrial fibrillation Echocardiographic abnormalities: Global LV dysfunction Global RV dysfunction Pericardial effusion Regional wall motion abnormalities LV hypertrophy Restrictive ventricular filling pattern Ventricular thrombi Radionucleotide abnormalities: Positive antimyosin antibody scan Positive gallium scan

FIGURE 9-28. Diagnostic criteria that may be helpful in identifying patients at high risk for myocarditis. Preceding symptoms may include fever, influenza-like symptoms (*eg*, cough, sore throat, general malaise, myalgia, arthralgia), gastrointestinal symptoms (*eg*, nausea, vomiting, anorexia, abdominal pain), and chest pain or discomfort. In a recent series of 58 consecutive patients with idiopathic myocarditis, however, only 52% of the 58 patients had an antecedent influenza-like illness within 3 months of presenting with congestive heart failure [32]. Serologic evidence of viral infections requires the demonstration of at least a fourfold rise in specific antibody in paired acute (less than 1 week) and convalescent (2 weeks or longer) serum specimens. Initially, IgM antibody is present, reaching peak titers by 2 to 3 weeks and declining to undetectable levels thereafter. IgG antibody production is the predominant immunoglobulin class after the first month of disease. Myocarditis should be clinically suspected in patients presenting with ischemic chest pain, particularly when electrocardiographic (ECG) changes are beyond a single vascular distribution or global left ventricular (LV) hypokinesis is present. In a study by Dec *et al.* [33], 34 patients who presented with ischemic chest pain syndromes but were found to have normal coronary anatomy on angiography underwent endomyocardial biopsy. Myocarditis was found in 11 patients and global LV hypokinesis in five. A variety of electrocardiographic changes were noted, such as ST elevations in six, ST depressions in two, and T-wave inversions in three. Although electrocardiographic changes were usually localized to the anterior precordium, diffuse changes were found in three patients. AV—atrioventricular; CPK—creatine phosphokinase; CHF—congestive heart failure; ESR—erythrocyte sedimentation rate; LBBB—left bundle branch block; LVH—left ventricular hypertrophy; RV—right ventricular.

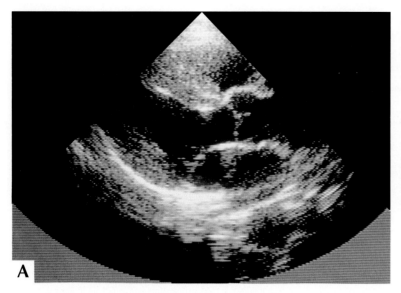

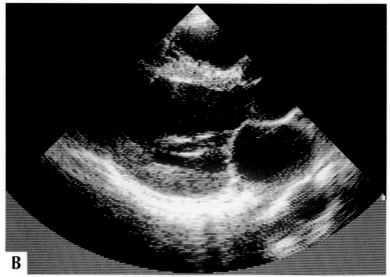

FIGURE 9-29. Two-dimensional echocardiographic images from two patients with acute myocarditis evidenced by endomyocardial biopsy. **A,** This patient had a history of rapid-onset congestive heart failure 3 weeks after an influenza-like illness and presented with hypotension and left-sided congestive heart failure. The two-dimensional echocardiogram reveals severe, global left ventricular (LV) hypokinesis associated with marked, concentric LV hypertrophy; cavity dimensions are normal. **B,** In contrast, this patient had no history of antecedent influenza-like illness but had a history of coughing and dyspnea for 1 to 2 months before admission with biventricular heart failure. The two-dimensional echocardiogram shows moderate, global LV hypokinesis associated with a dilated, nonthickened LV and a dilatated left atrium and right ventricle. Echocardiographic features of myocarditis are polymorphous and nonspecific [34]. LV dysfunction is common with or without cavity dilatation, while right ventricular dysfunction is less common. Pericardial effusion, regional wall motion abnormalities, ventricular hypertrophy, and restrictive ventricular filling patterns are not infrequently found. Ventricular thrombi may also be found and, in our experience, are more prevalent in fulminant presentations of myocarditis.

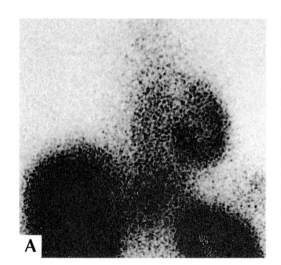

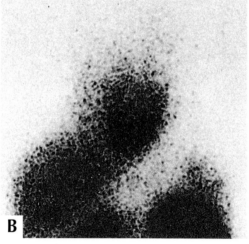

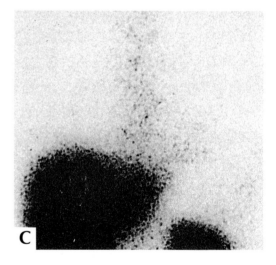

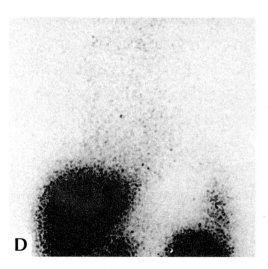

FIGURE 9-30. Myocardial images in anterior (**A** and **C**) and left anterior oblique (LAO; **B** and **D**) projections 48 hours after injection of indium-111 antimyosin in a patient with biopsy-proven myocarditis [35]. Diffusely positive scans are seen in the acute stage (*A* and *B*) 14 days after the onset of symptoms but become negative at follow-up 1 year later (*C* and *D*). Noninvasive imaging techniques, such as antimyosin and gallium scans, have been used successfully to detect myocarditis. In a study by Dec *et al.* [36] comparing the utility of antimyosin scanning with endomyocardial biopsy to diagnose myocarditis, 82 patients were studied with a mean ejection fraction of 30%. A positive antimyosin scan provided a sensitivity of 83% and a specificity of 53%, while the predictive value of a normal scan was 92%. Improvement in left ventricular function occurred within 6 months of treatment in 54% of patients with a positive antimyosin scan compared with 18% of those with a normal scan. O'Connell *et al.* [37] demonstrated that in 15 patients with positive gallium scans (all treated with immunosuppressive drugs), those with unchanged scans (*n*=9) did not improve hemodynamically, while those with improved scans (*n*=6) improved clinically. Although the precise clinical significance of noninvasive imaging is still being debated, it is evident that positive scans may help identify patients at high risk for myocarditis.

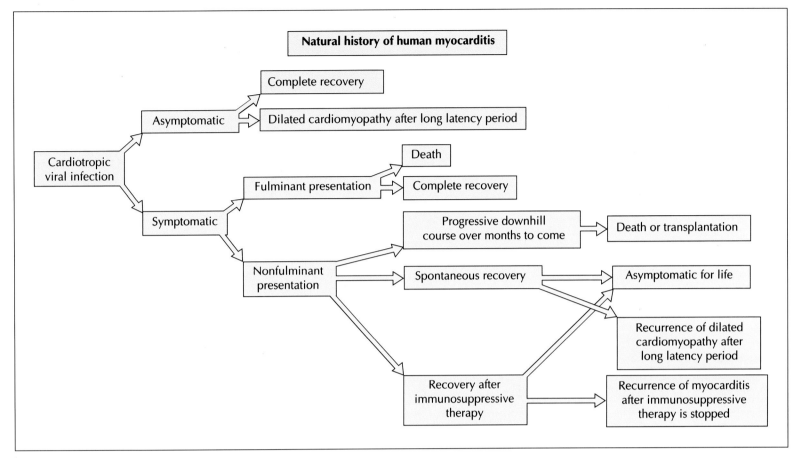

FIGURE 9-31. The natural history of human myocarditis. Most patients with mild symptoms of acute myocarditis are not seen by cardiologists and most of these patients appear to recover fully. Of the patients with symptomatic heart disease typically seen by cardiologists, a small number have fulminant presentations and either die in the acute stage or appear to recover fully. Of the remaining patients with myocarditis, a few are characterized by a progressive downhill course over a period of months to years that ends in death from heart failure or intractable arrhythmias [38,39]. Some spontaneously recover and remain asymptomatic for life, and others have an asymptomatic period followed by development of dilated cardiomyopathy. The heterogeneity of clinical presentations and natural history in human myocarditis probably reflect the genetic predisposition of the individual, the virulence of the cardiotropic virus, and environmental factors. With the advent of molecular viral probes, it will be critical to relate the presence of persistent enterovirus RNA with the patterns of the natural history of myocarditis.

FINAL DIAGNOSIS IN PATIENTS UNDERGOING ENDOMYOCARDIAL BIOPSY AT THE JOHNS HOPKINS HOSPITAL FROM JANUARY 1985 THROUGH DECEMBER 1990

SPECIFIC DIAGNOSES	FREQUENCY, n(%)
Idiopathic active myocarditis	49(9)
Idiopathic borderline myocarditis	9(2)
Primary (idiopathic) cases of cardiomyopathy	207(39)
Secondary cases of cardiomyopathy	
Occult coronary artery disease	44(8)
Peripartum and postpartum	27(5)
Human immunodeficiency virus cardiomyopathy	23(4)
Cocaine cardiomyopathy	6(1)
Other	53(10)
Restrictive cardiomyopathy	21(4)
Arrhythmias	31(6)
Miscellaneous	64(12)
Total	534

FIGURE 9-32. The final diagnostic categories of 534 consecutive patients undergoing endomyocardial biopsy at The Johns Hopkins Hospital. Fifty-eight of 534 (11%) patients presenting with heart dysfunction of recent onset (mean duration of heart failure symptoms, 58 days) were found to have either active (n=49) or borderline (n=9) myocarditis [32]. It is interesting to note that while idiopathic dilated cardiomyopathy remained the most common final clinical diagnosis, secondary causes of cardiomyopathy including those associated with metabolic disorders, neuromuscular diseases, and connective tissue diseases were not uncommon. Preliminary data from the multicenter Myocarditis Treatment Trial [40] described a 9% prevalence of active myocarditis in 2242 adult patients. In addition, Parrillo *et al.* [41] diagnosed lymphocytic myocarditis in two of 102 patients with idiopathic dilated cardiomyopathy who were symptomatic for a median of 8 months before entering the study. These findings may reflect a low prevalence of myocarditis in patients with chronic dilated cardiomyopathy, whereas a prevalence of 40% to 60% has been suggested in patients with acute onset of symptoms less than 4 weeks, duration [42–44]. Although the true incidence of this pattern of chronic disease is not yet known, these studies suggest that the prevalence of myocarditis in patients with recent onset (<12 months) of congestive heart failure is approximately 10% to 15%.

CLINICOPATHOLOGIC DESCRIPTION

A. CLINICAL CLASSIFICATION OF MYOCARDITIS

	FULMINANT
Initial presentation	Cardiogenic shock; severe LV dysfunction
Initial endomyocardial biopsy	Multiple foci of active myocarditis
Clinical natural history	Complete recovery or death
Immunosuppressive therapy	No likely benefit

FIGURE 9-33. Recently published classification of myocarditis based on both clinical and pathologic information, analogous to the accepted classification of viral hepatitis [43]. Four categories of myocarditis are described: fulminant (**A**), acute, chronic active, and chronic persistent (**B**). CHF—congestive heart failure; DCM—dilated cardiomyopathy; LV—left ventricular.

B. CLINICAL CLASSIFICATION OF MYOCARDITIS

	ACUTE	CHRONIC ACTIVE	CHRONIC PERSISTENT
Initial presentation	CHF; LV dysfunction	CHF; LV dysfunction	No CHF; normal LV function
Initial endomyocardial biopsy	Active or borderline myocarditis	Active or borderline myocarditis	Active or borderline myocarditis
Clinical natural history	Incomplete recovery or DCM	DCM	Non-CHF symptoms; normal LV function
Immunosuppressive therapy	Sometimes beneficial	May be of temporary benefit	No benefit

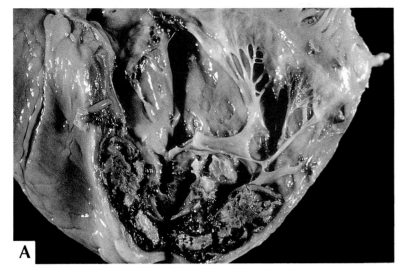

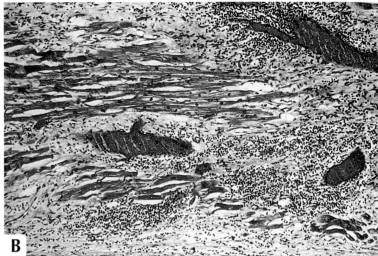

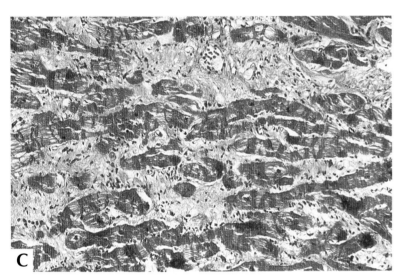

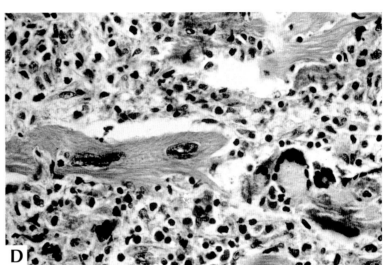

FIGURE 9-34. **A,** Gross autopsy specimen of a heart with fulminant myocarditis. The right ventricle is cut along the long axis to demonstrate an apical mural thrombus. **B,** Low-power photomicrograph of the myocardium revealing extensive mononuclear inflammation, which has replaced large clusters of myocytes that have undergone necrosis. Fulminant myocarditis is characterized by a nonspecific, severe influenza-like illness and the distinct onset of cardiac involvement. The patient's condition deteriorates rapidly, and the disorder frequently results in profound hemodynamic compromise and multisystem failure. Endomyocardial biopsies from fulminant myocarditis patients demonstrate unequivocal active myocarditis and are particularly notable for very extensive inflammatory infiltrates and numerous foci of myocyte necrosis. Within 1 month, the patients usually recover left ventricular function completely or die [45]. In contrast, acute myocarditis describes the clinical spectrum of the largest group of patients with active or borderline myocarditis. These patients have minimally dilated, hypokinetic left ventricles on presentation. The onset of cardiac symptoms is frequently indistinct, and some patients provide a vague history consistent with (but not diagnostic of) an antecedent viral illness. Active or borderline myocarditis is present on initial (but not subsequent) endomyocardial biopsies. Some patients in this group appear to respond to immunosuppressive therapy [46], while others experience either partial recovery of ventricular function or continue to deteriorate to end-stage dilated cardiomyopathy. **C,** Masson's trichrome (which stains collagen blue) of an endomyocardial biopsy of a patient with chronic active myocarditis. Note the extensive collagen deposition characteristically seen in end-stage dilated cardiomyopathy. Patients with chronic active myocarditis usually have a vague clinical presentation. Such patients have a slowly progressive course that inevitably deteriorates but may be punctuated by brief, often-dramatic but unsustained responses to immunosuppressive therapy. Serial endomyocardial biopsies demonstrate ongoing myocarditis with the development of extensive interstitial fibrosis. Inflammatory infiltrates in this subgroup of myocarditis patients may contain multinucleated giant cells. **D,** High-power photomicrograph taken from an explanted heart sample during transplant. The patient had a long-standing history of repeated episodes of myocarditis. Intense myocarditis with extensive myocyte lysis and multinucleated giant cells is seen. The photomicrograph is consistent with the histologic diagnosis of giant cell myocarditis.

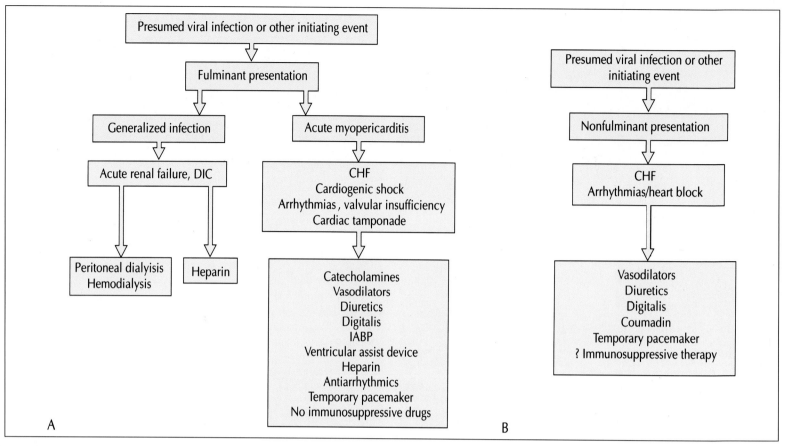

FIGURE 9-35. Clinical treatment strategies for myocarditis presenting in the fulminant (**A**) and nonfulminant (**B**) forms. Although viral gene expression has been documented in human myocarditis, such expression probably reflects persistent, nonpermissive infection rather than replicating virus. Clinical experience has shown that immunosuppression does not appear to cause acute exacerbation of myocarditis in most patients. Individuals presenting with fulminant myocarditis are one possible exception. It is therefore suggested that immunosuppressive agents be avoided in such patients, despite their profound contractile dysfunction. CHF—congestive heart failure; DIC—disseminated intravascular coagulopathy; IABP—increased arterial blood pressure.

IMMUNOSUPPRESSIVE THERAPY IN PATIENTS WITH CONGESTIVE HEART FAILURE AND BIOPSY OR GALLIUM-DIAGNOSED MYOCARDITIS

STUDY	PATIENTS TREATED, n	IMPROVED, n(%)
Mason et al. [49]	10	5(50)
Edwards et al. [50]	4	2(50)
Fenoglio et al. [51]	19	8(42)
Daly et al. [52]	9	7(78)
O'Connell et al. [53]	15	6(40)
Zee-Cheng et al. [54]	11	5(45)
Dec et al. [42]	9	4(44)
Hosenpud et al. [55]	6	1(17)
Jones et al. [46]	16	8(50)
Total	99	46(46)

FIGURE 9-36. Nonrandomized studies that have reported very different success rates for immunosuppressive therapy in myocarditis. Many studies did not evaluate biopsies using the Dallas criteria; thus, immunosuppressive drug therapy as well as methods for evaluation of clinical benefit were not standardized. Jones et al. [46] found that short-term immunosuppressive therapy (6 to 8 weeks of prednisone, 1.0 mg/kg/d, and azathioprine, 1.5 mg/kg/d) improved left ventricular contractile function in a subgroup of patients, particularly those with borderline myocarditis. The possibility that borderline myocarditis may represent immune-mediated cardiac injury is also supported by the study by Dec et al. [47]. Their study demonstrated that on repeat biopsy, many patients do, in fact, have active myocarditis, thereby reflecting problems with sampling error rather than a different disease. In terms of immunologic parameters, the prevalence of anti–heart antibodies and aberrant major histocompatibility expression by immunohistochemistry appear to be the same in patients with active myocarditis and borderline myocarditis [28,37,40,48–53]. (*Adapted from* Hosenpud and coworkers [55]; with permission.)

SPONTANEOUS IMPROVEMENT IN PATIENTS WITH CLINICAL DILATED CARDIOMYOPATHY WITH OR WITHOUT MYOCARDITIS

STUDY	PATIENTS TREATED, n	IMPROVED, n(%)
McDonald et al. [56]	31	19(61)
Fuster et al. [57]	104	18(17)
O'Connell et al. [53]	20	6(30)
Dec et al. [42]	18	6(33)
Figulla et al. [58]	18	7(39)
Taliercio et al.. [59]	24	7(39)
Total	215	62(29)

FIGURE 9-37. Reported spontaneous remission rates of histologically proven myocarditis. Frequent spontaneous remissions make the interpretation of noncontrolled treatment studies of myocarditis more difficult [37,47,54–57]. (*Adapted from* Hosenpud [60]; with permission.)

REFERENCES

1. Aretz HT: Myocarditis: the Dallas criteria. *Hum Pathol* 1987, 18:619–624.

2. Aretz HT, Billingham ME, Edwards WD, et al.: A histopathologic definition and classification. *Am J Cardiovasc Pathol* 1986, 1:3–14.

3. Tazelaar HD, Billingham ME: Myocardial lymphocytes: fact, fancy, or myocarditis. *Am J Cardiovasc Pathol* 1987, 1:47–50.

4. Gore I, Saphir O: Myocarditis: a classification of 1402 cases. *Am Heart J* 1947, 34:827–830.

5. Gravanis MB, Sternby NH: Incidence of myocarditis: a 10-year autopsy study from Malmo, Sweden. *Arch Pathol Lab Med* 1991, 115:390–392.

6. Bandt CM, Staley NA, Noren GR: Acute viral myocarditis: clinical and histologic changes. *Minn Med* 1979, 62:234–237.

7. Woodruff JF: Viral myocarditis: a review. *Am J Pathol* 1980, 101:427–429.

8. Grist NR: Epidemiology and pathogenicity of coxsackievirus. In *New Concepts in Viral Heart Disease*, ed 1. Edited by Schultheiss HP. New York: Springer Verlag; 1988:26–32.

9. Herskowitz A, Wolfgram LJ, Rose NR, et al.: Coxsackievirus B3 murine myocarditis: a pathologic spectrum of myocarditis in genetically defined inbred strains. *J Am Coll Cardiol* 1987, 9:1311–1319.

10. McManus BM, Chow LH, Wilson JE, et al.: Direct myocardial injury by enterovirus: a central role in the evolution of murine myocarditis. *Clin Immunol Immunopathol* 1993, 68:159–169.

11. Sole MJ, Liu P: Viral myocarditis: a paradigm for understanding the pathogenesis and treatment of dilated cardiomyopathy. *J Am Coll Cardiol* 1993, 22(suppl A):99A–105A.

12. Wilson FM, Miranda QR, Chason JL, et al.: Residual pathologic changes following murine coxsackie A and B myocarditis. *Am J Pathol* 1969, 55:253–266.

13. Woodruff JF, Woodruff JJ: Involvement of T lymphocytes in the pathogenesis of coxsackievirus B3 heart disease. *J Immunol* 1974, 113:1726–1734.

14. Lawson CM, O'Donoghue H, Bartholomaeus WN, et al.: Genetic control of mouse cytomegalovirus-induced myocarditis. *Immunology* 1990, 69:20–26.

15. Chow LH, Beisel KW, McManus BM: Enteroviral infection of mice with severe combined immunodeficiency evidence for direct viral pathogenesis of myocardial injury. *Lab Invest* 1992, 66:24–31.

16. Kishimoto C, Hung G-L, Ishibashi M, et al.: Natural evolution of cardiac function, cardiac pathology and antimyosin scan in a murine myocarditis model. *J Am Coll Cardiol* 1991, 17:821–827.

17. Neumann DA, Wulff SM, Leppo MK, et al.: Pathologic changes in the cardiac interstitium of mice infected with encephalomyocarditis virus. *Cardiovasc Pathol* 1993, 2:117–126.

18. Wolfgram LJ, Beisel KW, Rose NR: Heart-specific autoantibodies following murine coxsackievirus B3 myocarditis. *J Exp Med* 1985, 161:1112–1121.

19. Neu N, Rose NR, Neisel KW, et al.: Cardiac myosin induces myocarditis in genetically predisposed mice. *J Immunol* 1987, 139:3630–3636.

20. Neumann DA, Rose NR, Ansari AA, et al.: Induction of heart auto-antibodies in mice with coxsackievirus B3- and cardiac myosin-induced autoimmune myocarditis. *J Immunol* 1994, 152:343–350.

21. Huber SA, Moraska A: Cytolytic T lymphocytes and antibodies to myocytes in adriamycin-treated BALB/c mice. *Am J Pathol* 1992, 140:233–242.

22. Lane JR, Neumann DA, Lafond-Walker A, et al.: Interleukin 1 or tumor necrosis factor can promote coxsackievirus B3-induced myocarditis in resistant B10.A mice. *J Exp Med* 1992, 175:1123–1129.

23. Lane JR, Neumann DA, Lafond-Walker A, et al.: Role of IL-1 and tumor necrosis factor in coxsackie virus-induced autoimmune myocarditis. *J Immunol* 1993, 151:1682–1690.

24. Finkel MS, Oddis CV, Jacob TD, et al.: Negative inotropic effects of cytokines on the heart mediated by nitric oxide. *Science* 1992, 257:387–389.

25. Gulick T, Chung ML, Pieper SJ, et al.: Interleukin 1 and tumor necrosis factor inhibit cardiac myocyte beta-adrenergic responsiveness. *PNAS USA* 1989, 86:6753–6757.

26. Kuo L, Chilian WM, Davis MJ, et al.: Endotoxin impairs flow-induced vasodilation of porcine coronary arterioles. *Am J Physiol* 1992, 262:H1838–H1845.

27. Seko Y, Matsuda H, Kato K, et al.: Expression of intercellular adhesion molecule-1 in murine hearts with acute myocarditis caused by coxsackievirus B3. *J Clin Invest* 1993, 91:1327–1336.

28. Herskowitz A, Ansari AA, Neumann DA, et al.: Induction of major histocompatibility complex (MHC) antigens within the myocardium of patients with active myocarditis: a nonhistologic marker of myocarditis. *J Am Coll Cardiol* 1990, 15:624–632.

29. Ansari AA, Wang YC, Kanter K, et al.: Host T-cell primary allosen-sitization to MHC class 1- and class-II expressing human cardiac myocytes requires the presence of a second signal. *Hum Immunol* 1993, 37:108–118.

30. Ansari AA, Kanter K, Wang YC, *et al.*: Major histocompatibility complex-expressing human cardiac myocytes are not the direct target of host cardiac infiltrating cells: evidence for a prominent role of the indirect pathway in human cardiac allograft rejection. *Transplant Proc* 1993, 25:89–93.

31. Ansari AA, Sundstrom B, Runnels H, *et al.*: The absence of constitutive and induced expression of critical cell-adhesion molecules on human cardiac myocytes. *Transplantation* 1994, 57:942–949.

32. Herskowitz A, Campbell S, Deckers J, *et al.*: Demographic features and prevalence of idiopathic myocarditis in patients undergoing endomyocardial biopsy at The Johns Hopkins Hospital. *Am J Cardiol* 1993, 71:982–986.

33. Dec GW, Waldman H, Southern J, *et al.*: Viral myocarditis mimicking acute myocardial infarction. *J Am Coll Cardiol* 1992, 20:85–90.

34. Pinamonti B, Alberti E, Cigalotto A, *et al.*: Echocardiographic findings in myocarditis. *Am J Cardiol* 1988, 62:285–291.

35. Matsumori A, Kawai C, Yamada T, *et al.*: Mechanism and significance of myocardial uptake of antimyosin antibody in myocarditis and cardiomyopathy: clinical and experimental studies. *Clin Immunol Immunopathol* 1993, 68:215–219.

36. Dec GW, Palacios I, Yasuda T, *et al.*: Antimyosin antibody cardiac imaging: its role in the diagnosis of myocarditis. *J Am Coll Cardiol* 1990, 16:97–104.

37. O'Connell JB, Henkin RE, Robinson JA, *et al.*: Gallium-67 imaging in patients with dilated cardiomyopathy and biopsy-proven myocarditis. *Circulation* 1984, 70:58–62.

38. Strain JE, Grose RM, Factor SM, *et al.*: Results of endomyocardial biopsy in patients with spontaneous ventricular tachycardia but without apparent structural heart disease. *Circulation* 1983, 68:1171–1181.

39. Smith WG: Coxsackie B myopericarditis in adults. *Am Heart J* 1980, 80:34–36.

40. Mason JW: Incidence and clinical characteristics of myocarditis [abstract]. *Circulation* 1991, 84(suppl 2):2.

41. Parrillo JE, Cunnion RE, Epstein SE: A prospective, randomized, controlled trial of prednisone for dilated cardiomyopathy. *N Engl J Med* 1989, 321:1061–1068.

42. Dec GW Jr, Palacios IF, Fallon JT, *et al.*: Active myocarditis in the spectrum of acute dilated cardiomyopathies: clinical features, histologic correlates, and clinical outcome. *N Engl J Med* 1985, 312:885–890.

43. Lieberman EB, Hutchins GM, Herskowitz A, *et al.*: A clinico-pathologic description of myocarditis. *J Am Coll Cardiol* 1991, 18:1617–1626.

44. Midei MG, DeMent SH, Feldman AM, *et al.*: Peripartum myocarditis and cardiomyopathy. *Circulation* 1990, 81:922–928.

45. Rockman HA, Adamson RM, Dembitsky WP, *et al.*: Acute fulminant myocarditis: long-term follow-up after circulatory support with left ventricular assist device. *Am Heart J* 1991, 121:922–926.

46. Jones SR, Herskowitz A, Hutchins GM, *et al.*: Effects of immuno-suppressive therapy in biopsy-proved myocarditis and borderline myocarditis on left ventricular function. *Am J Cardiol* 1991, 68:370–376.

47. Dec GW, Fallon JT, Southern JF, *et al.*: "Borderline" myocarditis: an indication for repeat endomyocardial biopsy. *J Am Coll Cardiol* 1990, 15:283–289.

48. Neumann DA, Burek CL, Baughman KL, *et al.*: Circulating heart-reactive antibodies in patients with myocarditis or cardiomyopathy. *J Am Coll Cardiol* 1990, 16:839–846.

49. Mason JW, Billingham ME, Ricci DR: Treatment of acute inflammatory myocarditis assisted by endomyocardial biopsy. *Am J Cardiol* 1980, 45:1037–1045.

50. Edwards WD, Holmes Jr DR, Reeder GS: Diagnosis of active lymphocytic myocarditis by endomyocardial biopsy: quantitative criteria for light microscopy. *Mayo Clin Proc* 1982, 57:419–425.

51. Fenoglio Jr JJ, Ursell PC, Kellogg CF: Diagnosis and classification of myocarditis by endomyocardial biopsy. *N Engl J Med* 1983, 308:12–18.

52. Daly K, Richardson PJ, Olsen EGJ, *et al.*: Acute myocarditis: role of histological and virological examination in the diagnosis and assessment of immunosuppressive treatment. *Br Heart J* 1984, 51:30–35.

53. O'Connell JB, Robinson JA, Henkin RE, *et al.*: Immunosuppressive therapy in patients with congestive cardiomyopathy and myocardial uptake of gallium-67. *Circulation* 1981, 64:780–786.

54. Zee-Cheng CS, Tasi CC, Palmer DC, *et al.*: High incidence of myocarditis by endomyocardial biopsy in patients with idiopathic congestive cardiomyopathy. *J Am Coll Cardiol* 1984, 3:63–70.

55. Hosenpud JD, McAnulty JH, Niles NR: Lack of objective improvement in ventricular systolic function in patients with myocarditis treated with azathioprine and prednisone. *J Am Coll Cardiol* 1985, 6:797–801.

56. McDonald CD, Burch GE, Walsh JJ: Prolonged bed rest in the treatment of idiopathic cardiomyopathy. *Am J Med* 1972, 52:41–50.

57. Fuster V, Gersh BJ, Giuliani ER, *et al.*: The natural history of idiopathic dilated cardiomyopathy. *Am J Cardiol* 1981, 47:525–531.

58. Figulla HR, Rahlf G, Nieger M, *et al.*: Spontaneous hemodynamic improvement or stabilization and associated biopsy findings in patients with congestive cardiomyopathy. *Circulation* 1985, 71:1095–1104.

59. Taliercio CP, Seward JB, Driscoll DJ, *et al.*: Idiopathic dilated cardiomyopathy in the young: clinical profile and natural history. *J Am Coll Cardiol* 1985, 6:1126–1131.

60. Hosenpud JD: Chronic idiopathic myocarditis: controversies in causes and therapy. *Cardiovasc Rev Report* 1988, 5:32–38.

RHEUMATIC FEVER AND RHEUMATIC CARDITIS

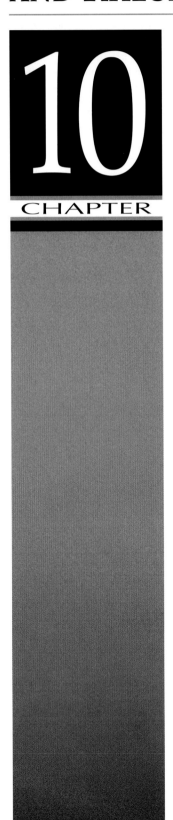

10

CHAPTER

Benedict F. Massell and Jagat Narula

Rheumatic fever is important because it is frequently a precursor of heart disease. In the early part of this century it was a leading cause of death and disability among children and young adults. Since then the mortality rate has gradually declined, with a fourfold accelerated decline during the penicillin era, which began about 1946. A recent localized resurgence of rheumatic fever in the United States and Europe remains unexplained. The disease also continues to be common in most developing countries.

Rheumatic fever may affect the endocardium, myocardium, and pericardium. Rheumatic endocarditis produces verrucous valvulitis along the closing edges of the valves. Acute rheumatic pericarditis produces serofibrinous effusion with shaggy deposition of fibrin on the epicardium. The myocardial inflammation is characterized by the interstitial presence of Aschoff nodules. Although Aschoff nodules are pathognomonic of rheumatic carditis, it is the endocarditis that may lead to permanent valve damage. The etiology of rheumatic fever is always an antecedent group A, hemolytic streptococcal throat infection, followed by a silent latent period before the onset of rheumatic fever. Its pathogenesis is still not understood completely.

Diagnosis of rheumatic fever rests on assessment of clinical findings combined with evidence of a recent streptococcal infection and signs of systemic inflammation (fever or a rapid sedimentation rate). Rheumatic fever is generally a poststreptococcal polyarthritis or carditis, or both. Chorea may develop in patients who have had joint symptoms or who have carditis, or it may be an isolated manifestation (pure chorea). Subcutaneous nodules and erythema marginatum are usually manifestations of severe rheumatic fever with carditis and are therefore of prognostic importance.

Joint manifestations usually respond dramatically to treatment with aspirin. ACTH and the adrenocortical hormones are highly suppressive of rheumatic inflammation and may be life-saving in critically ill patients who usually have a pancarditis. There is no agreement as to whether they may prevent or lessen permanent valve damage. The most important part of treatment in those who already have carditis from previous or current rheumatic fever is prevention of recrudescences or recurrences of rheumatic fever by the appropriate use of penicillin or other chemotherapeutic agents. Such treatment may be used to prevent streptococcal throat infection or, in the presence of such infection, to eradicate the group A streptococci from the throat flora. With this management, newly acquired significant murmurs often lessen and even disappear completely.

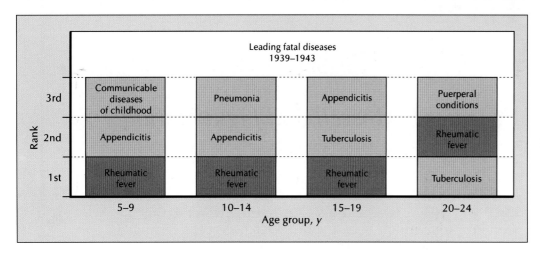

FIGURE 10-1. Leading fatal diseases among policyholders of the Metropolitan Life Insurance Company from 1939 to 1943. These data show that as recently as 1943, rheumatic fever was the leading fatal disease among 5- to 19-year-olds and the second leading fatal disease among 20- to 24-year-olds. (*Adapted from* Armstrong and Wheatley [1]; with permission.)

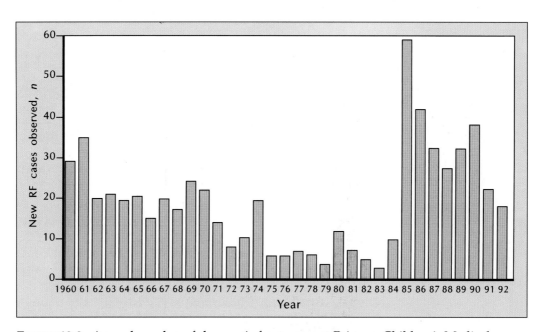

FIGURE 10-2. Annual number of rheumatic fever cases at Primary Children's Medical Center in Salt Lake City from 1960 to 1992 [2,3]. Beginning in 1985, there was an abrupt increase in the number of rheumatic fever cases diagnosed at the center. The number of cases observed in 1985 represented an eightfold increase over the average annual number of cases diagnosed in the previous decade [2]. Between 1985 and 1992, 274 cases of acute rheumatic fever were diagnosed [3], and the level of rheumatic fever admissions has not yet decreased to the pre-1985 level. Similar outbreaks of rheumatic fever have been reported in Pennsylvania, Ohio, Colorado, Texas, and Hawaii [4]. The cause for changes in severity (*see* Fig. 10-3) and incidence of rheumatic fever are poorly understood, but is likely related to the rheumatogenicity of the prevalent strains of group A streptococci, which in turn seems related to the content of M protein and the size of the hyaluronic acid capsule (and possibly to the serologic type). Factors influencing rheumatogenicity include rapidity of person-to-person spread, which is increased by crowding, especially in the home, and decreased by less crowding and by the widespread use of penicillin. Although the cases of rheumatic fever in Salt Lake City were mainly from middle class families, family size averaged 6.5 persons, which is approximately twice the average for the state of Iowa. Furthermore, a recent study of rheumatic fever in Dade County, Florida found the disease to be confined almost exclusively to black inner-city residents, who presumably lived under crowded conditions [5]. (*Adapted from* Veasy and coworkers [2,3]; with permission.)

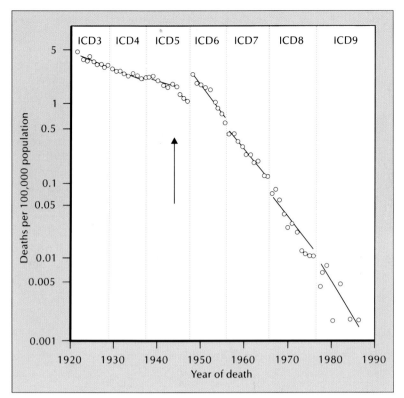

FIGURE 10-3. National mortality due to rheumatic fever from 1921 to 1988 in persons 5 to 19 years of age. Mortality rates are plotted both logarithmically and separately for each period covered by the International Classification of Diseases (ICD). Slope of the trend lines within each ICD (separated by vertical lines) indicates changes in mortality rates. Abrupt changes (up or down) from one ICD to another are due to changes in classification and can be disregarded. As indicated by the trend lines, mortality gradually declined until the beginning of the penicillin era in 1946 (*arrow*), when the rate of decline in mortality increased about fourfold. In the years not represented (1984, 1985, and 1987), no deaths were reported. (*Adapted from* Massell and coworkers [6]; with permission.)

ETIOLOGY

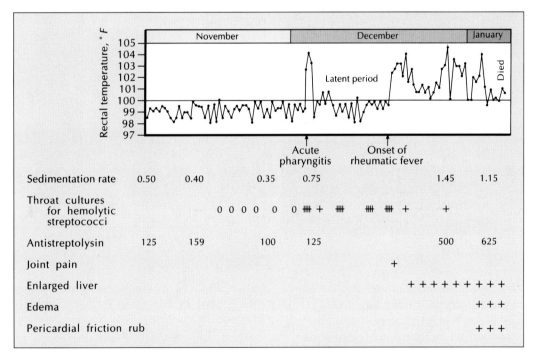

FIGURE 10-4. Clinical chart of a child who died from a severe recurrence of rheumatic fever at the House of Good Samaritan (Boston) during the prepenicillin era. This child had been convalescing quite satisfactorily from a previous attack of rheumatic fever. Despite residual rheumatic heart disease, he seemed clinically well with a normal temperature and sedimentation rate when he contracted acute pharyngitis with a sharp rise in temperature to 104°F. Frequent throat cultures that had been consistently negative for hemolytic streptococci became strongly positive for this organism. The patient soon recovered spontaneously from the pharyngitis and again seemed well even though his throat cultures remained strongly positive for hemolytic streptococci. The antistreptolysin-O titer, which had been at a low level of 100 to 125 units, subsequently rose to 500 to 625 units. Two weeks later his condition suddenly changed due to a severe recurrence of rheumatic fever that was characterized by fever, joint pain for only 1 day, a rapid sedimentation rate, congestive heart failure, pericarditis, and death about 3 weeks later. This case illustrates the etiologic role of hemolytic streptococcal throat infection in the development of recurrences of rheumatic fever, a role believed to be the same as its role in causing initial attacks of rheumatic fever. (*Adapted from* Massell and coworkers [7]; with permission.)

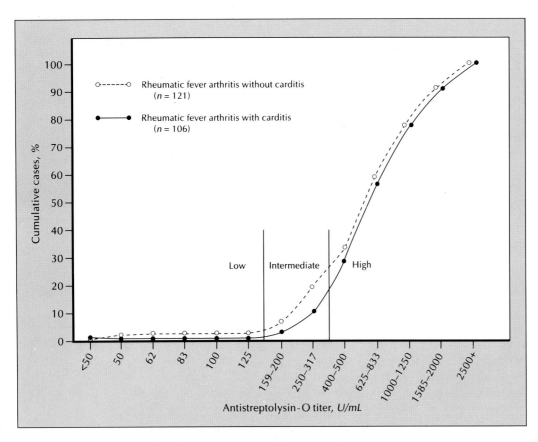

FIGURE 10-5. Distribution of the antistreptolysin-O titer in 227 patients with rheumatic fever below the age of 17 years whose symptoms included significant joint pain. Note the similar distribution curves for 106 patients who also had carditis and 121 patients who showed no signs of cardiac involvement. The antistreptolysin-O titer was definitely elevated (400 units or higher) in 89.7% of patients with carditis and in 80.9% of those with joint symptoms but no carditis. If 200 units were to be accepted as the upper limits of normal for the antistreptolysin-O titer, the corresponding figures would be 97.2% and 93.4%, respectively. The high incidence of the antistreptolysin-O titer in these patients indicates that they had a recent streptococcal infection and thus provides important support for the hemolytic streptococcus hypothesis for the etiology of rheumatic fever. (*Adapted from* Roy and coworkers [8]; with permission.)

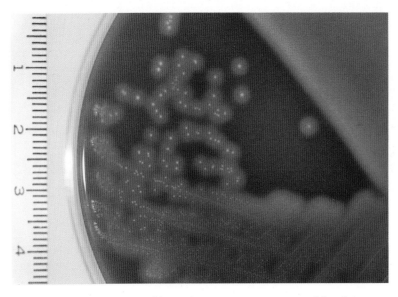

FIGURE 10-6. A culture of hemolytic streptococcus on blood agar (only part of the blood agar plate is shown). The colonies of streptococcus are surrounded by a large zone of complete hemolysis. Freshly isolated virulent group A strains usually have a large hyaluronic acid capsule and are rich in M protein. Rheumatic fever is always caused by an antecedent group A streptococcal throat infection. (Courtesy of the Bacteriology Laboratory, Children's Hospital, Boston.)

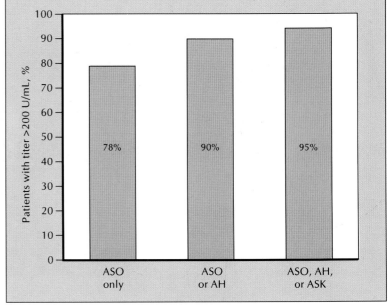

FIGURE 10-7. Three streptococcal antibodies (antistreptolysin O [ASO], antihyaluronidase [AH], and antistreptokinase [ASK]) in 88 rheumatic fever patients observed at the Irvington House (New York) within 2 months of their first symptoms. The failure of ASO to be elevated in a small number of patients with rheumatic fever (*see also* Fig. 10-5) has raised the question of whether there may be other nonstreptococcal causes of rheumatic fever. But in this study, when the ASO titer was not elevated, one or both of the other two antibody tests were usually diagnostic. The ASO titer was abnormally high in 78% of the 88 patients but at least one of the three antibodies studied was elevated in 95%. This figure approached 100% when sera for tests could be obtained earlier than 2 months from the onset of the rheumatic fever attack. (*Adapted from* Stollerman and coworkers [9]; with permission.)

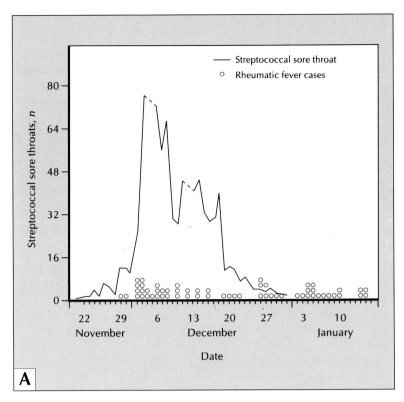

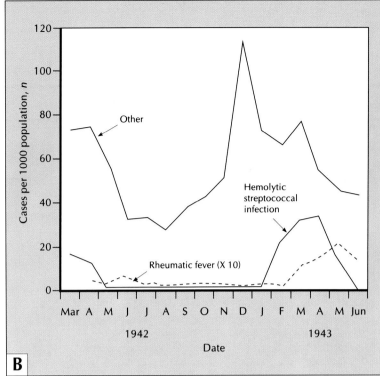

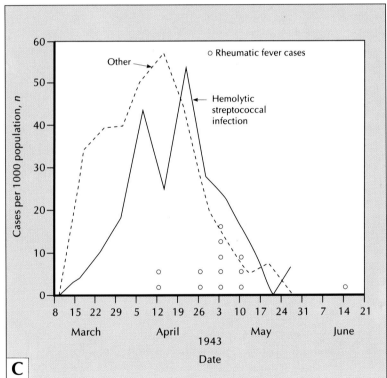

FIGURE 10-8. A, An explosive milk-borne epidemic of hemolytic streptococcal throat infection in Kölding, Denmark. Of 840 cases under medical treatment, 3.6% developed rheumatic fever after a silent latent period of 1 to 5 weeks (mostly 2 to 3 weeks). This figure shows additional cases of rheumatic fever related to streptococcal infection that were apparently not reported until rheumatic fever had developed. This is one example of many instances in which rheumatic fever has been associated with milk- and other food-borne epidemics of group A hemolytic streptococcal throat infections, epidemics of group A streptococcal throat infections in military training centers, and outbreaks of similar infection in schools, hospitals, and other closed-population groups. The frequent association of rheumatic fever with these epidemics provides important support for the hemolytic streptococcus hypothesis for the etiology of rheumatic fever. **B,** An outbreak of rheumatic fever associated with an epidemic of hemolytic streptococcal throat infections at the United States Naval Training Station in Newport, Rhode Island during World War II. Data are for the entire personnel of the center. Note that the peak for incidence of rheumatic fever follows that for streptococcal infections by about 3 to 4 weeks. **C,** Data for a single battalion of recruits within this naval training station. Note the much higher incidence of streptococcal infections among the recruits than for the station as a whole (B). (Part A *adapted from* Madsen and Kalbak [10]; parts B and C *adapted from* Massell and Jones [11]; with permission.)

RHEUMATIC MYOCARDITIS

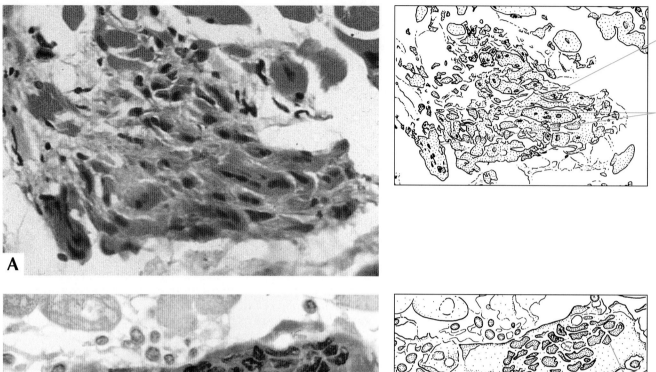

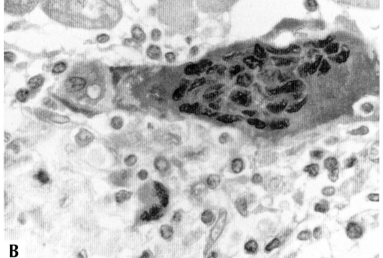

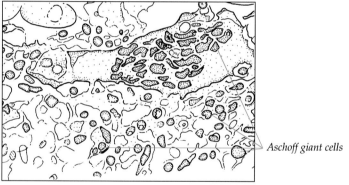

FIGURE 10-9. **A,** An Aschoff nodule in a right ventricular endomy-ocardial biopsy specimen from a 17-year-old girl with congestive heart failure due to recurrence of rheumatic fever. This fully developed Aschoff nodule (hematoxylin and eosin, × 330) has a central ill-defined area of edematous interstitial connective tissue with fraying, fragmentation, and disintegration of collagen fibers that stain deeply eosinophilic (fibrinoid necrosis). The interstitial alteration is associated with infiltration of mononuclear cells including large modified fibrohistiocytic Anitschkow's or Aschoff cells. Some of these histiocytes are multinucleated and form Aschoff giant cells. The Aschoff cells have vaguely defined borders, abundant amphophilic cytoplasm, and a large ovoid nucleus containing a large central chromatin mass. **B,** Aschoff giant cells are stained brown by immunoperoxidase staining with anti-α_1-antichy-motrypsin antibody indicating monocyte-macrophage lineage (× 500). (*continued*)

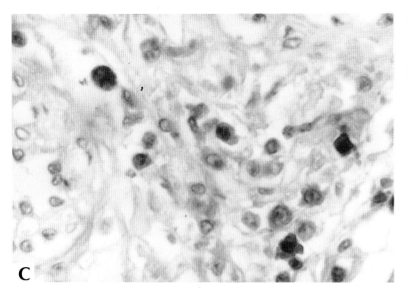

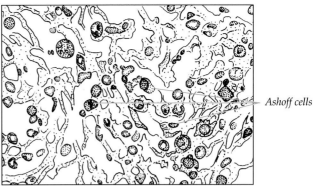

Ashoff cells

C

FIGURE 10.9 *(continued)* **C,** A similar staining pattern is seen for mononuclear Aschoff cells with anti-α_1-antitrypsin antibody ($\times 500$). The Aschoff nodules in the proliferative stage are regarded as pathognomonic of rheumatic carditis since this lesion has not been demonstrated in any other disease entity. Although they have been described almost invariably in the autopsies of patients dying of rheumatic carditis, we have observed such characteristic myocardial lesions in only 30% to 40% of biopsies of patients presenting with primary or recurrent episodes of rheumatic fever [12]. All of our patients demonstrating Aschoff nodules had overt clinical congestive heart failure. This is consistent with the higher prevalence of Aschoff nodules in autopsy material, which represents carditis severe enough to account for mortality. With time, the Aschoff bodies are eventually replaced by nondescript perivascular scars. Apart from the Aschoff lesions, a nonspecific inflammatory reaction in the edematous interstitial connective tissue is often observed. Some biopsy fragments demonstrate varying degrees of myocyte degenerative changes. Neither characteristic Aschoff nodules nor nonspecific interstitial or myocyte degeneration have been found in the biopsies from patients with chronic quiescent heart disease [12]. Also, Aschoff nodules have rarely been reported in the ventricular myocardium in autopsy specimens from patients with chronic rheumatic heart disease [13]. However, Aschoff nodules reported in left atrial appendages removed at the time of mitral valve surgery are of questionable significance. (Part A courtesy of Jagat Narula, P. Chopra, and James F. Southern, Massachusetts General Hospital, Boston and the All India Institute of Medical Sciences, New Delhi; parts B and C courtesy of James Gulizia and Bruce McManus, Cardiovascular Registry, University of Nebraska Medical Center, Omaha.)

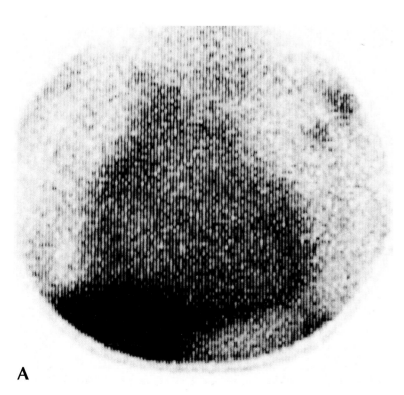

A

Antimyosin antibody uptake

Liver

FIGURE 10-10. A, Indium-111–labeled antimyosin antibody scan from an 11-year-old girl with recurrent rheumatic activity. Her clinical manifestations included congestive heart failure, pericarditis, and subcutaneous nodules, as well as mitral stenosis and mitral, aortic, and tricuspid incompetence. This planar gamma image was obtained 48 hours after intravenous injection of antimyosin Fab (R11D10-DTPA; Centocor, Malvern, PA), 500 µg, labeled with 1.8 mCi of indium-111 chloride. A diffuse uptake of antimyosin antibody in the cardiac region is consistent with active myocardial involvement. Hepatic activity reflects the normal distribution of indium-111–labeled antimyosin antibody. *(continued)*

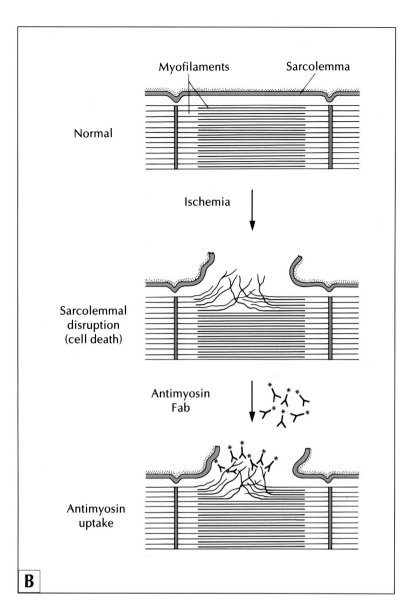

FIGURE 10.10 *(continued)* **B,** The principle of antimyosin imaging. The intact sarcolemma surrounding a normal cardiac myocyte does not permit extracellular macromolecules (such as antibody or their fragments) to enter the cells (*top*). This barrier no longer exists in injured myocytes after the loss of integrity of their sarcolemma, which exposes the intracellular contents to extracellular milieu through the breeches in the cell membrane (*middle*). An antibody specific for an intracellular protein, such as myosin, if administered intravenously, will localize at the site of myocardial sarcolemmal disruption (*bottom*). Thus if this antibody is appropriately radiolabeled, the areas of myocyte necrosis can be located by determining the areas of radioactivity. Therefore, indium-111–labeled antimyosin has been used for the noninvasive localization of acute myocardial infarction. Since myocyte degeneration may occur in active rheumatic myocarditis, indium-111– labeled antimyosin antibody can also be used for the detection of some cases of cardiac involvement in acute rheumatic fever. It should be noted, however, that antimyosin uptake in the myocardium would occur in myocyte necrosis of any cause and the diagnosis of rheumatic fever will have to be made only on the basis of other clinical findings. (Part A courtesy of Jagat Narula, Arun Malhotra, and Ban-An Khaw, All India Institute of Medicine, New Delhi and Massachusetts General Hospital, Boston; part B *adapted from* Khaw and coworkers [14]; with permission.)

RHEUMATIC PERICARDITIS

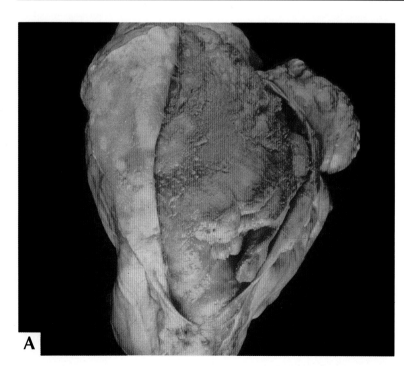

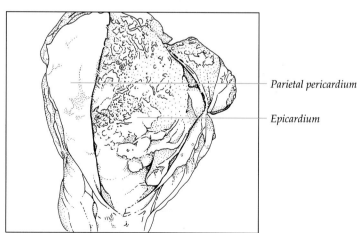

FIGURE 10-11. A, Gross pathologic specimen obtained from a patient who died of rheumatic fever. The outer, or parietal, layer of the pericardium has been partially reflected away, revealing the epicardium, which is covered with shaggy fibrinous exudate as if a butter sandwich had been pulled apart, hence the term "bread and butter pericarditis." *(continued)*

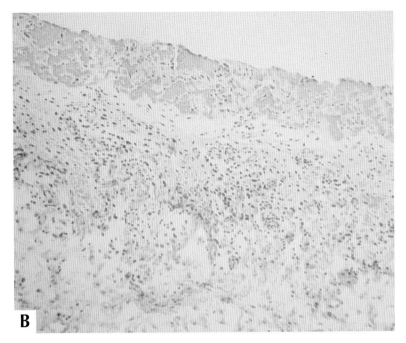

B

FIGURE 10.11 *(continued)* **B,** Photomicrograph of the pericardium from a similar case of rheumatic pericarditis showing fibrin deposits associated with a cellular infiltrate containing lymphocytes, histiocytes, and plasma cells (hematoxylin and eosin, × 100). Occasionally, characteristic Aschoff bodies may also be encountered with a pallisading arrangement of fibroblasts and Aschoff cells about the foci of fibrinoid degeneration. Rheumatic pericarditis is typically accompanied by small effusions not sufficient to result in tamponade. Although adhesions between the layers of pericardium may occur due to heavy fibrinous exudate, they usually do not result in constrictive pericarditis. (Courtesy of Jesse Edwards, Jesse E. Edwards Registry of Cardiovascular Diseases, St. Paul, MN.)

RHEUMATIC ENDOCARDITIS

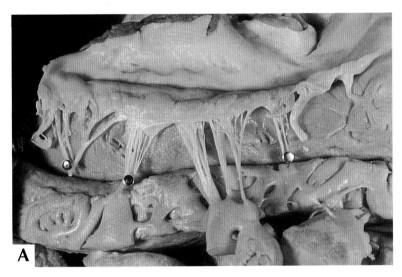

A

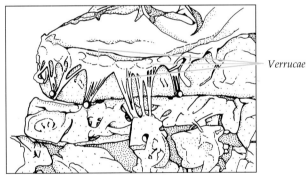

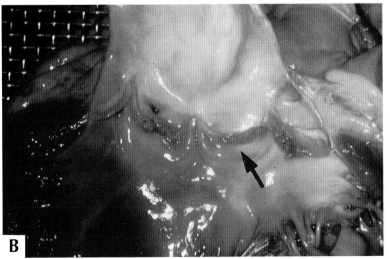

B

FIGURE 10-12. Pathologic specimens obtained at autopsy from patients who died of acute rheumatic fever. **A,** Gross appearance of the mitral valve showing characteristic tiny, wartlike verrucae or vegetations on its inflow side (atrial surface). **B,** Similar verrucae on the ventricular surface of the aortic valve *(arrow).* The verrucae are sterile and small and only rarely result in embolization (unlike vegetations of bacterial endocarditis). Reflection of light has resulted in some white shining areas; they do not represent any pathologic abnormality. *(continued)*

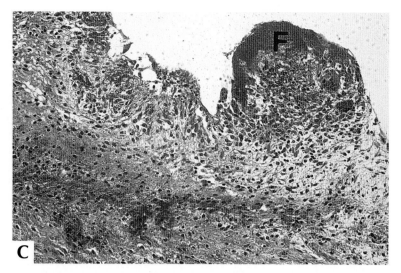

FIGURE 10.12 *(continued)* **C,** Part of mitral valve leaflet with a small thrombotic vegetation. Alteration in the collagen and fibrinoid change (F) are associated with pallisading mononuclear cell infiltration and occasional Aschoff cells at the base of the fibrinoid areas. The inflammation usually extends throughout the valve leaflet and is not limited to the endocardium. Edema, an increase in the number of capillaries, and mononuclear cell infiltration begin at the valve rings and gradually extend throughout the valve. (Courtesy of Renu Virmani, Department of Cardiovascular Pathology, Armed Forces Institute of Pathology, Washington, DC.)

DIAGNOSIS

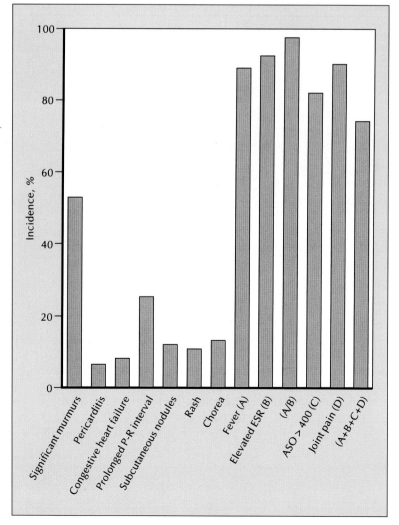

FIGURE 10-13. The various clinical and laboratory manifestations of rheumatic fever and their incidence in 457 patients observed in an initial attack at the House of Good Samaritan. Since there is no specific test for rheumatic fever, diagnosis depends on evaluation of these manifestations. The syndrome of joint pain, fever, and elevated antistreptolysin-O titer was present in 74% of all 457 patients. (*Adapted from* Massell and coworkers [15]; with permission.)

JONES CRITERIA, 1992 UPDATE

MAJOR MANIFESTATIONS
Carditis
Polyarthritis
Chorea
Erythema marginatum
Subcutaneous nodules

MINOR MANIFESTATIONS
Clinical findings
  Arthralgia
  Fever
Laboratory findings
  Elevated acute phase reactant
    Erythrocyte sedimentation rate
    C-reactive protein
  Prolonged P-R interval

SUPPORTING EVIDENCE OF STREPTOCOCCAL INFECTION
Elevated or rising streptococcal antibody titer
Positive throat culture or rapid streptococcal antigen test

FIGURE 10-14. Jones criteria, 1992 update. This is the fourth revision by the American Heart Association of criteria originally proposed by Jones in 1944. The guidelines divide the manifestations of rheumatic fever into major and minor categories. A high probability of rheumatic fever is indicated by the presence of two major manifestations, or one major and two minor manifestations supported by evidence of a preceding group A streptococcal infection, with certain exceptions (such as some cases of chorea). We think it is perhaps less complicated to consider the diagnosis of rheumatic fever when one or more of the following are present: poststreptococcal arthritis, poststreptococcal carditis, or chorea. (*Adapted from* the American Heart Association [16]; with permission.)

POSTSTREPTOCOCCAL ARTHRITIS

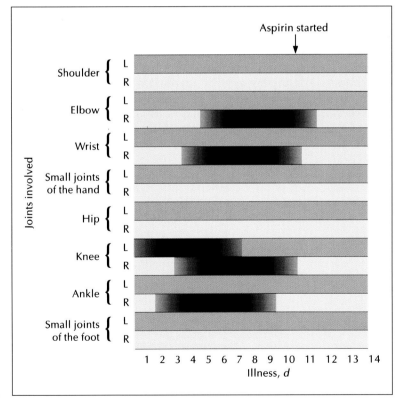

FIGURE 10-15. The time course of migratory polyarthritis of rheumatic fever. Notice that even in the absence of treatment, the involvement of each joint is short-lived, but the cumulative involvement of all joints is less so, and the arthritis rapidly responds to aspirin. Joint pain is of diagnostic importance because it is a frequent manifestation of rheumatic fever (90% of 457 initial attacks in Fig. 10-13) and because it nearly always occurs at the onset of the attack, thus calling attention to the patient's illness. It is typically a migratory polyarthritis, but in children joint symptoms are often mild. Even in these milder cases there usually has been pain in at least two joints, and examination of the patient usually reveals tenderness or other objective evidence of joint involvement. When joint symptoms are due to rheumatic fever, there nearly always is fever or a rapid sedimentation rate. There should also be evidence of a recent streptococcal infection, best indicated by a high titer of antistreptolysin-O or other antistreptococcal antibody. L—left; R—right. (*Adapted from* Taranta and Markowitz [17]; with permission.)

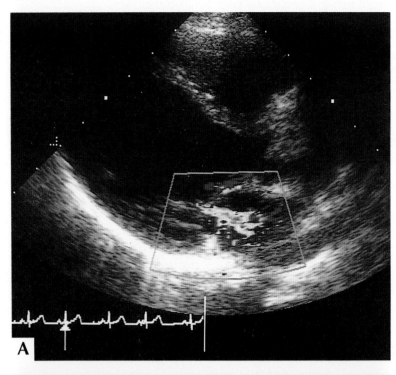

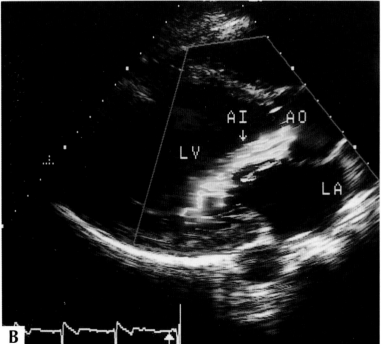

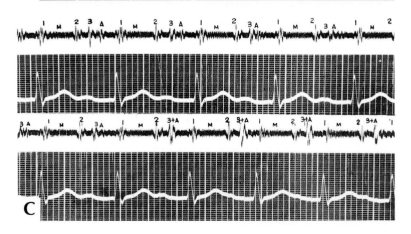

FIGURE 10-16. Endocarditis. Significant murmurs are the most common and the earliest clinical signs of carditis in acute rheumatic fever. As shown in Fig. 10-13, 240 (53%) of the 457 patients with an initial attack of rheumatic fever had significant murmurs indicative of valvular involvement. The usual early signs are mitral regurgitation alone or mitral plus aortic regurgitation. Pure aortic regurgitation is rare. Valvular stenosis never occurs early. Early endocarditis may also be detected by echocardiogram and Doppler studies. **A,** Two-dimensional echocardiogram with Doppler color flow imaging (parasternal long-axis view) obtained in a 12-year-old girl with acute rheumatic fever. Note that there is a high-velocity systolic turbulence (represented as a color mosaic on flow imaging) in the left atrium (LA) due to jet of mitral regurgitation, which is central and extends back up to half of the LA. **B,** Two-dimensional echocardiogram with Doppler color flow imaging (parasternal long-axis view) obtained in a 10-year-old boy with acute rheumatic fever. Note the high-velocity retrograde early diastolic turbulent jet of aortic insufficiency (AI; represented as a color mosaic). The AI jet is eccentric, strikes the anterior mitral leaflet, and extends beyond it. The left ventricle (LV) and LA are dilated. **C,** Simultaneously recorded phonocardiogram and electrocardiogram in a child with acute rheumatic carditis, mitral regurgitation, a mid-diastolic murmur (Carey Coombs murmur [18]), sinus arrhythmia, and a prolonged P-R interval. Upper and lower records are continuous. The acoustic effect of a mid-diastolic murmur is not uncommon in early acute rheumatic endocarditis with a systolic murmur of at least moderate intensity. It does not indicate mitral stenosis, which never occurs early. Although other explanations have been suggested, we believe it is due to a prolonged third sound that occurs during rapid inflow or a combination of a third sound and an atrial sound. This tracing shows the atrial sound either definitely separated from the third sound, immediately after the third sound, or superimposed on the third sound, depending on the duration of the diastole. A—atrial sound; M—systolic murmur; 1—first heart sound; 2—second heart sound; 3—third heart sound. (Parts A and B courtesy of L. George Veasy, Primary Children's Medical Center, The University of Utah School of Medicine, Salt Lake City; Part C *adapted from* Taquini and coworkers [19]; with permission.)

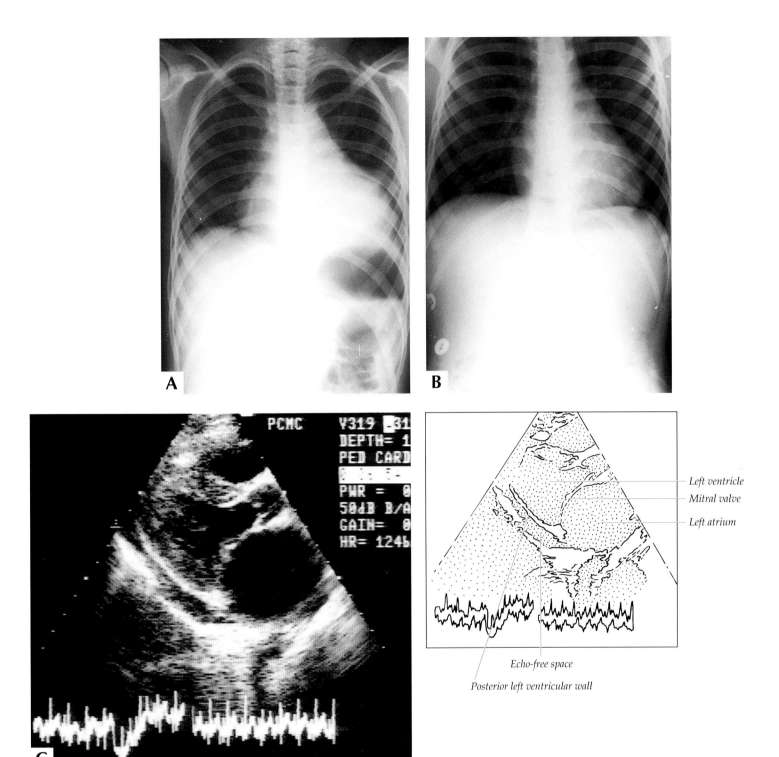

FIGURE 10-17. Pericarditis. **A,** Chest radiograph of an 11-year-old girl with severe rheumatic carditis taken soon after admission to the House of Good Samaritan (Boston). Cardiac enlargement is due mainly to pericarditis with effusion. A marked friction rub was also present. **B,** Radiograph taken after improvement, showing marked diminution in size of the cardiac silhouette. **C,** Two-dimensional echocardiogram (freeze-frame of the parasternal long-axis view) obtained in a 10-year-old boy with acute rheumatic fever. Note the echo-free space posterior to the left ventricle due to a small pericardial effusion. The left atrium is dilated. (Parts A and B *adapted from* Massell and coworkers [20]; with permission; part C is courtesy of L. George Veasy, Primary Children's Medical Center, University of Utah School of Medicine, Salt Lake City.)

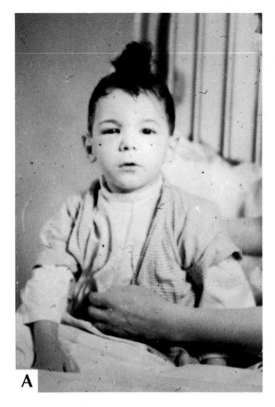
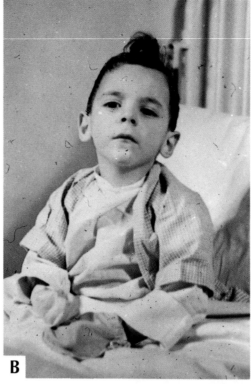

FIGURE 10-18. Congestive heart failure. A 3-year-old boy with severe rheumatic carditis showing facial swelling due to heart failure (**A**) and his appearance 48 hours after marked diuresis (**B**). In young people with rheumatic fever the development of congestive heart failure is almost always due to active rheumatic myocarditis in addition to valvular damage. Such patients always have significant murmurs and not infrequently pericarditis, indicated by the presence of friction rub. In very young children, such as this child, the first apparent change marking the development of heart failure may be swelling of the face. When the puffiness is marked, it may resemble that seen in the nephrotic syndrome. In the series of 457 patients with initial attacks of rheumatic fever (*see* Fig. 10-13), congestive heart failure developed in 7% of all 457 patients, in 15% of the 240 patients with significant murmurs, and in 46% of those with significant murmurs and pericarditis. (*Adapted from* Walsh and Sprague [21]; with permission.)

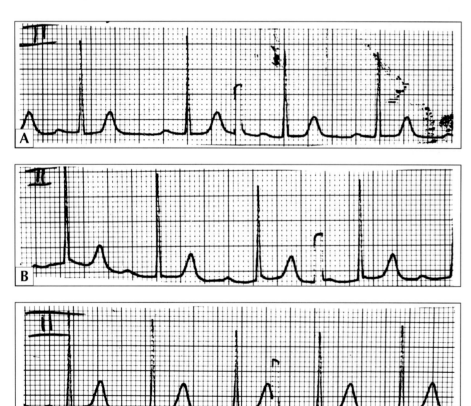

FIGURE 10-19. Prolonged P-R interval. Lead II of electrocardiograms of a patient with rheumatic fever. **A,** First tracing shows P-R interval of 0.20 s. **B,** Three days later the P-R interval prolonged to 0.26 s. **C,** Six days later it decreased to 0.22 s. In the study of the initial attack of rheumatic fever in 457 patients (*see* Fig. 10-13), a prolonged P-R interval was observed in 115 cases (25%). Since many infections and a variety of cardiac conditions may cause prolongation of the P-R interval, this finding is by no means specific for rheumatic fever. Conversely, the incidence of an abnormally long P-R interval in rheumatic fever is a great deal more common than that observed in other diseases and, therefore, this electrocardiographic manifestation has considerable importance as a confirmatory sign in the diagnosis of rheumatic fever. From the data in Fig. 10-13, it is evident that prolongation of the P-R interval was approximately as common in patients without significant murmurs (24% of 217 patients) as in those with significant murmurs (26% of 240 patients). Therefore, this manifestation has no apparent prognostic significance with regard to the development of valvular damage. (Courtesy of L. George Veasy, Primary Children's Medical Center, University of Utah School of Medicine, Salt Lake City.)

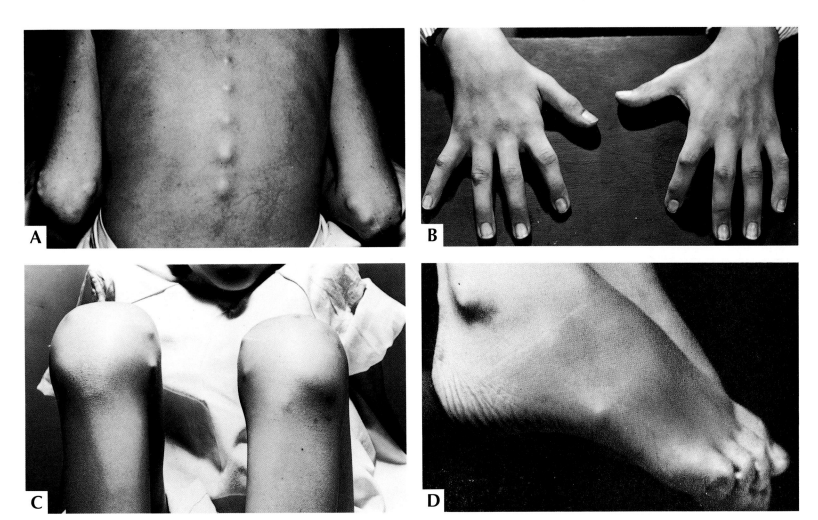

FIGURE 10-20. Subcutaneous nodules on the spine and elbows (**A**), proximal interphalangeal joints (**B**), medial condyles of the tibia (**C**), and lateral malleolus and outer aspect of the foot (**D**). Subcutaneous nodules, which are a sign of severe rheumatic fever, are nontender subcutaneous nodular structures located most commonly over bony prominences such as the olecranon process and lateral condyles of the elbow, the edge of the patella, the tips of the spinous processes over the back, and the occiput. They sometimes are attached to tendons such as the flexor tendons of the palm. They vary in number from one or two to many and they usually vary in size from that of a small seed to that of an almond. They are not attached to the underlying bone. Unless looked for they are easily missed. Nodules that are clinically indis-

tinguishable from those of rheumatic fever may occur in rheumatoid arthritis, but nodules of rheumatoid arthritis are almost always seen in adults whereas those of rheumatic fever are generally confined to children. When nodules develop in patients with rheumatic fever, they usually do not appear until 3 weeks or longer after onset of the attack. Therefore, they are not helpful in making an early diagnosis but are an important confirmatory sign. In the 457 initial attacks shown in Fig. 10-13, nodules were present in 12%, but in 240 patients with significant murmurs the incidence was 20%. Twenty-nine (91%) of 54 patients with nodules also had significant murmurs. When nodules are multiple, valvular involvement is almost invariable. (*Adapted from* Massell and coworkers [20] and Massell [22]; with permission.)

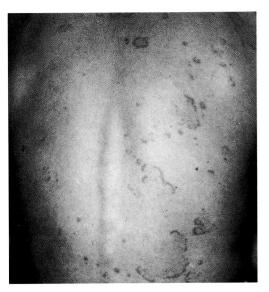

FIGURE 10-21. Erythema marginatum on the back of a patient with acute rheumatic fever. Erythema marginatum is an evanescent, pink, or faintly red, circinate, nonitching rash that occurs on various parts of the body but practically never on the face. The colored margins are usually thin and the clear centers relatively large. The lesions, which are quite variable in size and number, are usually macular but, when extensive, may be very slightly papular. The rash may be seen at one time but not at another, only to return later. For this reason, the incidence of erythema marginatum depends to some extent on the care and frequency with which the patient is examined. Like nodules, erythema marginatum is a useful confirmatory sign of rheumatic fever. This rash has some prognostic significance but not to the same extent as subcutaneous nodules. Thus in the series of patients in Fig. 10-13, the incidence of significant murmurs indicative of valvular involvement was 69% in patients with this rash compared with 53% for the entire series of 457 patients. To some extent, erythema marginatum and subcutaneous nodules tend to be correlated with each other. Thus the incidence of erythema marginatum was 26% in the 54 patients with nodules compared with 11% in the entire group of 457 patients. Similarly, the incidence of nodules in 48 patients with erythema marginatum was 29% compared with a 12% incidence in the total group of 457 patients. (*Adapted from* Massell [22]; with permission.)

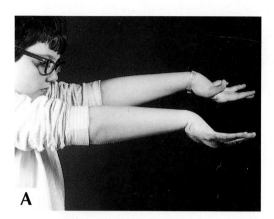

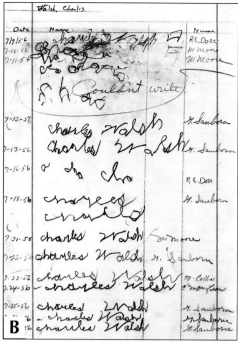

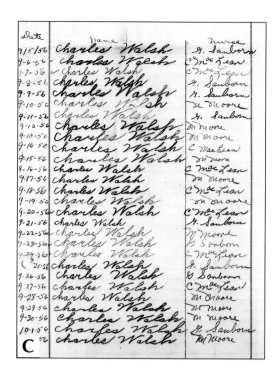

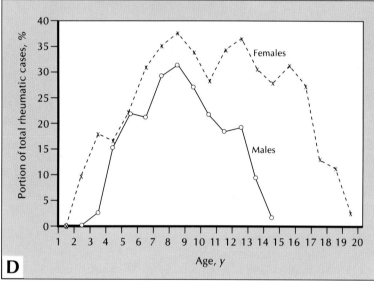

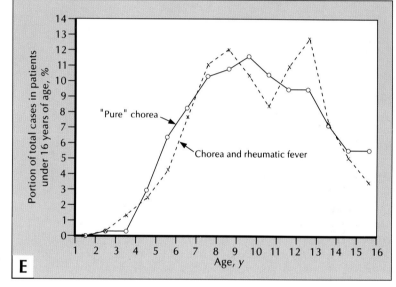

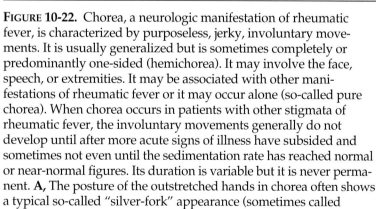

FIGURE 10-22. Chorea, a neurologic manifestation of rheumatic fever, is characterized by purposeless, jerky, involuntary movements. It is usually generalized but is sometimes completely or predominantly one-sided (hemichorea). It may involve the face, speech, or extremities. It may be associated with other manifestations of rheumatic fever or it may occur alone (so-called pure chorea). When chorea occurs in patients with other stigmata of rheumatic fever, the involuntary movements generally do not develop until after more acute signs of illness have subsided and sometimes not even until the sedimentation rate has reached normal or near-normal figures. Its duration is variable but it is never permanent. **A,** The posture of the outstretched hands in chorea often shows a typical so-called "silver-fork" appearance (sometimes called

"spooning"). **B,** Handwriting in a patient with severe chorea. **C,** Handwriting in the same patient after recovery. Keeping a record of handwriting is a good objective way to follow the progress of patients with chorea. Chorea is usually confined to childhood and is rarely seen long after adolescence. Statistics from the medical literature show this condition to be more common in girls than boys. **D,** This sex difference is due largely to a more rapid decrease in the incidence in boys after adolescence than in girls. Chorea in either sex is extremely rare after the age of 20 years. Pure chorea is always or nearly always due to rheumatic fever. **E,** Evidence for this conclusion is the similar age distribution of patients with pure chorea compared with those with chorea and other manifestations of rheumatic fever. (Parts B and C *adapted from* Massell [22]; with permission.)

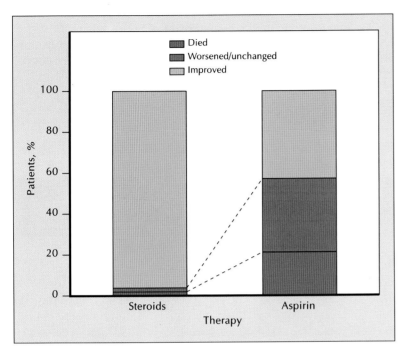

FIGURE 10-23. Results of therapy with aspirin or adrenocorticosteroids in 95 patients with severe rheumatic carditis. Of these 95 patients admitted to the House of Good Samaritan (Boston) with acute rheumatic fever and congestive heart failure, 42 patients were treated with aspirin and 53 with steroids. The death rate was markedly lower and the recovery rate significantly faster and greater in the steroid-treated group. Furthermore, no patients developed a pericardial friction rub while on steroids. Worsening of congestive heart failure also occurred much more rarely during steroid therapy. Steroids were more effective than aspirin regardless of concomitant penicillin therapy or whether the admission was for an initial or recurrent attack of rheumatic carditis. Failure of the demonstration of superiority of steroids by some other studies can be explained by the inclusion of mildly symptomatic cases. Steroids in large doses are the treatment of choice in severe rheumatic carditis with congestive heart failure or pericarditis. In fact, steroids may be life-saving in very ill patients. However, there is no agreement as to whether steroids will prevent or lessen the valve damage. (*Adapted from* Czoniczer and coworkers [23]; with permission.)

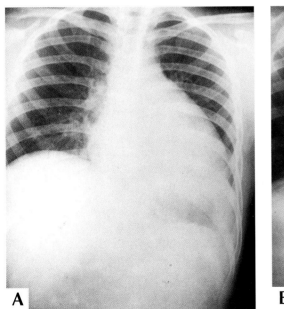
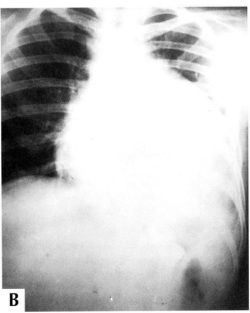
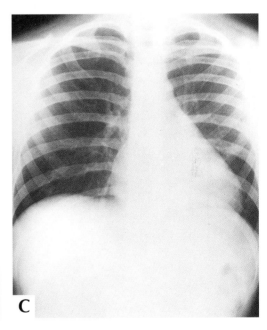

FIGURE 10-24. Chest radiographs showing the change in size of cardiac silhouette in a girl with rheumatic pericarditis. **A,** Radiograph taken soon after the onset of rheumatic fever. **B,** Radiograph taken 8 days later while the patient was being treated with aspirin. Heart size is obviously larger, presumably due to pericardial effusion. There also was a loud to-and-fro pericardial friction rub. Treatment was changed to cortisone. **C,** Radiograph taken after another 8 days shows a striking diminution in heart size. The friction rub had almost disappeared. As illustrated here, although effective in suppressing the polyarthritis of rheumatic fever, aspirin has no appreciable effect on pericarditis. Adrenocorticotropic hormone (ACTH) and other adrenocortical hormones (*eg,* cortisone, prednisone) have a much more potent anti-inflammatory effect than aspirin and are especially useful in the treatment of severe rheumatic carditis. The diminution in heart size shown in Fig. 10-17*B* was due to treatment with ACTH.

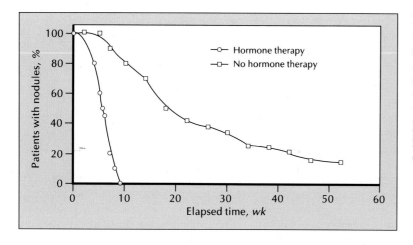

FIGURE 10-25. Duration of subcutaneous nodules in rheumatic fever patients treated with adrenocorticotropic hormone, cortisone, or other adrenocortical hormones compared with the duration in patients not so treated. These two groups may not be entirely comparable because most of those not given hormones were observed at the House of Good Samaritan (Boston) prior to 1949 when hormone therapy was first used at this hospital. Nevertheless, the difference in duration of nodules is striking and is consistent with other evidence for the highly suppressive effect of the hormones on the rheumatic inflammatory process.

PREVENTION AND PROGNOSIS

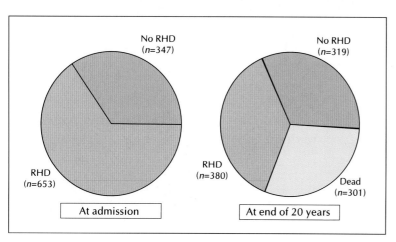

FIGURE 10-26. Prognosis of rheumatic fever and rheumatic carditis prior to the use of penicillin and adrenocorticosteroids. Data are from a 20-year follow-up study of 1000 patients with rheumatic fever and rheumatic heart disease who were admitted to the House of Good Samaritan (Boston) between 1921 and 1931 and who were 20 years of age or less at the time of admission. On admission, 653 (65%) patients were classified as having rheumatic heart disease and 347 (35%) as having no cardiac involvement. By the end of 20 years, 301 patients had died, nearly all of whom initially had rheumatic heart disease. This poor prognosis contrasts strikingly with the good prognosis after penicillin use began in 1945, when there was a marked decrease in mortality and a marked increase in disappearance of murmurs. (*Data from* Bland and Jones [24]; with permission.)

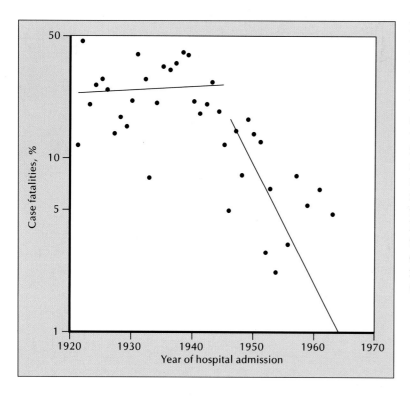

FIGURE 10-27. Case fatality rates for rheumatic carditis in patients who were 15 years old or younger at the time of admission to the House of Good Samaritan (Boston) from 1921 to 1970 and who were followed up for 5 years. Fitted trend lines are superimposed on the annual values. Note that the ordinate is logarithmic. From 1921 to 1945 there was a fluctuating pattern with little overall trend and a great deal of year-to-year variation, apparently due to variation in the incidence of rheumatic fever recurrences, a major factor in mortality. An abrupt change occurred in 1946 when a rapid decline in the case fatality rate began with an average annual decrease of 13.2%. There were no deaths in 1955, 1958, or 1960 and none after 1963. This decline started after penicillin began to be used in 1945 both for prophylaxis and treatment of recognized hemolytic streptococcal throat infections. It may be pertinent that the year 1946, the beginning of the decline of mortality at the House of Good Samaritan, is also the year when the decline in national mortality from rheumatic fever accelerated fourfold (*see* Fig. 10-3). (*Adapted from* Massell and coworkers [6]; with permission.)

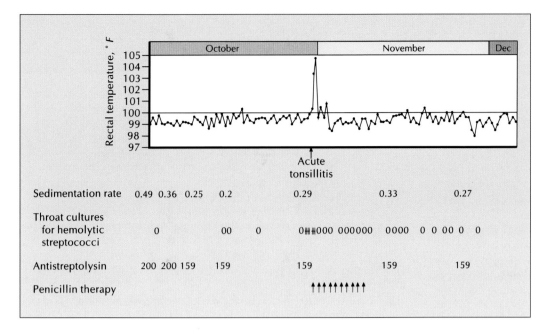

FIGURE 10-28. Clinical chart of a patient similar to that of the patient in Fig. 10-4. This patient also developed a hemolytic streptococcal throat infection but was treated orally with penicillin for 10 days. The throat culture, which was strongly positive for hemolytic streptococci, became negative and remained negative even after penicillin was discontinued. The anti-streptolysin-O titer showed no increase in level, and the patient remained well without any evidence of active rheumatic fever. This patient is from the original study [25] of 1948, which first demonstrated that rheumatic fever can be prevented by the eradication of the hemolytic streptococcus from the throat flora at the time of streptococcal infection. This observation also provides important confirmatory evidence for the hemolytic streptococcus hypothesis for the etiology of rheumatic fever. (*Adapted from* Massell and coworkers [7]; with permission.)

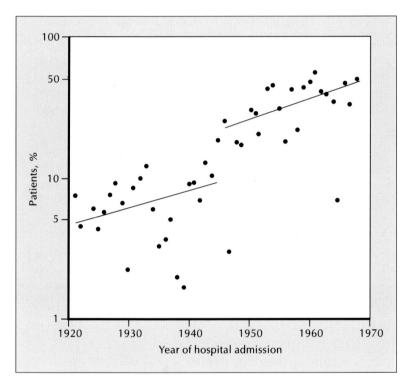

FIGURE 10-29. Proportion of patients with rheumatic carditis in whom all murmurs disappeared during follow-up. Plotted points are for the year of admission to the House of the Good Samaritan (Boston). There is no point for 1923 because none of the patients with carditis admitted in that year lost their murmurs. Trend lines are fitted separately for 1921 to 1945 and 1945 to 1970. Note that the ordinate is logarithmic. Before 1945 the rate at which murmurs disappeared was low and variable with an average rate of 3%. In 1946 there was a jump of 143% in the probability of resolution of a murmur. By 1970 the probability that significant murmurs in children hospitalized with active rheumatic carditis would subsequently disappear exceeded 40%. This favorable change beginning in 1945 seems to be related to the prevention of recurrences of rheumatic fever through the use of penicillin. (*Adapted from* Massell and coworkers [6]; with permission.)

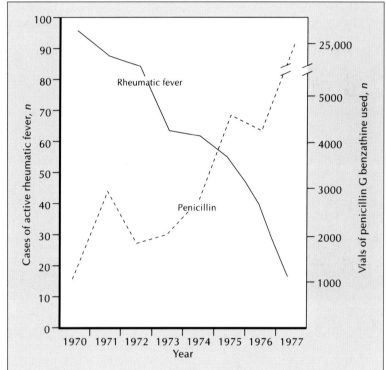

FIGURE 10-30. Number of patient admissions with rheumatic fever compared with the number of vials of benzathine penicillin G used for treatment of patients with sore throats in National Children Hospital in San Jose, Costa Rica. National Children Hospital catered to a population of 6 to 9 million during the study period (1970 to 1977), and treated liberally with penicillin all patients in whom a sore throat was clinically suspected to be of streptococcal origin. Laboratory confirmation of the diagnosis was not required. It is evident that with a progressive increase in the use of penicillin, there was a constant decrease in the number of rheumatic fever patients admitted to the hospital. (*Adapted from* Nelson and Mohs [26]; with permission.)

REFERENCES

1. Armstrong DB, Wheatley GM, eds: *Studies in Rheumatic Fever*. New York: Metropolitan Life Insurance Company; 1944:2.

2. Veasy LG, Wiedmeier SE, Orsmond GS, *et al.*: Resurgence of rheumatic fever in the intermountain area of the United States. *N Engl J Med* 1987, 316:421-427.

3. Veasy LG, Tani LY, Hill HR: Persistence of acute rheumatic fever in the intermountain area of the United States. *J Pediatr* 1994, 124:9–16.

4. Stollerman GH: Rheumatogenic group A streptococci and the return of rheumatic fever. *Adv Intern Med* 1990, 35:1–26.

5. Ferguson GW, Schultz JM, Bisno AL: Epidemiology of acute rheumatic fever in a multi-ethnic, multi-racial US urban community. *J Infect Dis* 1991, 164:720–725.

6. Massell BF, Chute CG, Walker AM, *et al.*: Penicillin and the marked decrease in morbidity and mortality from rheumatic fever in the United States. *N Engl J Med* 1988, 318:280-286

7. Massell BF, Sturgis GP, Knobloch JD, *et al.*: Prevention of rheumatic fever by prompt penicillin therapy of hemolytic streptococcic respiratory infections: progress report. *JAMA* 1951, 146:1469–1474.

8. Roy SB, Sturgis GP, Massell BF: Application of the antistreptolysin-O titer in the evaluation of joint pain and in the diagnosis of rheumatic fever. *N Engl J Med* 1956, 254:95–102.

9. Stollerman GH, Lewis AJ, Schultz I, *et al.*: Relationship of immune response to group A streptococci to the course of acute, chronic and recurrent rheumatic fever. *Am J Med* 1956, 20:163–169.

10. Madsen TH, Kalbak K: Investigations on rheumatic fever subsequent to some epidemics of septic sore throat (especially milk epidemics). *Acta Pathol Microbiol Scand* 1940, 17:305–327.

11. Massell BF, Jones TD: *Studies in Rheumatic Fever*. Edited by Armstrong DB, Wheatley GM. New York: Metropolitan Life Insurance Company; 1944:11.

12. Narula J, Chopra P, Talwar KK, *et al.*: Does endomyocardial biopsy aid in the diagnosis of active rheumatic carditis? *Circulation* 1993, 88:2198–2205.

13. Roberts WC, Virmani R: Aschoff bodies at necropsy in valvular heart disease: evidence from an analysis of 543 patients over 14 years of age that rheumatic heart disease, at least anatomically, is a disease of mitral valve. *Circulation* 1978, 57:803–807.

14. Khaw BA, Homcy CH, Fallon JT, *et al.*: Irreversible ischemic injury in anoxiccultured myocytes: demonstration by cell sorting with anti-myosin-fluorescent beads and scanning electron microscopy. In: *Cardiology*. Edited by Chazov EI, Smirnov VN, Oganov RG. New York: Plenum Publishing Corporation, 1984:1135–1147.

15. Massell BF, Fyler DC, Roy SB: The clinical picture of rheumatic fever. *Am J Cardiol* 1958, 1:436–449.

16. Special Writing Group of the Committee on Rheumatic Fever, Endocarditis, and Kawasaki Disease of the Council on Cardiovascular Disease in the Young, American Heart Association: Guidelines for the diagnosis of rheumatic fever: Jones' criteria 1992 update. *JAMA* 1992, 268:2069–2073.

17. Taranta A, Markowitz M: *Rheumatic Fever*, ed 2. London: Kluwer Academic Publishers; 1989.

18. Coombs CF: *Rheumatic Heart Disease*. New York: William Woods and Company; 1924:190–191.

19. Taquini AC, Massell BF, Walsh BJ: Phonocardiographic studies of early rheumatic mitral disease. *Am Heart J* 1940, 20:295–303.

20. Massell BF, Warren J, Sturgis G, *et al.*: The clinical response of rheumatic fever and acute carditis to ACTH. *N Engl J Med* 1950, 242:641–647.

21. Walsh BJ, Sprague HB: Characteristics of congestive heart failure in children with acute rheumatic fever. *Am J Dis Child* 1941, 61:1003–1011.

22. Massell BF: The diagnosis and treatment of rheumatic fever and rheumatic carditis. *Med Clin North Am* 1958, 42:1343–1360.

23. Czoniczer G, Amezcua F, Pelargonio S, *et al.*: Therapy of severe rheumatic carditis: comparison of adrenocortical steroids and aspirin. *Circulation* 1964, 29:813–819.

24. Bland EF, Jones TD: Rheumatic fever and rheumatic heart disease: a twenty-year report on 1000 patients followed since childhood. *Circulation* 1951, 4:836–843.

25. Massell BF, Dow JW, Jones TD: Orally administered penicillin in patients with rheumatic fever. *JAMA* 1948, 138:1030–1035.

26. Nelson JD, Mohs EA: Socioeconomic and behavioral residua of antibiotic therapy in infancy and childhood. In *New Trends in Antibiotics*. Edited by Geraldoroni GG, Sabath LD. New York: Elsevier/North Holland Biomedical Press; 1981:247–254.

EXPERIMENTAL CARDIOMYOPATHIES

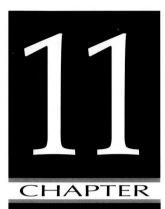

CHAPTER

Judith K. Gwathmey

What attributes should an animal model of human heart disease possess? It should mimic the disease state in humans without causing additional unrelated multisystemic disease. Ideally, the model should be reproducible and easily made without toxic risk to the investigator. There are naturally occurring models of heart failure in companion and domestic animals that mimic many of the clinical signs noted in humans. There are also experimentally induced models of heart failure in several animal species. Although all models, including those of spontaneous dilated cardiomyopathy, result in clinical heart failure, it is unclear whether similar pathophysiologic changes are shared between species and animal models. Differences have been demonstrated in contractile response to changes in frequency of stimulation, extracellular calcium concentrations, and receptor stimulation. Furthermore, differences reside at the level of the contractile proteins and intracellular calcium concentrations. Histopathologically, there are differences in myocytolysis, cellular hypertrophy, and the connective tissue matrix. With these differences in mind, investigators must carefully address the aspects of human heart failure that they are interested in studying and must determine whether experimental findings can be extrapolated to humans.

There is clinical overlap between veterinary medical cardiology and clinical cardiology. In this series of illustrations, we present primarily large animal models of heart failure, which demonstrate clinical presentations similar to those seen in humans. Despite varying causes, the end results of myocardial damage are often dilated cardiomyopathy and congestive heart failure. The goal of this series is to present several clinical syndromes seen in domestic and companion animals that share similarities with human disease. Therefore, diseases common to both humans as well as to the species reported have been selected. The use of large animal models for human disease provides the opportunity for monitoring hemodynamic changes using both noninvasive and invasive techniques. In addition, experimental findings in large animals may more closely reflect diseases seen in humans. Presented are postmortem findings, histopathologic findings, angiograms, radiographs, ventriculograms, and echocardiograms. By providing these selected examples, it is hoped that the reader will gain sufficient background knowledge of available animal models of human heart failure.

CATS

DISTINGUISHING CLINICAL FEATURES

TYPE OF CAT	INCIDENCE OF HCM, n/n(%)
Domestic shorthair	21/31(67.7)
Domestic longhair	9/31(29)

CLINICAL FEATURE	INCIDENCE, n(%)
Male:female ratio (% male)	6.75(87.1)
Murmur cardiac apex	13(41.9)
Diastolic gallop rhythm	12(38.7)
Ventricular premature beats	11(35.5)
Left axis deviation	8(25.8)

FIGURE 11-1. Distinguishing clinical features of hypertrophic cardiomyopathy (HCM) in cats. HCM appears to occur commonly in related cats, similar to human HCM. HCM has therefore been considered to be familial in domestic shorthair cats; however, linkage analysis has not been performed, unlike for human cases of the disorder. Similar to human disease, there is a significantly shortened life span in cats. The animals sometimes die of progressive left ventricular heart failure, but they die most commonly from atrial thromboemboli. HCM in cats has been considered primarily to be a model of diastolic dysfunction, again similar to human disease. Human dilated HCM is associated with sudden death that is sometimes preceded by syncope. As demonstrated here and in the following illustrations, there is considerable overlap in the manifestations of feline HCM and the disorder in humans. Values presented are based on analysis of clinical data from 73 cats during a period of 3.5 years. The diagnosis was made by nonselective angiography. Thirty-one cats had HCM. (*Adapted from* Harpster [1]; with permission.)

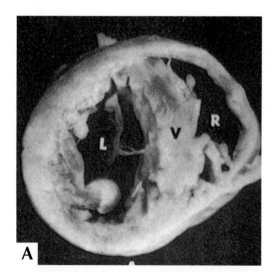

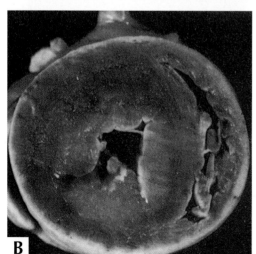

FIGURE 11-2. Gross pathology of feline hypertrophic cardiomyopathy in transverse sections. **A,** Normal heart of an 8-year-old male domestic shorthair cat. **B,** Symmetric hypertrophic cardiomyopathy in a 9-year-old domestic shorthair cat. Uniform hypertrophy of the left ventricular free wall, papillary muscles, and ventricular septum resulted in narrowing of the left ventricular cavity. L—left ventricular cavity; R—right ventricular cavity; V—ventricular septum. (*Adapted from* Liu [2]; with permission.)

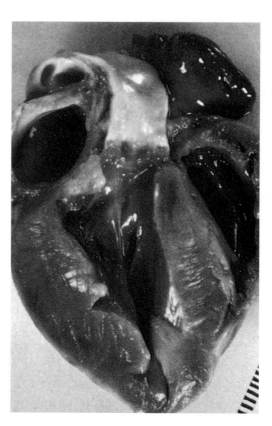

FIGURE 11-3. Gross pathology of feline hypertrophic cardiomyopathy in the heart of a 5-year-old male domestic shorthair cat with symmetric hypertrophic cardiomyopathy. As in Fig. 11-2, hypertrophy of the left ventricular free wall, papillary muscles, and ventricular septum resulted in narrowing of the left ventricular cavity. (*Adapted from* Liu [2]; with permission.)

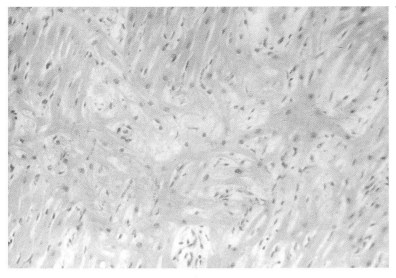

FIGURE 11-4. Histopathologic characteristics of hypertrophic cardiomyopathy in cats. Low-power magnification of microscopic fiber disarray in a case of feline hypertrophic cardiomyopathy in a domestic shorthair cat. A pathognomonic sign of hypertrophic cardiomyopathy is fiber disarray, the clinical significance of which is unknown. It is thought that the fiber disarray reflects mutations in the DNA encoding β-cardiac myosin heavy chain. Linkage analysis has suggested that chromosome 14 may be involved and is linked to the myosin locus, suggesting that myosin defects cause hypertrophic cardiomyopathy.

M-MODE ECHOCARDIOGRAPHY

FINDING	HCM	MEAN±SD NORMAL	RANGE
LVFW thickness, *cm*	0.92	0.37±0.08	0.32–0.56
LVIDd, *cm*	1.0	1.51±0.21	1.12–2.18
LVIDs, *cm*	0.2	0.69±0.22	0.64–1.68
FS, %	80	55.0±10.2	23–56
HW/BW	0.0073±0.0023	0.0042±0.006	—

FIGURE 11-5. Results of M-mode echocardiography of cats with hypertrophic cardiomyopathy (HCM). The incidence of HCM in domestic shorthair cats is high, followed by domestic longhair cats. Persians may be predisposed. The disorder is rare in Siamese, Burmese, and Abyssinian cats, which tend to be predisposed to dilated cardiomyopathy. Male cats are more commonly affected than females, representing 23% to 87% of reported cases. A familial genetic basis has been suggested. Calcium channel blockers have been beneficial in the treatment of HCM. FS—fractional shortening; HW/BW—heart weight: body weight ratio; LVFW—left ventricular free wall; LVIDd—left ventricular diastolic internal dimension; LVIDs—left ventricular systolic internal dimension.

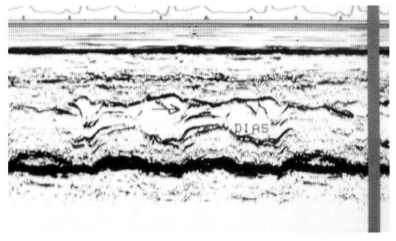

FIGURE 11-6. M-mode echocardiogram of hypertrophic cardiomyopathy in cats shows hypertrophy of the left ventricle and interventricular septum as well as systolic motion of the anterior mitral valve (*arrow*).

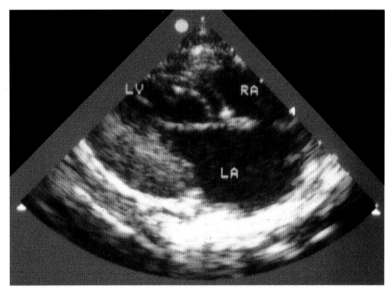

FIGURE 11-7. This two-dimensional echocardiogram of feline hypertrophic cardiomyopathy shows asymmetric hypertrophy of the left ventricular (LV) free wall with normal septal thickness and dilatation of the left atrium (LA). RA—right atrium.

DOGS

DISTINGUISHING CLINICAL FEATURES

High incidence in Boxer and Doberman Pinscher breeds

Etiology unknown

S_3 gallop

Irregular cardiac rhythm

Atrioventricular valve insufficiency murmur

Syncope

Hepatosplenomegaly or ascites

Dyspnea and cough

FIGURE 11-8. Distinguishing clinical features of canine dilated cardiomyopathy. Dogs with dilated cardiomyopathy generally develop the disorder at 1 to 2 years of age, thereby shortening their life spans. As demonstrated here and in the following illustrations, these clinical features in dogs closely mimic those of the disorder in humans. The incidence of dilated cardiomyopathy is particularly high in boxers and Doberman pinschers. (*Adapted from* Ware and Bonagura [3]; with permission.)

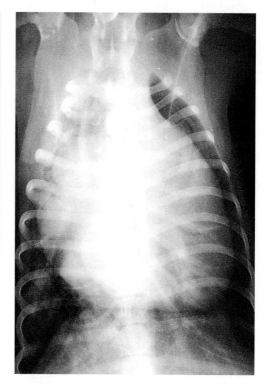

FIGURE 11-9. Dilated cardiomyopathy in Doberman Pinschers. Doberman Pinschers have a high incidence of idiopathic dilated cardiomyopathy accompanied by high mortality. A genetic basis has been suggested. This chest radiograph of a Doberman pinscher with dilated cardiomyopathy demonstrates generalized cardiomegaly, pulmonary venous congestion, and pulmonary interstitial and alveolar edema.

M-MODE ECHOCARDIOGRAPHY

	NORMAL	CARDIOMYOPATHY
LVIDd, *mm*	46.8±4.16	57.6±10.9*
LVIDs, *mm*	30.8±3.31	46.9±11.84*
LVFW thickness, *mm*	14.1±0.84	10.1±1.1*
FS, %	34.2±1.81	18.3±5.91*

FIGURE 11-10. M-mode echocardiographic measurements in 21 clinically normal and 26 cardiomyopathic Doberman pinschers. Mean ± SD of the left ventricular diastolic internal dimension (LVIDd) and the systolic dimension (LVIDs) as well as left ventricular free wall (LVFW) thickness at systole. Fractional shortening (FS) was calculated as (LVIDd-LVIDs/LVIDd × 100). *Asterisks* indicate $P < 0.0001$. These data demonstrate the marked cardiac dilatation with cardiac chamber enlargement and associated reduced systolic performance. These echocardiography-determined parameters of cardiac dilatation and impaired contractile function (*ie*, reduced wall thickening during systole and enlarged end-systolic dimension) are similar to findings in humans with dilated cardiomyopathy. (*Adapted from* Calvert and Brown [4]; with permission.)

CARDIAC CATHETERIZATION DATA (MEAN VALUE ± 1 SD)

	PA, *mm Hg*	PCWP, *mm Hg*	LVEDP, *mm Hg*	LVESP, *mm Hg*	LVESV, *mL*	LVEDV, *mL*	LVEF, %
Dobermans (*n*=16)	25/12±7/4	10±3	13±7	126±18	50±14	79±19	0.38±0.11
Mongrels (*n*=12)	29/15±4/4	13±8	14±5	150±22*	31±12*	77±20	0.63±0.09*

*$P < 0.01$.

FIGURE 11-11. Cardiac catheterization data for 16 Doberman pinschers with dilated cardiomyopathy compared with 12 healthy mongrels. This study demonstrated that clinically healthy Doberman pinschers can have left ventricular dysfunction. Subjects were weight-matched. LVEDP—left ventricular end-diastolic pressure; LVEDV—left ventricular end-diastolic volume; LVEF—left ventricular end-systolic fraction; LVESP—left ventricular endsystolic pressure; LVESV—left ventricular end-systolic volume; PA—pulmonary artery pressure; PCWP—pulmonary capillary wedge pressure. (*Adapted from* Smucker and coworkers [5]; with permission.)

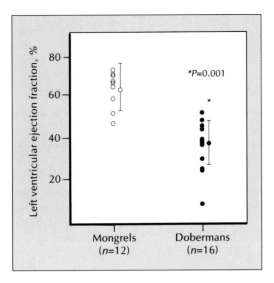

FIGURE 11-12. Cineangiographic left ventricular ejection fraction in Doberman pinschers compared with mongrels. Dobermans had a lower mean ejection fraction, which reflects impaired systolic function as a result of cardiac chamber enlargement and reduced myocardial contractility. Studies of myocardial tissue homogenates have demonstrated an imbalance between calcium cycling activity and energy supply, which have been proposed to result in the reduced myocardial contractility. (*Adapted from* Smucker and coworkers [5]; with permission.)

TURKEYS

IDIOPATHIC DILATED CARDIOMYOPATHY IN TURKEY POULTS

	LVFWth, *mm*	LVvol, *mL*	EJECTION FRACTION, %	SYSTOLIC BP, *mm Hg*
Control	5.8±0.4	1.0±0.1	67±5	128±5.8
IDCM	3.9±1.0*	7.7±3.7*	42±4*	66±10.5*

FIGURE 11-13. Idiopathic dilated cardiomyopathy (IDCM) in turkey poults compared with control animals. In this illustration, *in vitro* left ventricular free wall thickness (LVFWth) as well as left ventricular volume (LVvol) with the heart arrested in diastole are shown. *In vivo* ejection fraction (EF) was calculated as LVEDV-LVESV/LVEDV. Peak systolic blood pressure (BP) was measured using a transcutaneous Doppler technique. *Asterisks* indicate a significant difference from control animal measurements. (*Adapted from* Gwathmey and Hajjar [6] and Gruver and coworkers [7]; with permission.)

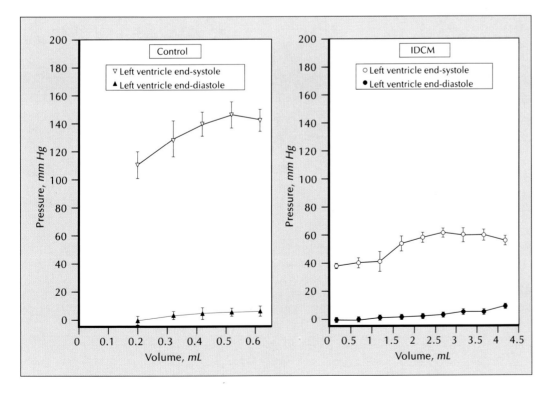

FIGURE 11-14. Pressure-volume relationship in cases of idiopathic dilated cardiomyopathy (IDCM) in turkey poults (*right*) compared with controls (*left*). Approximately 20% of the poults studied developed detectable IDCM by 14 days of age. Hearts were Langendorff perfused at 83 mm Hg pressure. A latex balloon was placed in the left ventricle for recording of pressure. The volume of the balloon was incrementally increased until there was no further increase in systolic pressure. Experiments were performed at 41°C. *In vitro* heart rates were the same for both groups. Markedly depressed maximal pressure is evident in the IDCM hearts. The occurrence of idiopathic IDCM in poults seems to be different from the genetic inbred type documented in turkey poults. (*Adapted from* Gwathmey and Hajjar [6] and Gruver and coworkers [7]; with permission.)

VIRAL AND PROTOZOAN MYOCARDITIS AND CARDIOMYOPATHY

PARVOVIRUS MYOCARDITIS IN DOGS

CLINICAL AND POSTMORTEM FINDINGS

High incidence in 4- to 8-week-old puppies

Necrotizing infection

Sudden death

Milder forms heart failure, arrhythmias, death at 19 weeks
    to 6 months of age

Chronic myocarditis, cardiomegaly, pleural effusion,
    ascites, systolic murmurs, gallops, and arrhythmias

Histopathology

    Mostly left ventricle affected

    Diffuse infiltrates of lymphocytes and plasma cells

    Interstitial fibrosis

    Degenerative changes in myocytes

    Basophilic intranuclear inclusion bodies

FIGURE 11-15. Clinical and postmortem findings of parvovirus myocarditis in dogs. Except for parvovirus myocarditis, clinically significant myocarditis caused by other viruses is rare in dogs. Parvovirus myocarditis is encountered most commonly in 4- to 8-week-old puppies. As demonstrated in the following illustrations, cellular infiltration occurs, leading to dilated cardiomyopathy. This necrotizing infection has an acute clinical onset and causes sudden death. The clinical syndrome in dogs is similar to that noted in infants and young children with myocarditis. Milder forms of parvovirus myocarditis in dogs cause arrhythmias and heart failure, which more closely resemble myocarditis in adult humans. Diagnosis can be made in dogs by serologic and histologic tests; in humans serologic tests can be used. Infection in adult humans is mild or asymptomatic; however, arthralgia, especially in women, is a well-known sequela of infection. Erythropoietic effects of parvovirus infection are likely to be clinically unrecognized except in patients with secondary hemolytic anemia and immunosuppressed hosts.

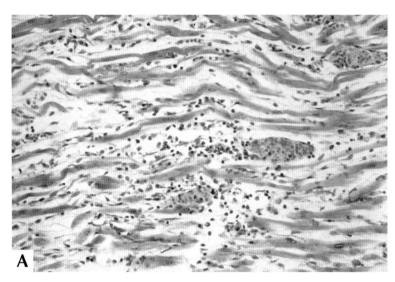

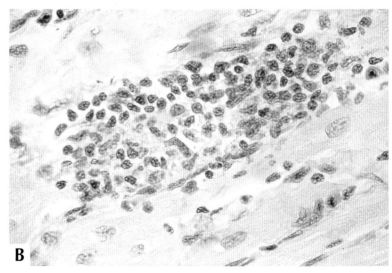

FIGURE 11-16. Histopathology of parvovirus myocarditis. A, Low-power magnification of the myocardium of a 3-week-old Collie with myocarditis secondary to canine parvovirus infection. Note the myocardial necrosis with muscle fraying, and cellular infiltrates. B, High-power histologic section of the myocardium of a 3-week-old collie with myocarditis secondary to canine parvovirus infection. Note the severe myocytolysis and mononuclear cellular infiltrates.

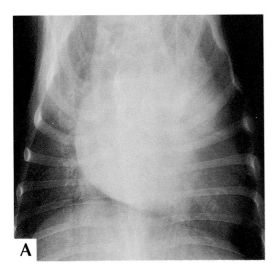
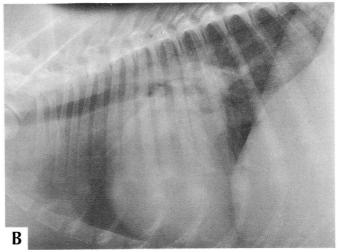

FIGURE 11-17. Dorsoventral (**A**) and lateral (**B**) radiographs of a dog with post-parvovirus myocarditis. Note the enlargement of the heart, which is a common radiographic finding in dogs with the disorder, and the presence of pulmonary edema.

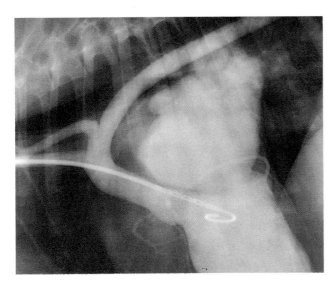

FIGURE 11-18. Ventriculogram of the left atrium and left ventricle of a dog with postparvovirus myocarditis. The angiogram demonstrates severe dilatation of the left atrium and left ventricle as well as mitral regurgitation.

MYOCARDITIS IN SWINE

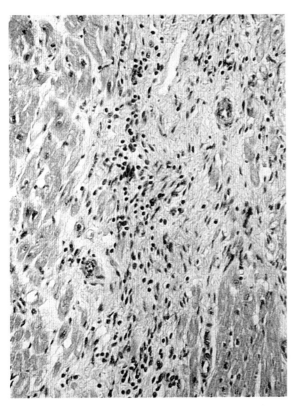

FIGURE 11-19. A significant number of human patients who present within 1 month of developing symptoms of heart failure without coronary disease have been found to have myocarditis. A large percentage of cases of idiopathic dilated cardiomyopathy is thought to have viral origins. It is therefore important for a large animal model to demonstrate histopathologic features and a natural history similar to that of humans. The existence of such a model would allow diagnostic techniques, such as endomyocardial biopsy and gallium imaging, to be tested in the setting of known disease. Such a model may be found associated with the encephalomyocarditis virus, which is myotrophic in the hearts of swine. This virus has also been known to produce epidemic outbreaks in swine herds. Encephalomyocarditis is rare in humans. This illustration depicts histopathologic findings of early myocarditis 5 days after infection with encephalomyocarditis virus; myocardial fibrosis and interstitial infiltration with mononuclear cells are demonstrated (hematoxylin and eosin, × 40). (*Adapted from* Gwathmey and coworkers [8]; with permission.)

PREVALENCE OF ELECTROCARDIOGRAPHIC ABNORMALITIES IN PIGS INFECTED WITH ENCEPHALOMYOCARDITIS VIRUS

	PREVALENCE, %
T-wave inversions in two or more leads	76
Premature ventricular complexes	60
Supraventricular tachycardia	24

FIGURE 11-20. Prevalence of electrocardiographic abnormalities in swine infected with encephalomyocarditis virus. One or more abnormalities were present in all infected animals (eight females, 18 males). Perhaps one of the most serious clinical consequences of encephalomyocarditis virus in swine is arrhythmia, which can result in sudden death. Animals often demonstrate runs of supraventricular tachycardia that can progress to ventricular fibrillation. This large animal model similarly demonstrates early nonspecific T-wave inversions, which are often seen in humans. Nonspecific arrhythmias similar to those reported in humans are associated with viral infections in these animals. A higher mortality is also associated with the ocurrence of ventricular arrhythmias in this model of dilated cardiomyopathy. Histopathologic study of the myocardium often demonstrates pyknosis and diffuse eosinophilia of the Purkinje fiber system. (*Adapted from* Gwathmey and coworkers [8]; with permission.)

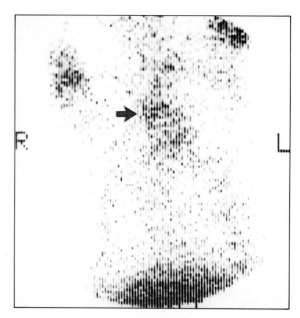

FIGURE 11-21. Gallium imaging for encephalomyocarditis virus in swine. A pig was experimentally infected with encephalomyocarditis virus. Five days after infection, the pig was lightly sedated and scanned with an Elscint Apex 410 gamma camera (72 hours post 6 mCi intravenous gallium-67 nitrate). Anterior-posterior, posterior-anterior, oblique, and lateral images were obtained. Pigs that are positive for myocardial inflammation on histologic examination may be negative on gallium scan. There appears to be a window of approximately 5 days after infection in which a positive gallium image can be obtained. *Arrow* denotes positive gallium scan for myocardial inflammation. Later gallium scans (*ie*, longer durations after infection) may be negative despite positive histologic documentation of myocarditis. (*Adapted from* Gwathmey and coworkers [8]; with permission.)

MURINE MODEL OF MYOCARDITIS

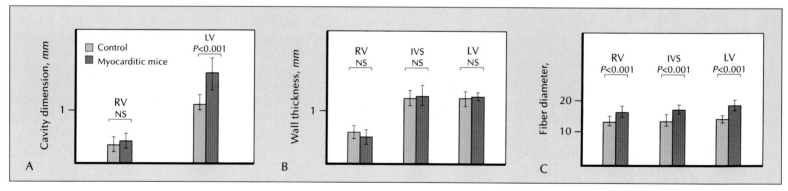

FIGURE 11-22. Myocarditis caused by coxsackievirus B is a well-recognized clinical problem in humans; encephalomyocarditis (EMC) virus infection in mice closely resembles this disease. In the experiment reflected in this illustration, DBA/2 mice were inoculated intraperitoneally with the M variant of the EMC virus and were observed for 90 days. At the end of the 90-day period, cavity dimension (**A**) and wall thickness (**B**) in 11 mice with myocarditis were measured and compared with the values in 20 control mice. The cavity dimension of the left ventricle (LV) was larger in infected mice than in controls; however, wall thickness did not differ from controls. Myocyte diameters

(**C**) were significantly larger in the right ventricle (RV), LV, and interventricular septum (IVS), thereby reflecting hypertrophy. Values are mean ±SD. In addition to pigs and mice, EMC-induced myocarditis also occurs in baboons, African green monkeys, and squirrel monkeys, but because the disorder is not pathogenetic in humans, it is a good experimental model. In mice, there is a strain-dependent occurrence of acute myocarditis with associated heart failure as well as a strain-dependent chronic myocarditis; this type of myocarditis results in dilated cardiomyopathy in the absence of active myocarditis and inflammation. NS–not significant. (*Adapted from* Matsumori and Kawai [9]; with permission.)

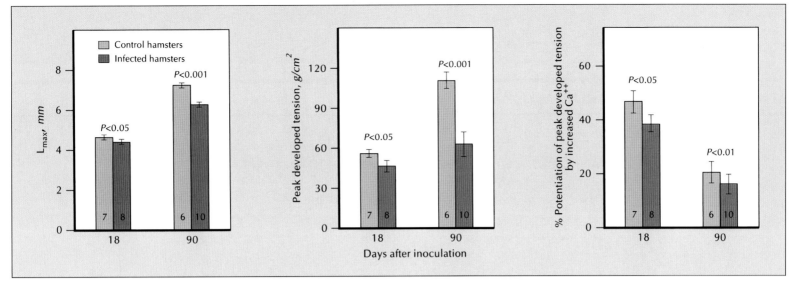

FIGURE 11-23. Coxsackievirus has been shown experimentally to induce myocarditis and cardiac failure. In this illustration, coxsackievirus B3 was originally isolated from a human with coxsackievirus infection and was serially propagated in cultures of Vero (African green monkey kidney) cells. Syrian golden hamsters were inoculated intraperitoneally with 10^6 placque-forming units of virus. Muscle mechanics were evaluated at 18 and 90 days after inoculation. Left ventricular trabeculae carneae were isolated and studied in temperature-regulated baths of $32.0\pm0.1°C$. The trabeculae carneae were stimulated to contract isometrically once every 4 seconds with a biphasic stimulus of 6-ms duration set at 10% above threshold. The infected hamsters had a shorter muscle length and developed less force at the point of maximal contractile activation as a result of stretching (L_{max}). Addition of external calcium increased peak twitch force, but the potentiation was less in the muscles of the infected group. The number of experiments is shown in each bar. Histologic changes and myocardial fibrosis were absent in the subjects of the study; therefore, this experiment clearly demonstrates that contractile abnormalities from coxsackievirus do occur despite the absence of histologic changes. (*Adapted from* Adesanya and coworkers [10]; with permission.)

CHAGAS' DISEASE IN DOGS

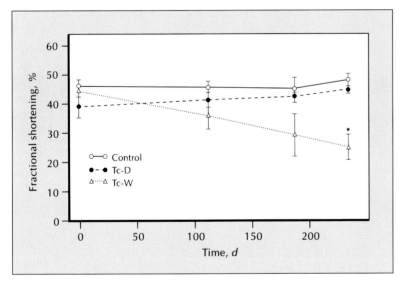

FIGURE 11-24. Chagas' disease is widespread in Central and South America and commonly affects young people (*see* Chapter 8). This form of cardiomyopathy starts as acute myocarditis that is often clinically undetected and may later be followed by progressive dilated cardiomyopathy. No effective vaccine is yet available. Dogs have also been found to have Chagas' disease. In this illustration, the mean (±SEM) change in the percentage of fractional shortening from each dog group, as measured from M-mode echocardiograms, was taken from the inoculation date (day 0) to 237 days after inoculation for control dogs, dogs inoculated with a canine *Trypanosoma cruzi* isolate (Tc-D), and dogs inoculated with wild *T. cruzi* isolate (Tc-W). Control, $n=4$; Tc-D, $n=6$; Tc-W, $n=8$. *Asterisk* indicates $P < 0.05$ compared with control values. All Tc-D–inoculated dogs fulfilled the criteria for the indeterminate stage. In other words, these dogs were serologically positive for *T. cruzi*; had parasitemia; and had minimal clinical, electrocardiographic, or echocardiographic abnormalities. A small percentage of humans in the indeterminate stage of disease develop a chronic form; however, none of the Tc-D–inoculated dogs developed chronic disease. All the Tc-W–inoculated dogs that survived the acute phase developed premature ventricular contractions, which became multiform and progressed to ventricular tachycardia. In Tc-W–inoculated dogs that developed chronic disease, the percentage of left ventricular ejection fraction and fractional shortening also decreased. These changes occurred late in the study and coincided with hypokinesis and decreases in left ventricular free wall thickness. Tc-W–inoculated dogs developed electrocardiographic, anatomic, and functional cardiac abnormalities during chronic disease that were similar to the abnormalities seen in humans with *T. cruzi*–induced heart disease. This model may represent a valuable animal model for the study of aspects of chronic *T. cruzi*–induced heart disease in humans, particularly chronic cardiac dilatation. (*Adapted from* Barr and coworkers [11]; with permission.)

ETHANOL-INDUCED CARDIOMYOPATHY IN TURKEYS

ETHANOL-INDUCED DILATED CARDIOMYOPATHY IN TURKEY POULTS

	CONTROL	ETHANOL
Body weight, *kg*	2.99±0.52	2.68±0.52
HW/BW, *g/kg*	3.88±0.27	4.92±1.34*
LVEDD, *mm/kg*	3.3±0.5	4.7±0.7*
LVESD, *mm/kg*	0.6±0.2	2.2±0.5*

FIGURE 11-25. Birds have been used extensively in developmental biology studies. Furthermore, birds have afforded investigators the opportunity to observe naturally occurring disease as well as to develop several models of human disease. Such diseases include alcohol-induced dilated cardiomyopathy, atherosclerosis, hypertension with dissecting aneurysm, cardiomyopathy induced by such drugs as doxorubicin and furazolidone, dietary deficiencies, and spontaneous idiopathic dilated cardiomyopathy. Presented in the following illustrations are discussions of two turkey models of dilated cardiomyopathy: alcohol-induced and furazolidone-induced dilated cardiomyopathy. These two syndromes in turkeys share many of the functional and biochemical deficits demonstrated in failing human hearts and class IV heart failure. Alcohol-induced cardiomyopathy is induced in turkey poults with 5% ethanol. This is one of the earliest and few animal models of alcohol-induced cardiomyopathy that clearly demonstrates heart failure. Beginning at 1 day of age and continuing until 56 days of age, turkeys were randomized into a control group (*n*=115) and an ethanol group (*n*=86). Turkeys that received ethanol demonstrated cardiac dilatation and congestive heart failure. Ultrastructural features included accumulation of glycogen, swollen mitochondria, myofibrillar lysis, increased number of lysosomes, and dilated sarcoplasmic reticulum. In these birds, arachidonic acid content was significantly decreased, as was linolic and linoleic acid content in the triglycerides. These alterations in myocardial phospholipid and fatty acid composition have been implicated in the electrophysiologic and functional derangements of the left ventricle. In humans, alcohol-induced cardiomyopathy has long been recognized. *Asterisks* indicate $P < 0.01$. HW/BW—heart weight/body weight ratio; LVEDD—left ventricular end-diastolic diameter; LVESD—left ventricular end-systolic diameter. (*Adapted from* Noren and coworkers [12]; with permission.)

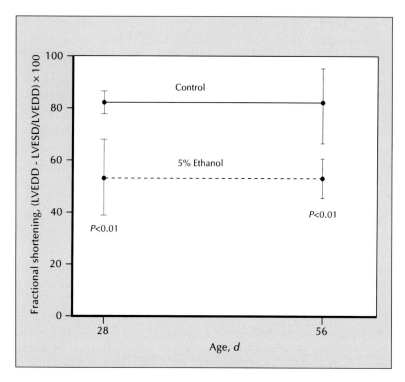

FIGURE 11-26. Results of echocardiograms at 28 and 56 days in ethanol-treated and control birds comparing fractional shortening between the two groups (calculated as [LVEDD-LVESD/LVEDD] × 100). Results are mean±SD. LVEDD—left ventricular end-diastolic diameter; LVESD—left ventricular end-systolic diameter. (*Adapted from* Noren and coworkers [12]; with permission.)

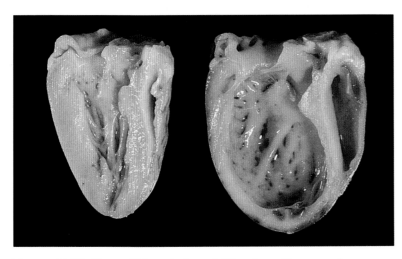

FIGURE 11-27. Furazolidone-induced dilated cardiomyopathy (Fz-DCM) in turkey poults demonstrated functional and biochemical abnormalities including decreased peak left ventricular pressure and peak systolic systemic blood pressure, reduced fractional shortening and ejection fractions, increased end-diastolic volume, tachycardia, and high mortality. Furazolidone, a nitrofuran, is an

antifungal and coccidiostat that is used as a growth promoter in turkeys. It is similarly used in humans to treat gastrointestinal tract pathogens including *Escherichia coli*, staphylococci, *Salmonella*, *Shigella*, *Proteus*, *Aerobacter aerogenes*, *Vibrio cholerae*, and *Giardia lamblia*. The agent is well tolerated in humans and has a low incidence of adverse reactions (*ie*, hypersensitivity). As occurs in human myocardium during Fz-DCM, there is a significant reduction in myofibril protein content, myofibrillar adenosine triphosphatase activity, and creatine kinase activity in the turkey model. This model has both the energy deficits and abnormal calcium mobilization (*ie*, impaired sarcoplasmic reticulum function) that are seen in end-stage heart failure in humans. Fz-DCM in turkeys has been shown to be responsive to β-receptor blocking agents. Turkeys can be handled easily during experiments, and echocardiograms and transcutaneous Doppler blood pressure can be obtained without the use of chemical restraint. This illustration shows a formalin-fixed, age-matched control heart (*left*) and a heart from a bird that received furazolidone in feed for 2 weeks (*right*). Note the enlarged right and left ventricles and the thin walls. (*Adapted from* Hajjar and coworkers [13]; with permission.)

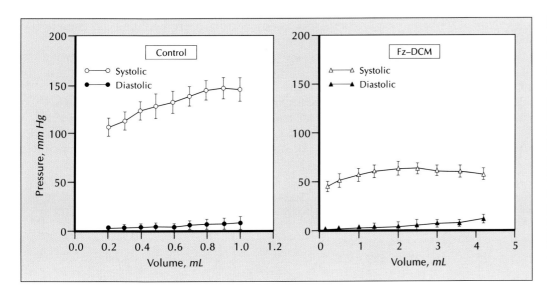

FIGURE 11-28. Pressure-volume relationship in furazolidone-induced dilated cardiomyopathy (Fz-DCM) as demonstrated in turkey poults. Hearts of controls and turkeys with Fz-DCM were Langendorff perfused at 83 mm Hg pressure. A latex balloon was placed in the left ventricle to record pressure. The volume of the balloon was incrementally increased until the systolic pressure reached a peak. Experiments were performed at 41°C. No difference between the *in vitro* heart rates of both groups was found; however, a blunted pressure-volume relationship in cardiomyopathic hearts was noted. (*Adapted from* Hajjar and coworkers [13]; with permission.)

FUNCTIONAL *IN VIVO* PARAMETERS

	LVIDd, mm	LVIDs, mm	FRACTIONAL SHORTENING, %	SYSTOLIC BP, mm Hg
Control	7.4±0.5	2.8±0.4	62.3±3.7	134±6
Fz-DCM	18.2±0.3*	16.6±0.7*	8.7±1.2*	67±14*

FIGURE 11-29. Functional *in vivo* parameters in furazolidone-induced dilated cardiomyopathy (Fz-DCM) in turkey poults. Echocardiographic long-axis parasternal views were obtained using a 7.5-MHz transducer on unsedated and hooded birds that were resting. Echocardiographically determined left ventricular internal dimension in diastole (LVIDd) and systole (LVIDs) are shown. Also shown are fractional shortening (FS), which was calculated as LVIDd-LVIDs/LVIDd × 100 and peak systolic blood pressure (BP), which was determined with a transcutaneous Doppler technique. *Asterisks* indicate a significant difference (*P* < 0.05) compared with controls. (*Adapted from* Hajjar and coworkers [13]; with permission.)

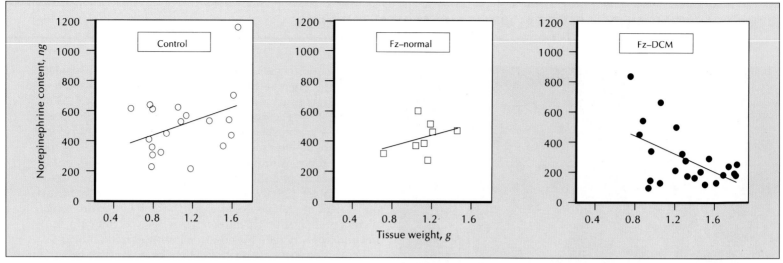

FIGURE 11-30. Norepinephrine content in furazolidone-induced dilated cardiomyopathy (Fz-DCM) in turkey poults. Avian myocardium has been used to facilitate study of basic cardiac physiology as well as calcium handling. Although it has been recognized that excessive catecholamine release occurs during heart failure and myocardial depletion of norepinephrine stores, it is not clear whether these adaptive changes (ie, elevated circulating catecholamines and depleted myocardial content) are in response to the heart failing or are causally related to the heart failure. After 2 weeks of Fz, approximately 78% of the birds had echocardiographically discernible heart failure. There was, however, a group of birds with borderline impairment of cardiac function. This illustration compares myocardial norepinephrine content (determined in myocardial samples from the left ventricle) in the hearts of control birds as well as Fz-treated birds with and without overt Fz-DCM. Fz had been added to the feed of treated animals for 14 days before the experiment. *Regression lines* illustrate group relationships between tissue weight and norepinephrine content; statistical analysis demonstrates a highly significant difference between this relationship in control and Fz-treated birds (P=0.0037). Despite the larger tissue samples from the myopathic birds, cardiac norepinephrine content was markedly reduced in these birds (-42%). Both left ventricle weight and cardiac norepinephrine content in Fz-treated birds with borderline impairment of cardiac function were similar to values obtained in controls. Moreover, the relationship between tissue weight and norepinephrine content also differed between normal and myopathic birds. In both control and Fz-treated birds with mild cardiac dysfunction, norepinephrine content was positively correlated to tissue weight while in Fz-DCM birds it was inversely related. Because of the intergroup difference in the relationship between norepinephrine content and tissue weight, comparisons of myocardial norepinephrine concentrations (ng/g) between normal and myopathic birds should not be performed. These data demonstrate that myocardial tissue hypertrophies with the development of the cardiomyopathic state in a manner independent of tissue norepinephrine content. The discordance between the ratio of myocardial norepinephrine to tissue weight is not a uniform index of cardiac norepinephrine storage in normal and myopathic hearts and should therefore be avoided. (*Adapted from* Hajjar and coworkers [13]; with permission.)

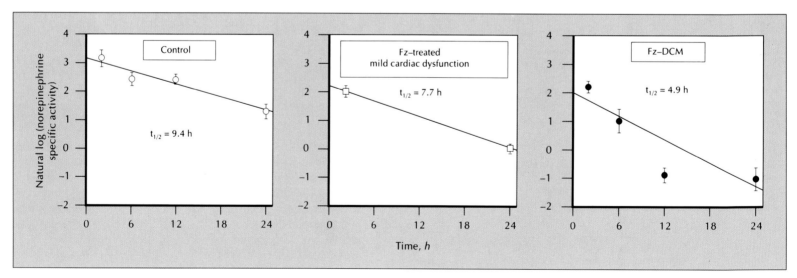

FIGURE 11-31. A comparison of norepinephrine turnover in the hearts of turkey poults with mild cardiac dysfunction and furazolidone-induced dilated cardiomyopathy (Fz-DCM) compared with control birds. Fz was added to the feed of treated birds for 14 days before norepinephrine injection. Data are plotted as mean±SD for specific activity of [³H] norepinephrine turnover from four to six animals in each group at 6-hour intervals. Fractional norepinephrine turnover was 7.4±1.4% and 14.0±2.4% per hour (P=0.03) for control and cardiomyopathic birds, respectively. Fractional turnover was 9.0±1.1% per hour in Fz-treated birds without gross cardiac dysfunction and did not differ radically from control birds. These studies demonstrate that the failing heart has increased adrenergic activity despite having depleted myocardial norepinephrine stores. Furthermore, with mild cardiac dysfunction there is normal norepinephrine turnover and myocardial norepinephrine content. Therefore, it is unlikely that increased sympathetic drive resulted in the contractile failure seen in this model. (*Adapted from* Hajjar and coworkers [13]; with permission.)

CHARACTERISTIC FINDINGS

Ascites
Hepatomegaly and congestion
Heart pallor and dilatation
Vacuolization and loss of myofibrils

FIGURE 11-32. The pathologic findings associated with doxorubicin-induced cardiomyopathy in swine. Chronic administration of doxorubicin in swine results in cardiotoxicity. Affected animals demonstrate classic signs of biventricular heart failure. Unlike the situation in dogs, heart failure through doxorubicin administration is easily induced in swine. Doxorubicin toxicity is also well recognized in humans and often results in congestive heart failure.

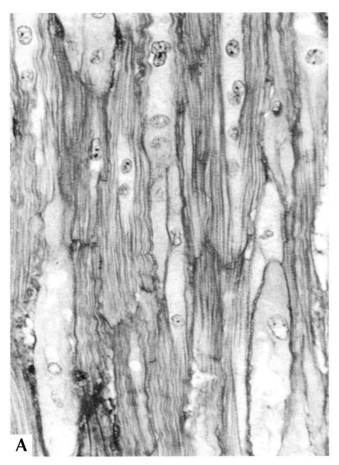

A

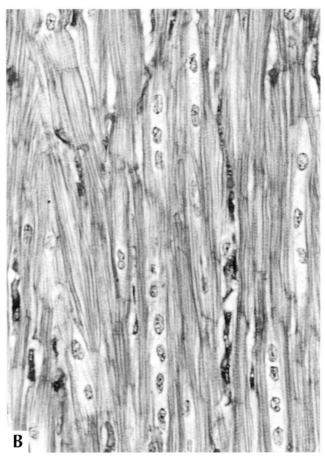

B

FIGURE 11-33. Doxorubicin, which is a valuable therapeutic agent against a variety of neoplasms, has been shown to induce cardiac lesions in rabbits, dogs, rats, and humans in addition to swine. Thirteen miniature swine received intravenous injections of 2.4 mg/kg of doxorubicin once a week for 3 weeks [14]. As shown in this illustration, animals had vacuolization and marked loss of myofibrils. Lesions were detected as early as 17 days after doxorubicin administration. **A,** Myocardium stained with alkaline toluidine blue from a pig treated with doxorubicin. **B,** Myocardium of a pig treated with doxorubicin and 12.5 mg/kg of ICRF-187 intraperitoneally. ICRF-187 is an agent reported to reduce the chronic cardiac toxicity seen with doxorubicin. Two of six pigs treated with doxorubicin alone died, and all six pigs demonstrated cardiac lesions. None of the seven pigs that received ICRF-187 died; five of the seven demonstrated cardiac lesions. (*Adapted from* Herman and Ferrans [14]; with permission.)

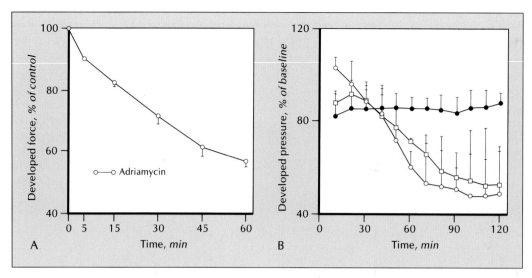

FIGURE 11-34. Doxorubicin-induced myocardial dysfunction *in vitro*. Doxorubicin (Adriamycin; Sigma, St. Louis, MO) cardiotoxicity is cumulative in dogs and humans. In humans, there is an acute effect followed by a chronic effect. In this illustration, the effect of acute administration of doxorubicin to the superfusate of isolated muscles and the perfusate of isolated Langendorff perfused hearts is demonstrated. Male Sprague-Dawley rats were decapitated, and the hearts were quickly removed. Hearts were used for isolated papillary muscle studies in temperature-regulated baths. The hearts were electrically stimulated to contract, and the effects of doxorubicin (100 μM) on developed force in isolated papillary muscles are shown (**A**). Values are mean±SE of five to seven experiments. Whole hearts were studied with Langendorff whole-heart perfusion techniques, and the effects of doxorubicin on left ventricular pressure in those hearts are shown (**B**). Points represent mean±SD for three to five hearts in each group. Untreated hearts are represented by *closed circles*; doxorubicin, 10 μM, is represented by *open boxes*; and doxorubicin, 20 μM, by *open circles*. Beginning at 60 minutes, the doxorubicin-treated group showed significantly decreased peak left ventricular pressure compared with the control group. Doxorubicin significantly decreased myocardial contractility in both experimental preparations (*ie*, papillary muscle and whole hearts), which clearly demonstrates the acute effect of doxorubicin toxicity. (Panel A *adapted from* Lee and coworkers [15]; Panel B *adapted from* Sato and coworkers [16]; with permission.)

WORK-INDUCED CARDIOMYOPATHY

PACING-INDUCED HEART FAILURE IN SWINE AND DOGS

EFFECTS OF SUPRAVENTRICULAR TACHYCARDIA ON HEART FUNCTION IN SWINE

	SWINE	
	CONTROL	HEART FAILURE
Heart rate, *bpm*	102±10	141±22*
LV/BW, *g/kg*	2.58±0.3	2.66±0.4
Catheterization		
LV pressure, *mm Hg*		
Peak	88±7	90±18
End-systole	75±11	80±16
+dP/dt, *mm Hg/s*	1.4±0.2	0.9±0.2*
Echocardiography dimension		
EDD, *cm*	3.5±0.4	4.9±0.5*
ESD, *cm*	2.5±0.3	4.3±0.6
Th$_{ed}$, *cm*	0.75±0.05	0.6±0.1*
FS, %	30±4	13±5*
-dD/dt/D, *s^{-1}*	1.9±0.3	0.9±0.3*
+dTh/dt/Th, *s^{-1}*		
Wall stress, *g/cm^2*		
Peak	90±15	180±49*
End-systole	39±8	142±37*
Myocyte fiber diameter, *μm*	26±2	28±2

FIGURE 11-35. Heart failure has been induced in swine via rapid ventricular pacing. There is some debate as to whether differences in the pathophysiology of failure occur dependent of the site from which the pacing is induced. This model was developed to mimic cardiac dysfunction induced by supraventricular tachycardia in children. It has several distinguishing features, which include the absence of myocyte hypertrophy. Contractile dysfunction is reversible with cessation of the pacing. Mechanisms proposed to explain the myopathy include changes in blood flow and capillary density, collagen remodeling, reduction in total myocyte volume, and myofibril content. Swine would also appear to make an excellent model of tachycardia-induced heart failure in adult humans because of similar cardiac anatomy and coronary supply. In this and the following illustrations, hemodynamic and functional parameters that result in tachycardia-induced heart failure are presented. The heart rate reported is postpacing (*ie*, after the pacemaker had been turned off). *Asterisks* indicate *P* < 0.05 versus control. -dD/dt/D—rate of increase in chamber dimension; +dP/dt— slope of increasing pressure (first derivative of pressure vs time); +dTh/dt/Th— rate of wall thickening; EDD—end-diastolic diameter; ESD—end-systolic diameter; FS—fractional shortening; LV—left ventricular; LV/BW—left ventricular weight at autopsy to body weight ratio; P—pressure; Th$_{ed}$—end-diastolic wall thickness. (*Adapted from* Tomita and coworkers [17]; with permission.)

EFFECTS OF SUPRAVENTRICULAR TACHYCARDIA ON HEART FUNCTION IN CANINES

VARIABLE	CONTROL	HEART FAILURE
Heart rate, *bpm*	96±5	117±6*
Catheterization		
LV systolic pressure, *mm Hg*	119±3	102±2*
LV end-diastolic pressure, *mm Hg*	8±1	28±2*
Mean arterial pressure, *mm H*	96±3	87±3*
LV end-systolic stress, *g/cm²*	58±3	87±4*
LV end-diastolic stress, *g/mm²*	56±2	79±3*
LV +dP/dt, *mm Hg/s*	2865±155	1539±103*

FIGURE 11-36. Like swine, heart failure has been induced in dogs via rapid ventricular pacing. This model suggests an importance of tachycardia-induced heart failure in humans. This model may mimic supraventricular tachycardia–induced cardiac dysfunction seen in humans. Mechanisms proposed to explain the myopathy in dogs include changes in calcium handling of the sarcoplasmic reticulum, myofilament calcium responsiveness, and myocardial energetics. The heart rate reported is postpacing (*ie,* after the pacemaker had been turned off). *Asterisks* indicate *P* < 0.001 versus control. LV—left ventricular. (*Adapted from* Komamura and coworkers [18]; with permission.)

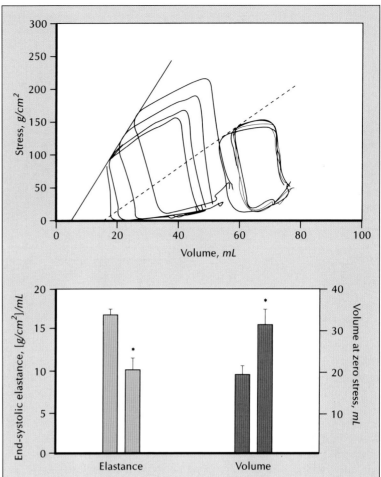

FIGURE 11-37. Top, Representative tracing of the stress-volume relationship generated by intravenous infusions of phenylephrine in a dog studied before (*solid line*) and after (*dashed line*) development of pacing-induced cardiomyopathy. **Bottom,** Average end-systolic elastance and extrapolated volume at zero stress for six dogs studied before and after development of pacing-induced cardiomyopathy. Independent of the load, marked contractile dysfunction still occurs [19]. Load dependency of heart failure in humans has not been closely studied in clinical settings. *Asterisks* indicate *P* < 0.05. (*Adapted from* Shannon and coworkers [19]; with permission.)

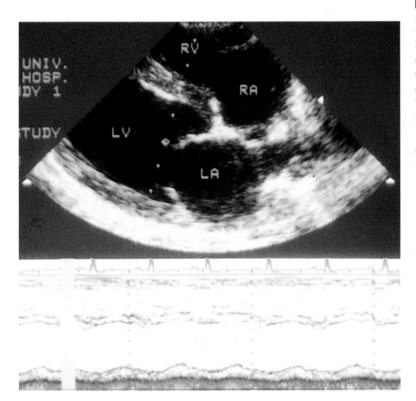

FIGURE 11-38. Two-dimensional M-mode echocardiogram of a dog with congestive heart failure induced by rapid pacing. Note the generalized cardiac dilatation and decreased left ventricular shortening fraction. LA—left atrium; LV—left ventricle; RA—right atrium; RV—right ventricle.

LEFT VENTRICULAR DYNAMICS IN CANINES AFTER 3 WEEKS OF RAPID VENTRICULAR PACING

	CONTROL	HEART FAILURE
LV ejection fraction, %	50±3	28±2*
LV end-diastolic volume, *mL*	56±2	79±3*
LV end-systolic volume, *mL*	28±2	56±2*
LV stroke volume, *mL*	28±2	22±2*

FIGURE 11-39. Heart failure was induced in 13 mongrel dogs that were paced 24 hours per day for 3 weeks at 240 bpm. A programmable model EV 4543 (Pace Medical Inc., Waltham, MA) was used. Left ventricular (LV) hemodynamics were recorded from the animals, which were constantly monitored. (*Adapted from* Komamura and coworkers [18]; with permission.)

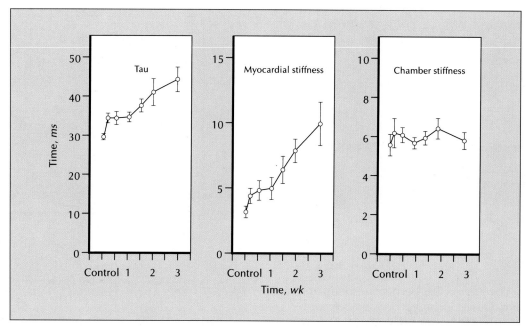

FIGURE 11-40. Changes in isovolumic relaxation and myocardial stiffness in dogs with pacing-induced heart failure. Data were taken during the same experiment described in Fig. 11-39. The time course of the changes in the isovolumic relaxation time constant (Tau) were obtained assuming a nonzero asymptote (T_D), myocardial stiffness, and the coefficient of chamber stiffness normalized to left ventricular wall volume (α_n). Tau and myocardial stiffness were increased 1 day after rapid ventricular pacing was initiated and increased progressively during the 3-week monitoring period. Chamber stiffness remained unchanged throughout the study. These data suggest that changes in radial myocardial stiffness are intrinsic to the myo-cardium and result in diastolic dysfunction. It should be noted that these measurements of stiffness are conceptually different because chamber stiffness depends on the size and geometry of the left ventricle, whereas radial myocardial stiffness reflects mechanical properties of the myocardium itself. In the calculation of chamber stiffness, the increase in myocardial stiffness is offset by the increase in operating volume of the ventricle. The increase in radial myocardial stiffness in the absence of increases in collagen during heart failure has been suggested to reflect myocyte slippage as well as other ultrastructural changes. (*Adapted from* Komamura and coworkers [18]; with permission.)

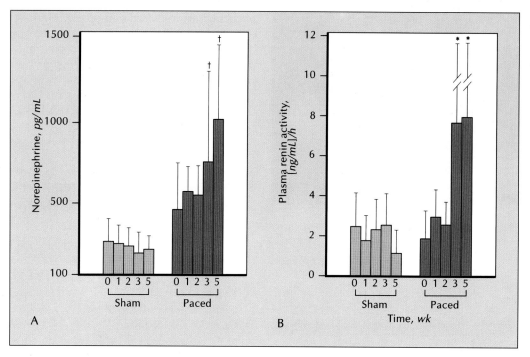

FIGURE 11-41. Plasma norepinephrine concentration (**A**) and renin activity (**B**) in dogs with pacing-induced heart failure. Six animals were paced until the biologic end-point of heart failure was reached (average 5.3±1.9 weeks). The presence of atrial natriuretic factor in the left atrium was inversely correlated with right atrial pressure in the paced group. Norepinephrine concentration in sham-operated dogs was significantly lower than that in dogs with heart failure 3 and 5 weeks after pacing. Similarly, plasma renin activity was significantly increased at these time points. With the recent suggested role of angiotensin in heart failure and the beneficial effects of angiotensin-converting enzyme inhibitors in the treatment of heart failure, models that demonstrate changes in the activation of the renin-angiotensin system might provide important insights into the natural history and pathogenesis associated with derangements of this system. Values are mean±SD; *asterisks* indicate $P < 0.05$; *daggers* indicate $P < 0.01$. (*Adapted from* Armstrong and coworkers [20]; with permission.)

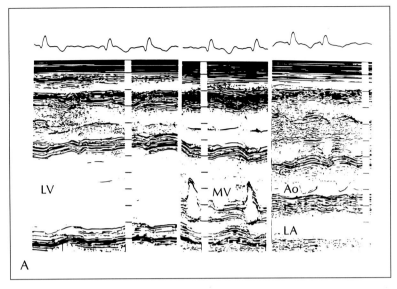

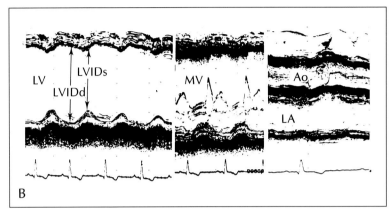

FIGURE 11-42. In humans, carnitine deficiency is a rare, usually familial cause of dilated cardiomyopathy. It is characterized by subendocardial fibrosis, and responds to carnitine supplementation. American cocker spaniels demonstrate a high incidence of dilated cardiomyopathy associated with very low levels of L-carnitine. **A,** M-mode echocardiogram from a dog before L-carnitine supplementation. Systolic ventricular dysfunction is severe (fractional shortening = 2%). The dog had atrial fibrillation.

B, M-mode echocardiogram from the same dog after 24 weeks of L-carnitine supplementation. Systolic ventricular function is improved, evidenced by the enhanced difference between end-diastolic diameter (LVIDd) and end-systolic diameter (LVIDs); fractional shortening is 24%. The dog had sinus rhythm. Both recordings were taken in standard positions at the level of the left ventricle (LV), mitral valve (MV), aorta (Ao), and left atrium (LA). (*Adapted from* Keene and coworkers [21]; with permission.)

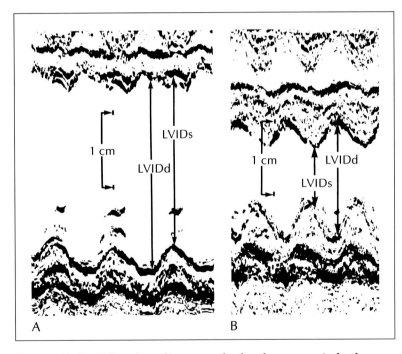

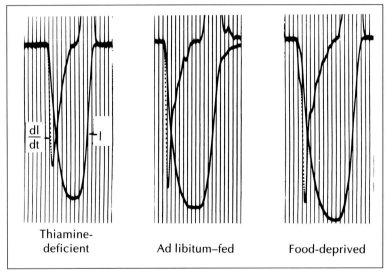

FIGURE 11-43. Dilated cardiomyopathy has been seen in both foxes and cats as a result of taurine deficiency. A direct link between decreased taurine concentration in the myocardium and decreased myocardial mechanical function has not been clearly demonstrated in humans. These M-mode echocardiograms are from the same cat before (**A**) and 10 weeks after (**B**) taurine supplementation. Left ventricular end-systolic (LVIDs) and end-diastolic (LVIDd) diameters are demonstrated. (*Adapted from* Pion and coworkers [22]; with permission.)

FIGURE 11-44. Thiamine is an essential vitamin for the metabolism of glucose. Dilated cardiomyopathy as a result of thiamine deficiency is seen clinically in dogs. In clinical thiamine deficiency and in experimental animal models, pyruvate and lactate are elevated in the blood. Lactate dehydrogenase in the heart is a marker of glycolytic flux. This was demonstrated in thiamine-deficient male Sprague-Dawley rats, which experienced isoform switching with a significant decrease in M-LDH. M-LDH is usually more prominent in anaerobic tissue. Male Sprague-Dawley rats that had observable neuromotor deficits as a result of thiamine deficiency of 53 days' duration demonstrated changes in isolated cardiac muscle mechanics. As shown here, time to peak tension and shortening was strikingly decreased. This was significantly different from food-deprived and ad libitum–fed age-matched rats. dl/dt—first derivative of shortening. (*Adapted from* Cohen and coworkers [23]; with permission.)

	FOOD-DEPRIVED	FOOD AD LIBITUM	THIAMINE-DEFICIENT
MUSCLE MECHANICS			
TPT, *ms*	158±3	142±6	123±7*
Time to peak shortening, *ms*	178±6*	149±5	125±8*
Maximum rate tension development, *g/mm²/s*	100.6±7.0	89.7±8.1	51.7±4.3*
Active tension, *g/mm²*	10.3±0.8*	7.3±0.6	4.7±0.9*

FIGURE 11-45. Mechanics in isolated muscle in thiamine-deficient rats compared with food-deprived and ad libitum–fed rats. In these male Sprague-Dawley rats, the time to peak shortening, as well as the maximum rate of tension development, was significantly less in thiamine-deficient rats than in the other two groups. Although no differences were noted in resting tension among the experimental groups, active tension was significantly lower in thiamine-deficient rats when compared by an unpaired *t* test. All muscle preparations were stretched to the apices of their length tension curve. *Asterisks* indicate $P < 0.05$ compared with ad libitum–fed rats. TPT—time to peak tension. (*Adapted from* Cohen and coworkers [23]; with permission.)

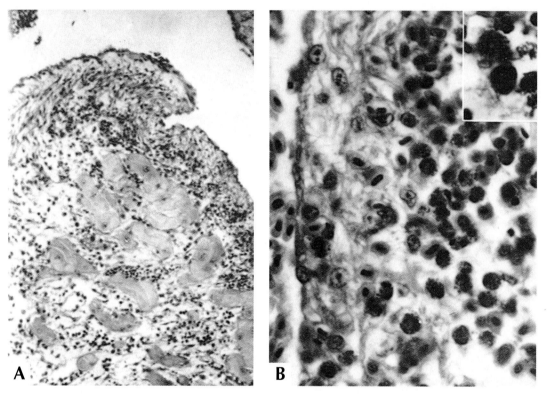

FIGURE 11-46. Selenium-responsive myopathy of the myocardium in turkey poults (*see also* Chapter 7 for human disease). Myopathy of the gizzard followed by myopathy of the heart muscle, particularly the atrium, are the first signs of selenium and vitamin E deficiency in turkey poults. Pericardial transudate apparently causes death in a high percentage of the cases. Death is typically associated with hemopericardium caused by epicardial effusion, which occurs in a high percentage of cases, as well as cardiac tamponade with rupture of the left atrium. If they survive these complications, poults may exhibit muscular dystrophy of the pectoral muscle. The earliest histologic finding is the appearance of hyaline bodies in the gizzard and heart. Selenium appears to be the key to prevention of the syndrome in poults. **A,** Acute Zenker's degeneration with muscle bundles separated by edema and hemorrhage in the left atrium of a turkey poult fed a selenium-deficient diet ($\times$ 120). **B,** Extensive intramural hemorrhage as well as subendothelial and subepicar-dial edema and hemorrhage with an admixture of heterophilic leukocytes. These disorders occurred in the heart of a selenium-deficient poult (hematoxylin and eosin, $\times$ 800; *inset,* $\times$ 1150). (*Adapted from* Scott and coworkers [24]; with permission.)

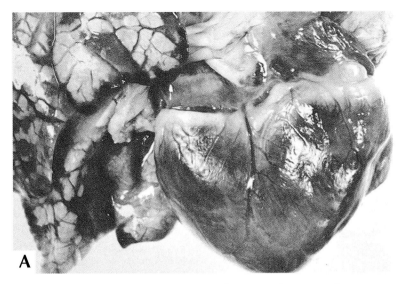

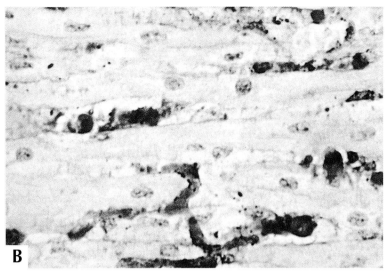

FIGURE 11-47. Keshan disease is an endemic cardiomyopathy in China that has been linked to deficiency of selenium, an essential nutrient that is present in many foods (*see also* Chapter 7). Selenium deficiency causes low activity of erythrocyte glutathione peroxidase as well as cardiomyopathy. Nutritional myodegeneration associated with dietary imbalances of selenium and vitamin E in farm animals is well recognized. In North America, the disease is a problem primarily in foals; fatal myopathy has no sex predilection, and may be clinically acute or chronic. The clinical syndrome varies and may appear in horses ranging in age from 1 day to several months. **A**, In swine, the syndrome is called mulberry heart disease and is associated with extensive cardiac hemorrhage as demonstrated in the illustration. Note the diffuse congestion of the myocardium and patched areas of necrosis and pulmonary edema. The characteristic lesion is a grossly distended pericardial sac that contains straw-colored fluid and fibrin strands with extensive hemorrhage throughout the myocardium. **B**, Microscopically, fibrin thrombi in capillaries, myocardial necrosis, and interstitial hemorrhage are noted. Capillary thrombi in the heart are also present (periodic acid-Schiff, × 400). (*Adapted from* Van Vleet and coworkers [25]; with permission.)

HEREDITARY OR CONGENITAL DEFICIENCIES

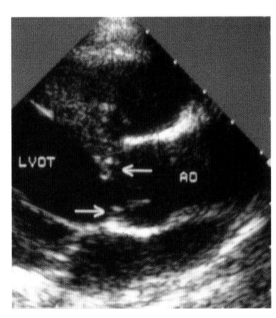

FIGURE 11-48. Subaortic stenosis in Newfoundland terriers provides a classic example of subaortic stenosis, as demonstrated in this two-dimensional echocardiogram. Subaortic stenosis in dogs is analogous to subvalvar aortic stenosis, which is a congenital lesion often associated with other congenital anomalies in humans. Such anomalies include ventricular septal defect, pulmonary stenosis, patent ductus arteriosus, and coarctation. *Arrows* in the left ventricular outflow tract (LVOT) demonstrate portions of the subaortic obstruction. AO–aorta.

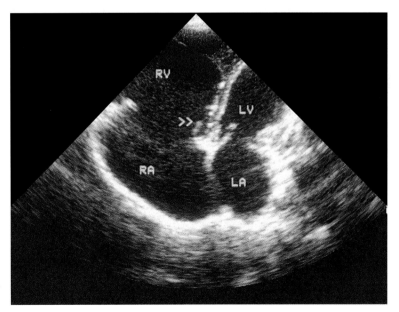

FIGURE 11-49. Silent atrium is a type of inherited muscular dystrophy; inflammatory infiltrates are also reportedly associated with this syndrome. Dogs with silent atrium typically have a loss of P waves and junctional or ventricular escape rhythms, and fine atrial fibrillation. There is severe dilatation of the right atrium and right ventricle. This disease is different from the clinical profile of a concealed form of arrhythmogenic right ventricular cardiomyopathy, also known as right ventricular dysplasia. Arrythmogenic right ventricular cardiomyopathy in humans presents as an idiopathic ventricular arrhythmia that commonly has a familial origin; in one study, 29% of 24 patients had a positive family history. LA—left atrium; LV—left ventricle; RA—right atrium; RV—right ventricle.

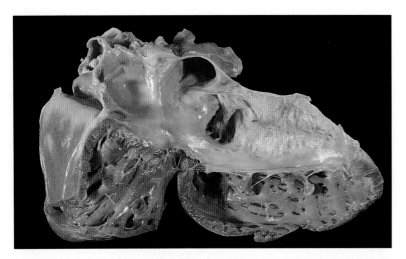

FIGURE 11-50. Findings at necropsy of a springer spaniel with silent atrium. Severe loss of atrial myocardium and replacement with fibrous connective tissue also was noted.

MISCELLANEOUS

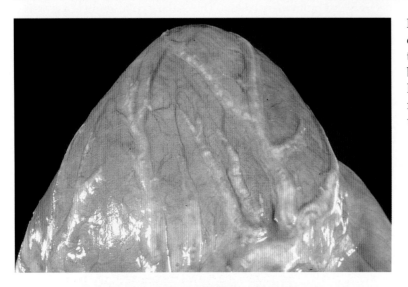

FIGURE 11-51. A few dogs develop severe and spontaneous coronary atherosclerosis. To induce the disorder in dogs, a diet that elevates serum cholesterol to more than 700 mg/dL must be fed. Atherosclerosis in dogs is commonly associated with hypothyroidism. This heart of a dog with severe hypothyroidism manifests atherosclerosis. The serum cholesterol for this animal was greater than 700 mg/dL.

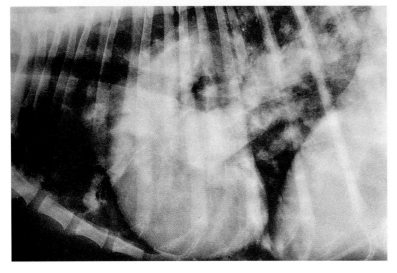

FIGURE 11-52. Heartworm disease, which is caused by the parasite *Dirofilaria immitis*, has historically been enzootic along the southeastern coastlands but is now recognized in most midwestern states and is spreading toward the west coast. Immature heartworms reach the pulmonary arteries, particularly those of the caudal lobe, between 90 to 100 days after infection. Heartworms can be found in the right atrium, right ventricle, and pulmonary artery, depending on the number of parasites. Disease of the pulmonary artery results from endothelial damage caused by adult worms and not per se from the obstruction caused by the worms. Diseased large arteries dilate, become tortuous, develop aneurysms, and lose normal tapering arborization. Morphologic changes in small pulmonary arteries increase pulmonary artery resistance and pressure, leading to increased right ventricular afterload. Pulmonary artery hypertension develops within a few months of heartworm infestation. This lateral thoracic radiograph demonstrates heartworm infection that resulted in cor pulmonale, dilatation of the pulmonary artery, and pulmonary infiltrates.

Many thanks to Dr. Skip Carmichael (James A. Baker Institute for Animal Health, New York State College of Veterinary Medicine, Cornell University, Ithaca, NY) for providing the myocarditis (parvovirus) slide. All other radiographs and echocardiograms were provided courtesy of John D. Bonagura, DVM, Department of Veterinary Clinical Sciences at the Ohio State University College of Veterinary Medicine.

REFERENCES

1. Harpster NK: Feline myocardial diseases. In: *Current Veterinary Therapy IX: Small Animal Practice*. Edited by Kirk RW. Philadelphia: WB Saunders; 1986:380–398.

2. Liu S-K: Pathology of feline heart diseases. *Vet Clin North Am Small Anim Pract* 1977, 7:323–339.

3. Ware WA, Bonagura JD: Canine myocardial diseases. In: *Current Veterinary Therapy IX: Small Animal Practice*. Edited by Kirk RW. Philadelphia: WB Saunders; 1986:370–380.

4. Calvert CA, Brown G: Use of M-mode echocardiography in the diagnosis of congestive cardiomyopathy in Doberman pinschers. *J Am Vet Med Assoc* 1986, 189:293–297.

5. Smucker ML, Kaul S, Woodfield JA, *et al.*: Naturally occurring cardiomyopathy in the Doberman pinscher: a possible large animal model of human cardiomyopathy? *J Am Coll Cardiol 1990,* 16:200–206.

6. Gwathmey JK, Hajjar RJ: Calcium-activated force in a turkey model of spontaneous dilated cardiomyopathy: adaptive changes in thin myofilament Ca^{2+} regulation with resultant implications on contractile performance. *J Mol Cell Cardiol* 1992, 24:1459–1470.

7. Gruver EJ, Glass MG, Marsh JD, Gwathmey JK: An animal model of dilated cardiomyopathy: characterization of dihydropyridine receptors and contractile performance. *Am J Physiol* 1993, 265:H1704–1711.

8. Gwathmey JK, Nakao S, Come PC, *et al.*: An experimental model of acute and subacute viral myocarditis in the pig. *J Am Coll Cardiol* 1992, 19:864–869.

9. Matsumori A, Kawai C: An animal model of congestive (dilated) cardiomyopathy: dilatation and hypertrophy of the heart in the chronic stage in DBA/2 mice with myocarditis caused by encephalomyocarditis virus. *Circulation* 1982, 66:355–360.

10. Adesanya CO, Goldberg AH, Phear WPC, *et al.*: Heart muscle performance after experimental viral myocarditis. *J Clin Invest* 1976, 57:569–575.

11. Barr SC, Holmes RA, Klei TR: Electrocardiographic and echocardiographic features of trypanosomiasis in dogs inoculated with North American *Trypanosoma cruzi* isolates. *Am J Vet Res* 1992, 53:521–527.

12. Noren GR, Staley NA, Einzig S, *et al.*: Alcohol-induced congestive cardiomyopathy: an animal model. *Cardiovasc Res* 1983, 17:81–87.

13. Hajjar RJ, Liao R, Young JB, *et al.* Pathophysiological and biochemical characterization of an avian model of dilated cardiomyopathy: comparison to findings in human dilated cardiomyopathy. *Cardiovasc Res* 1993, 27:2212–2221.

14. Herman EH, Ferrans VJ: Influence of vitamin E and ICRF-187 on chronic doxorubicin cardiotoxicity in miniature swine. *Lab Invest* 1983, 49:69–77.

15. Lee V, Arvinder K, Randhawa AK, Singal PK: Adriamycin-induced myocardial dysfunction in vitro is mediated by free radicals. *Am J Physiol* 1991, 261:H989–H995.

16. Sato Y, Eddy L, Hochstein P: Comparative cardiotoxicity of doxorubicin and a morpholino anthracycline derivative (KRN8602). *Biochem Pharmacol* 1991, 42:2283–2287.

17. Tomita M, Spinale FG, Crawford FA, Zile MR: Changes in left ventricular volume, mass, and function during the development and regression of supraventricular tachycardia-induced cardiomyopathy. *Circulation* 1991, 83:635–644.

18. Komamura K, Shannon RP, Pasipoularides A, *et al.*: Alterations in left ventricular diastolic function in conscious dogs with pacing-induced heart failure. *J Clin Invest* 1992, 89:1825–1838.

19. Shannon RP, Komamura K, Stambler BS, *et al.*: Alterations in myocardial contractility in conscious dogs with dilated cardiomyopathy. *Am J Physiol* 1991, 260:H1903–H1911.

20. Armstrong PW, Stopps TP, Ford SE, DeBold AJ: Rapid ventricular pacing in the dog: pathophysiologic studies of heart failure. *Circulation* 1986, 74:1075–1084.

21. Keene BW, Panciera DP, Atkins CE, *et al.*: Myocardial L-carnitine deficiency in a family of dogs with dilated cardiomyopathy. *J Am Vet Med Assoc* 1991, 198:647–650.

22. Pion PD, Kittleson MD, Rogers QR, Morris JG: Myocardial failure in cats associated with low plasma taurine: a reversible cardiomyopathy. *Science* 1987, 237:764–768.

23. Cohen EM, Abelmann WH, Messer JV, Bing OHL: Mechanical properties of rat cardiac muscle during experimental thiamine deficiency. *Am J Physiol* 1976, 231:1390–1394.

24. Scott ML, Olson G, Krook L, Brown WR: Selenium-responsive myopathies of myocardium and of smooth muscle in the young poult. *J Nutr* 1967, 91:573–583.

25. Van Vleet JF, Carlton W, Olander HJ: Hepatosis dietetica and mulberry heart disease associated with selenium deficiency in Indiana swine. *J Am Vet Med Assoc* 1970, 157:1208–1219.

ENDOMYOCARDIAL BIOPSY

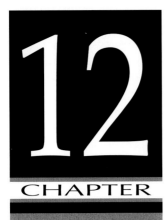

CHAPTER

Jagdish Butany and Frederick J. Schoen

Knowledge of disease is vastly enhanced by a thorough understanding of its morphologic basis. Until relatively recently, cardiac morphologic and pathologic studies were based almost entirely on tissues obtained at human autopsy; tissues from other mammalian hearts were also sometimes used. Biopsy is now, however, considered integral for histologic studies in the management of patients with cardiac disease. Cardiac biopsy has historically included a variety of techniques that involved open procedures as well as closed-chest percutaneous transthoracic needle biopsy. In 1962, Sakakibara and Konno [1] designed and reported the successful use of a transvenous endomyocardial bioptome, thus making small quantities of fresh human cardiac tissue readily available. A number of excellent cardiac biopsy catheters and bioptomes are now available, and transvenous endomyocardial biopsy is widely used throughout the world to diagnose and manage cardiac disease. Transarterial biopsy is occasionally used. A compilation of clinical and pathologic aspects of endomyocardial biopsy has recently been published [2].

Today, the most frequent clinical situations in which endomyocardial biopsy is performed are cases of heart failure of unknown or uncertain origin and postoperative surveillance of heart transplant patients. Other indications are unexplained arrhythmia, tumor diagnosis, and monitoring of the cardiotoxic effects of anthracycline chemotherapeutic agents. Despite controversy surrounding indications for and specificity of findings in the tissue generated by endomyocardial biopsy, diagnostic information is often provided by skilled interpretation of the tissue obtained [3–5]. In many clinical situations, an important contribution is provided not only when the pathologist renders a specific diagnosis but also when nonspecific findings (such as hypertrophy, cellular degenerative changes, and fibrosis) or normal findings are reported. Such findings can often rule out a number of conditions in a differential diagnosis, thereby precluding the need for therapies with deleterious side effects. Endomyocardial biopsy is most frequently used to study patients who have hearts with dilated or restrictive physiology. In contrast, endomyocardial biopsy is generally not considered useful for the diagnosis or exclusion of hypertrophic cardiomyopathy [6].

A major indication for endomyocardial biopsy is the monitoring of allograft hearts following transplantation, particularly for the presence of acute rejection. Cardiac transplant patients regularly undergo scheduled biopsies. Serious rejection is often clinically silent, and no other method is available to reliably detect rejection at a stage when it is reversible and serious cardiac damage has not yet occurred; endomyocardial biopsy remains the gold standard. For this and other clinical indications, it is assumed that pathologic features of the tissue obtained are representative of those of the whole heart and thereby reflect processes either causing dysfunction or requiring specific therapy. The extent to which this assumption is accurate may, however, vary in different situations. Therefore, while a positive biopsy is diagnostic, a negative biopsy must be viewed with caution, especially if clinical suspicion of underlying pathology is strong. Further investigation should be considered for negative biopsies.

Serious complications of endomyocardial biopsy are uncommon. Cardiac perforation and pulmonary or systemic embolism are the most feared potential hazards; however, biopsy of the right side of the heart diminishes the consequences of such complications as follows: 1) the consequences of intracardiac damage or perforation, should they occur, are minimized; and 2) the likelihood of systemic embolism is nearly eliminated in the event of the development of ventricular mural thrombus or catheter-associated thrombus. Although short runs of premature ventricular contractions occur frequently during biopsy, prolonged arrhythmia is uncommon. Pneumothorax may occasionally complicate internal jugular vein cannulation. Biopsy of the chordae tendineae or other parts of the tricuspid valve apparatus is infrequent and generally leads only to minor degrees of tricuspid insufficiency. Endomyocardial biopsy is usually contraindicated in patients with a severe bleeding disorder or other conditions that would contraindicate cardiac catheterization.

Endomyocardial biopsy is, therefore, a safe and useful tool for sampling the living heart. This technique currently has wide application. Many cardiac conditions remain to be investigated, however, and we anticipate that the endomyocardial biopsy will achieve increasing application in the future not only for morphologic examination but also to yield tissue whose study will elucidate the molecular and biochemical basis of cardiovascular disease.

GENERAL PATHOLOGIC CONDITIONS

SPECIFIC DIAGNOSES BY ENDOMYOCARDIAL BIOPSY

Acute allograft rejection

Myocarditis (including giant cell myocarditis)

Drug hypersensitivity

Catecholamine effect

Cardiotoxicity (eg, adriamycin)

Rheumatic carditis

Sarcoidosis and other granulomatous diseases

Cardiac infections (eg, fungus, toxoplasmosis, cytomegalovirus)

Lyme carditis

Ischemic damage or myocardial infarction

Systemic metabolic or immunologic abnormalities (eg, hemochromatosis, amyloidosis, Fabry's disease, glycogen storage diseases)

Cardiac tumor (intramyocardial or intraluminal, primary or metastatic)

Irradiation injury

Vascular processes (eg, vasculitis, small vessel disease, transplant graft arteriosclerosis)

Endocardial disease (eg, eosinophilic endomyocardial fibrosis, endocardial fibroelastosis, carcinoid endocardial fibrosis)

Miscellaneous processes (eg, carnitine deficiency, Whipple's disease, Kearns-Sayre syndrome, Chagas' disease, right ventricular dysplasia)

FIGURE 12-1. Diseases that are amenable to diagnosis by endomyocardial biopsy. Endomyocardial biopsy can also diagnose nonspecific abnormalities, including hypertrophic changes (*eg*, increased cell size, and nuclear enlargement, complexity, and hyperchromasia) and degenerative changes (*eg*, intracellular alterations, fibrosis). (*Adapted from* Schoen [7]; with permission.)

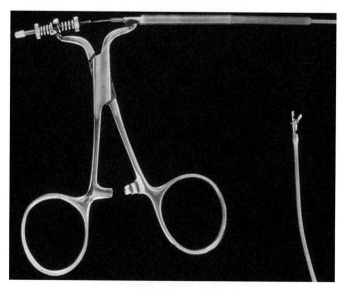

FIGURE 12-2. The modified Caves-Schultz bioptome developed at Stanford University. This is one of many bioptomes available today [8].

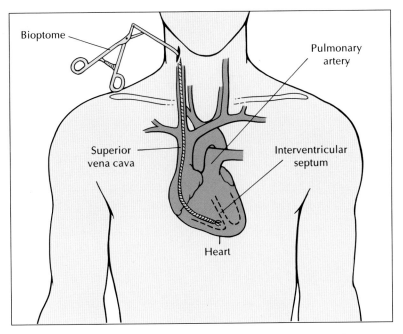

FIGURE 12-3. The commonly employed percutaneous right internal jugular approach to right ventricular endomyocardial biopsy. To obtain myocardium that is most representative of left-sided processes and to avoid the risk of right ventricular free-wall rupture, biopsy samples are taken preferentially from the right side of the interventricular septum near the apex. For diagnostic biopsies of left ventricular lesions, the approach is via the femoral artery using a longer bioptome that can extend to the left ventricle. Although fluoroscopic control has been used most extensively, two-dimensional echocardiography can be used to guide placement of the bioptome as well as to eliminate radiation exposure.

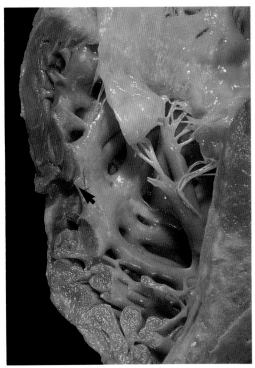

FIGURE 12-4. Right ventricular fat. Gross section of a heart with an opened right ventricle demonstrates the not unusual finding of patchy, multifocal, subendocardial fatty infiltration (*yellow patches, arrow*). An endomyocardial biopsy could include one of these foci. Clearly, a biopsy composed largely of adipose tissue does not necessarily indicate that a transmural perforation has occurred. Such a biopsy may be inadequate for diagnosis, but the possibility of arrhythmogenic right ventricular dysplasia (*see* Fig. 12-26) must be considered.

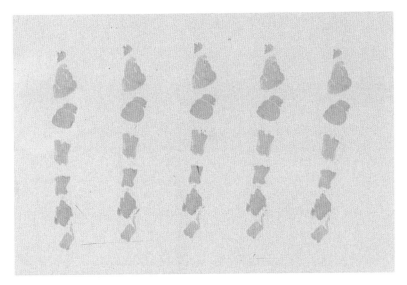

FIGURE 12-5. A typical biopsy specimen. The pieces of tissue are arranged in a linear array, and five consecutive cuts through the entire sample have been mounted on the slide. Three such slides are usually examined. An adequate biopsy sample usually comprises four or more pieces of myocardium, each measuring 1 to 2 mm, without excessive fibrosis, fat, or blood clot.

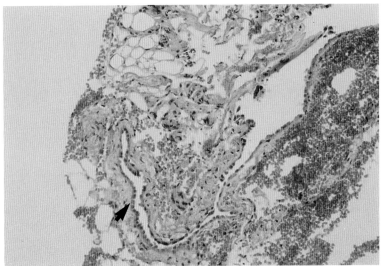

FIGURE 12-6. Biopsy indicating perforation. No myocardium is visible. Epicardial fat has acute hemorrhage, and there is a lining of mesothelial cells (*arrow*). Biopsies are taken from the right ventricular free wall fairly often; however, full-thickness biopsies are relatively rare.

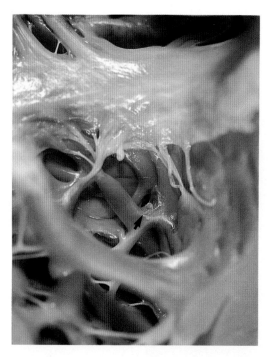

FIGURE 12-7.
Biopsy site demonstrated in a gross specimen showing the tricuspid valve and the inflow tract of the right ventricle. A recent biopsy site is revealed by a small mural thrombus on the trabeculae carneae near the septum (*arrow*).

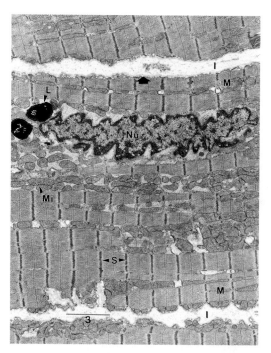

FIGURE 12-8.
Ultrastructure (electron microscopy) of human myocardium. Myocytes (M) and interstitium (I) are shown. Within the cell, sarcomeres (S) extending between dark Z-lines, the nucleus (Nu), mitochondria (Mi), and lysosomes containing lipofuscin (L) can be seen. The muscle cell membrane (*arrow*) is intact. Bar=3 µm.

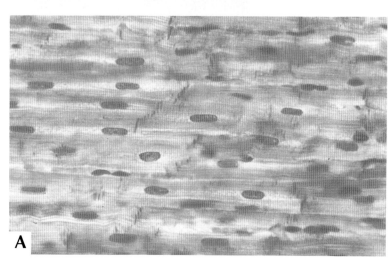

A

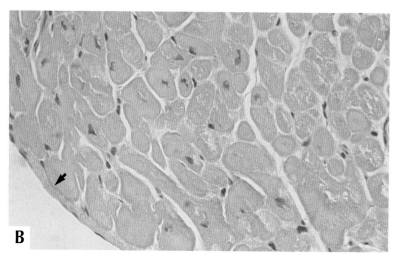

B

FIGURE 12-9. Histology of myocardium. Cardiac muscle fibers cut longitudinally (**A**) and transversely (**B**) are shown (hematoxylin and eosin). Normal myocardium has minimal interstitial and endocardial fibrous tissue, and inflammatory cells are absent. The interstitium is virtually invisible, except for an occasional endothelial cell or connective tissue cell nucleus. The muscle fibers are nearly uniform in size and shape, and the nuclei are similar in size and configuration. Normal tissue has approximately one capillary per muscle fiber. Although only approximately one quarter of all cells in the myocardium are myocytes, the overwhelming volume fraction is composed of cardiac myocytes. In *B*, the free surface (endocardium) is covered by a single layer of endothelium (*arrow*). In most pathologic states, observed abnormalities include cell degeneration, intracellular deposits (such as iron), endocardial thickening or interstitial widening (usually from fibrosis), infiltration of extraneous substances (such as amyloid), or increased inflammatory cells in the interstitium.

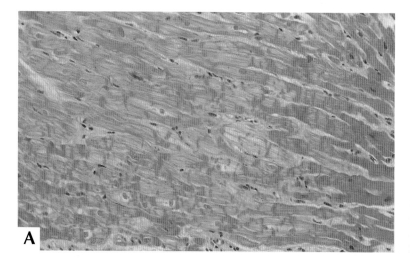

A

FIGURE 12-10. Artifactual contraction bands. When a biopsy is taken from functional myocardium, the specimen tends to contract. This leads to the formation of contraction bands, which are easily visible by both light (**A**) and electron (*between arrows* in **B**) microscopy. (*continued*)

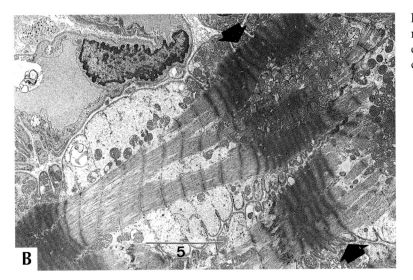

FIGURE 12-10. (*continued*) In contrast to with contraction bands, necrosis, an important pathologic condition [7], artifactual contraction bands often extend across many myocytes and the cells with contraction bands are otherwise normal. Bar=5 μm in *B*.

MYOCARDIAL DISEASE

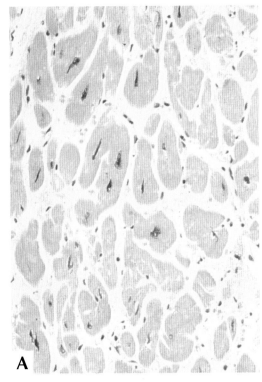

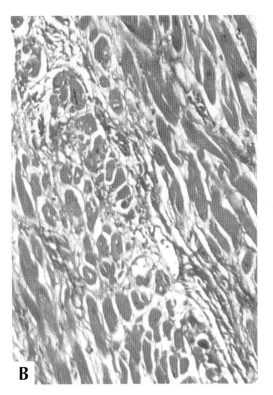

FIGURE 12-11. Nonspecific findings consistent with dilated cardiomyopathy (DCM). Generalized myocyte hypertrophy and patchy, interstitial fibrosis are illustrated. There is no evidence of an inflammatory or infiltrative process. **A,** Hematoxylin and eosin. **B,** Masson's trichrome (collagen blue). As discussed in Chapter 3, DCM is characterized by the gradual development of cardiac failure associated with four-chamber hypertrophy and dilatation of the heart. Although proof of a cause-and-effect relationship exists only in a small number of patients, the following patho-genetic pathways may be suspected: 1) genetic influences, 2) previous myocarditis, 3) alcohol or other toxicity, or 4) preg-nancy-related nutritional deficiency or immunologic reaction. No primary biochemical, functional, or structural abnormality of genetic origin can be identified in most cases; however, contemporary molecular analysis will probably reveal a genetic basis of cardiomyopathy in many patients [9]. Microscopic features of a biopsy from a patient with dilated cardiomyopathy are usually nonspecific, both at the light microscopic and the ultrastructural levels; moreover, no morphologic features distinguish among heart failure resulting from alcohol or toxins, myocarditis or its sequelae, or peripartum dysfunction. Endomyo-cardial biopsy tissue in dilated cardiomyopathy usually shows muscle fiber hypertrophy; variable interstitial, perivascular, and endocardial fibrosis; and muscle fiber degeneration. In addition, biopsies may show small foci of interstitial lymphocytes, which are usually limited to fibrous tissue and lack evidence of muscle fiber necrosis. These nonspecific features vary in severity, and their pathologic significance may not correlate with the severity of clinical or other cardiac dysfunction parameters, although this remains a controversial issue [10,11].

ENDOMYOCARDIAL BIOPSY DIAGNOSIS OF MYOCARDITIS

TERMINOLOGY

First biopsy

Myocarditis with or without fibrosis

Borderline myocarditis (rebiopsy may be indicated)

No myocarditis

Subsequent biopsies

Ongoing (persistent) myocarditis with or without fibrosis

Resolving (healing) myocarditis with or without fibrosis

Resolved (healed) myocarditis with or without fibrosis

DESCRIPTORS

Infiltrate type—lymphocytic, eosinophilic, neutrophilic, giant cell, granulomatous, or mixed

Infiltrate distribution—focal, confluent, or diffuse

Infiltrate severity—mild, moderate, or severe

Fibrosis type—endocardial, replacement, perivascular, or interstitial

Fibrosis severity—mild, moderate, or severe

FIGURE 12-12. Terminology and criteria for the diagnosis of myocarditis, according to the Dallas criteria [12]. (*See* also chapter 9.) Myocarditis (strictly, inflammation of the cardiac muscle) was loosely applied for a long time to a variety of illnesses or clinical symptom complexes, without confirmation by histopathologic evidence. Until recently, there were no broadly accepted criteria for the morphologic diagnosis of myocarditis; the diagnosis of myocarditis ranged from 5% to more than 50% of biopsies in some series of patients with unexplained cardiac dilatation and failure. Endomyocardial biopsy provides a repeatable test that can provide information about the progression of this disease. The Dallas criteria define *myocarditis* as an inflammatory infiltrate with necrosis or degeneration of adjacent myocytes not typical of the ischemic damage associated with coronary artery disease. The histologic changes can vary from diffuse, severe inflammation and myofiber destruction to small focal lesions. Myocarditis has a broad spectrum of clinical presentations, ranging from sudden death to congestive heart failure and arrhythmia to asymptomatic cases. (*Adapted from* Schoen [7]; with permission.)

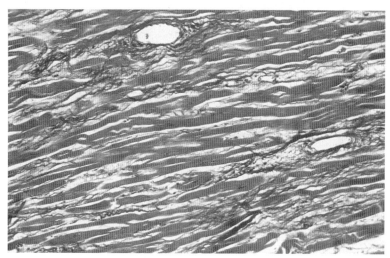

FIGURE 12-13. Restrictive cardiomyopathy from idiopathic interstitial fibrosis without prior irradiation. Extensive interstitial fibrosis, delineated by Masson's trichrome stain (collagen blue), is shown. The clinical features of restrictive cardiomyopathy can be mimicked by any disorder that produces restriction of ventricular filling, such as amyloidosis, constrictive pericarditis, or hypertrophic cardiomyopathy.

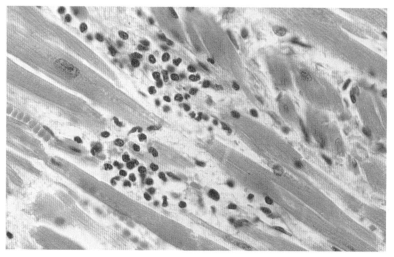

FIGURE 12-14. Focal myocarditis. Photomicrograph of the essential diagnostic lesion of myocarditis, which is a focus of interstitial lymphocytic inflammation with associated myocyte injury (hematoxylin and eosin).

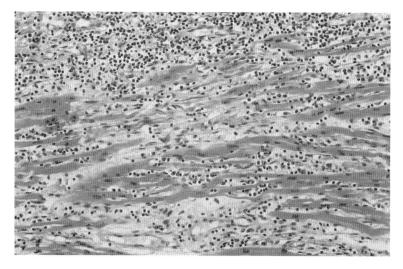

FIGURE 12-15. Diffuse myocarditis. A dense infiltrate of inflammatory cells, predominantly lymphocytes, with extensive destruction of muscle fibers, is shown (hematoxylin and eosin). Although myocarditis is believed to be initiated by a virus in most cases, direct viral cytotoxicity is probably infrequent, especially in adults. Instead, most myocarditis is probably a postinfectious T-cell mediated immunologic reaction directed against the heart and stimulated by either new myocardial antigens generated by the virus or cross-reacting antigens in the heart. Recent studies using the polymerase chain reaction show that coxsackievirus is associated with some cases of active myocarditis [13].

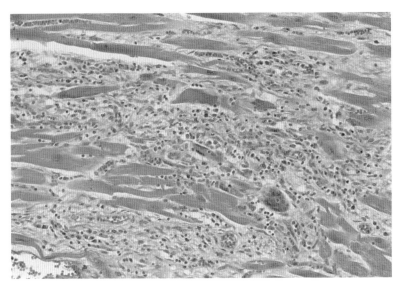

FIGURE 12-16. Giant cell myocarditis. Depicted are extensive loss of muscle, an infiltrate of lymphocytes and macrophages, and multinucleated giant cells (hematoxylin and eosin). Immunohistochemical studies have indicated that giant cells have a myogenic origin in some cases; in others, there is a clear derivation from monocytes. The cause of giant cell myocarditis is unknown in most cases. Recognition of giant cell myocarditis is clinically important because it often has a poor prognosis and can recur after transplantation.

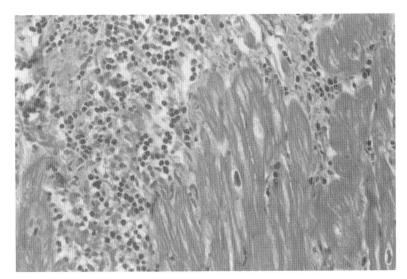

FIGURE 12-17. Hypersensitivity myocarditis. This form of myocarditis is characterized by a focal or diffuse interstitial inflammatory infiltrate composed of large numbers of eosinophils and mononuclear cells, mainly lymphocytes and plasma cells (hematoxylin and eosin). The infiltrate is usually predominantly localized to the perivascular and large interstitial spaces. Myocyte damage is generally focal and scant and may be difficult to identify. Myocarditis related to drug hypersensitivity was first reported to be associated with sulfonamide drug therapy. It is now known to be related to a very large number of drugs, including some antibiotics, vaccines (*eg*, tetanus toxoid), and diuretics [14]. Myocardial dysfunction or malignant ventricular arrhythmia can occur. Nevertheless, hypersensitivity myocarditis is generally a self-limiting disease that usually resolves with cessation of the causative drug. Residual myocardial damage is unusual. Hypersensitivity myocarditis occurs in up to 15% of patients undergoing transplantation and is considered an incidental finding in nearly all cases.

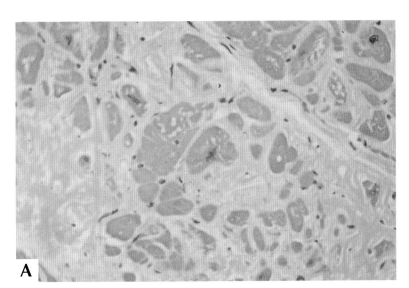

A

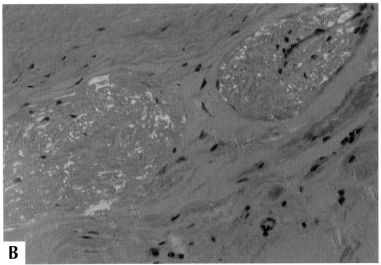

B

FIGURE 12-18. Cardiac amyloidosis. **A,** Interstitial amyloid (hematoxylin and eosin). **B,** Pericellular and perivascular amyloid. This tissue was stained with Congo red and examined under crossed polarizers to yield an apple green birefringence, which is virtually diagnostic of amyloid. (*continued*)

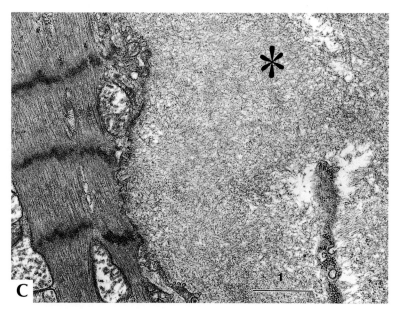

FIGURE 12-18. (*continued*) C, Electron photomicrograph showing the characteristic fibrillar appearance of amyloid in the extracellular space (*asterisk*). By immunohistochemical analysis of biopsy tissue, it is now possible to distinguish between isolated (senile) cardiac amyloidosis, systemic amyloidosis associated with a plasma cell dysplasia, and reactive (secondary) amyloidosis [15]. Bar=1 µm in C.

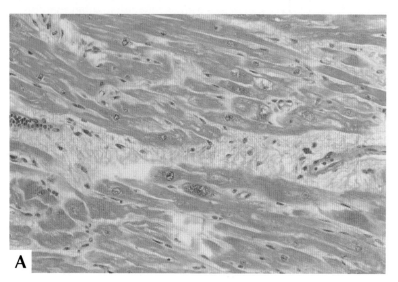

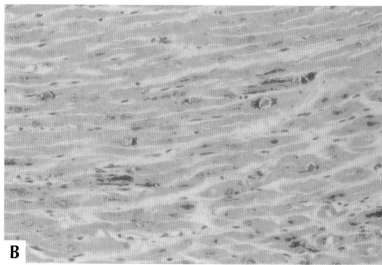

FIGURE 12-19. Cardiac hemochromatosis. A, Small, brown, iron granules in muscle fibers (hematoxylin and eosin). B, Iron stains blue and is easily demonstrated by the Prussian blue stain. Stainable quantities of iron, although not normally seen in cardiac myocytes, accumulate in the heart in primary and secondary hemochromatosis. It is impossible to distinguish these two conditions by morphologic criteria.

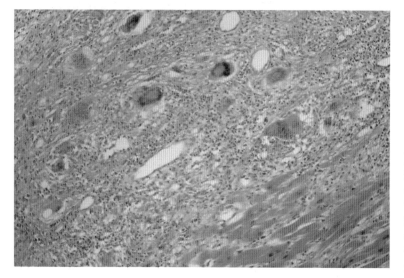

FIGURE 12-20. Cardiac sarcoid. The histologic features of myocardial involvement by active sarcoidosis are similar to those of other organs: active granulomas (as illustrated here) or large fibrotic areas with surrounding macrophages, lymphocytes, and scattered multinucleated giant cells (hematoxylin and eosin). It is important to emphasize that because lesions of cardiac sarcoidosis can be focal, they may be missed and the biopsy may show only interstitial fibrosis, small areas of healed granulomas, or no abnormality.

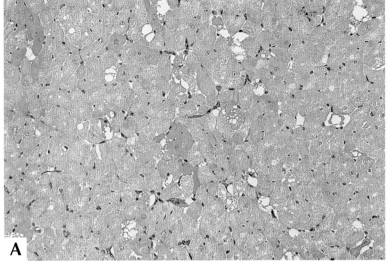

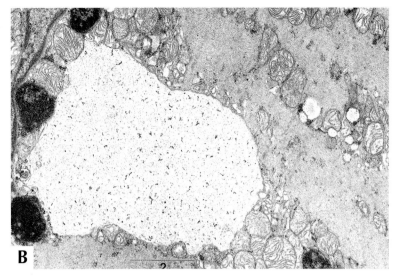

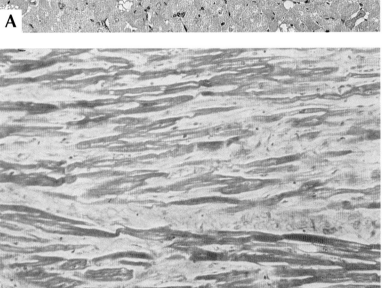

FIGURE 12-21. Anthracycline cardiotoxicity. The anthracyclines, most commonly doxorubicin, are antineoplastic agents that are effective against various solid and hematologic malignancies. A major side effect of these drugs is cardiotoxicity. Doxorubicin-induced cardiomyopathy is dose-dependent; it occurs infrequently with a total dose of less than 500 mg/m^2 but more consistently with a higher total dose. Toxicity may be potentiated by pre-existing cardiac disease or prior mediastinal irradiation. Characteristic morphologic features of doxorubicin cardiotoxicity are intracytoplasmic vacuolization and myofibrillar lysis. Endomyocardial biopsy is a sensitive method of monitoring histopathologic changes of anthracycline cardiotoxicity through a morphologic grading system [4] (see Fig. 12-22). **A,** Light microscopic appearance of biopsy in which scattered muscle cells have large vacuoles (hematoxylin and eosin). **B,** Ultrastructurally, cardiac myocytes show vacuolization and loss of myofibrils. With progressive muscle fiber damage, virtually all of the myofibrils are lost and the interstitium shows increasing fibrosis. **C,** The chronic stage is morphologically indistinguishable from idiopathic dilated cardiomyopathy (Masson's trichrome, collagen green). Bar=2 μm in B.

GRADING SYSTEM FOR ANTHRACYCLINE CARDIOTOXICITY

GRADE	MORPHOLOGY
0	Normal myocardial morphology
1.0	Isolated myocytes affected by distended sarcotubular system (vacuolization) or early myofibrillar loss; damage to <5% of all myocytes
1.5	Changes similar to those in grade 1 but with damage to 6%–15% of myocytes
2.0	Clusters of myocytes affected by myofibrillar loss or vacuolization, with damage to 16%–25% of myocytes overall
2.5	26%–35% of myocytes affected by vacuolization or myofibrillar loss
3.0	Severe and diffuse involvement with >35% of myocytes having vacuolization or myofibrillar loss

FIGURE 12-22. Grading system for adriamycin cardiotoxicity based on examination of 10 or more plastic blocks from an endomyocardial biopsy. Grading is based on the extent of myocyte alterations, as determined by the proportion of damaged cells, measured on light microscopy of semithin sections (0.5 to 1.0 μm) of myocardium. The sections are fixed in glutaraldehyde and embedded in epoxy, as for electron microscopy. The grading system is a combined assessment by light microscopy as well as confirmation of these qualitative findings by electron microscopy. Thus, for evaluation of doxorubicin cardiotoxicity, the entire specimen (ie, all pieces of tissue obtained) should be fixed in glutaraldehyde. At grade 2.5, more doses of anthracycline should not be given without further evaluation. At grade 3.0, no more anthracycline should be given. (*Adapted from* Billingham [4]; with permission.)

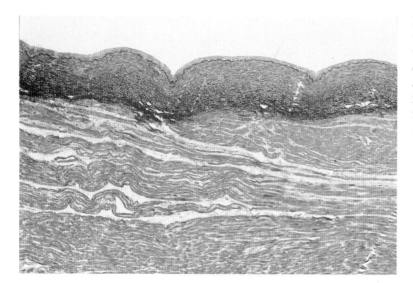

FIGURE 12-23. Endocardial fibroelastosis. Photomicrograph of tissue stained for elastin demonstrates marked endocardial thickening rich in highly layered elastic tissue (van Gieson's stain, elastin black) [16]. The subendocardium also shows some fibrosis, and the muscle fibers are mildly hypertrophied. Inflammatory infiltrates are usually absent. This rare disorder is typically seen in infants and children and is believed to be the result of fetal viral myocarditis or a manifestation of idiopathic dilated cardiomyopathy.

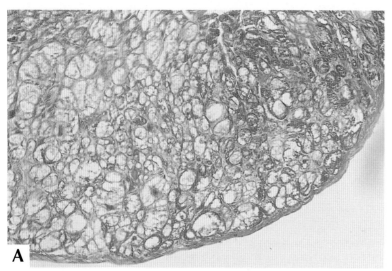

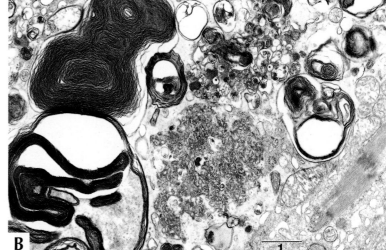

FIGURE 12-24. Fabry's disease. This is a storage disorder that results from a lysosomal enzyme deficiency that causes an inability to metabolize the glycosphingolipid ceramide trihexoside. **A,** Biopsy showing large, markedly vacuolated myocytes. Much of the deposited glycolipid material was dissolved during tissue processing in organic solvents. **B,** Transmission electron microscopic appearance of Fabry's disease, illustrating the characteristic intracellular deposits of lamellar or whorled, membrane-bound glycolipids. When a storage disease is clinically suspected, biopsy tissues should be taken and specially fixed in glutaraldehyde for electron microscopy. If a disorder involving a water-soluble storage substance is suspected (*eg,* glycogen storage disease), some tissue should be fixed in absolute ethyl alcohol and specially processed to retain deposits. Bar=1 μm in *B.*

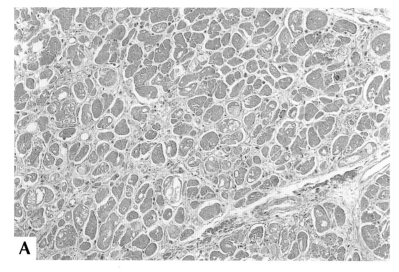

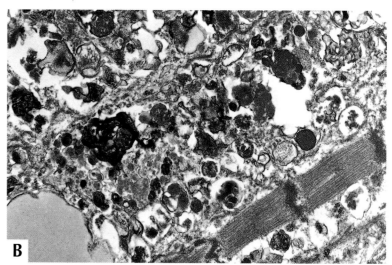

FIGURE 12-25. Chloroquine cardiotoxicity. **A,** Light micrograph showing large muscle fibers with numerous variably sized vacuoles, representing phospholipids that were lost during fixation for light microscopy. **B,** Electron micrograph showing large lamellar structures bound to phospholipid membranes [17]. The accumulation of such membranes is related to chloroquine use. Bar=1 μm in *B.*

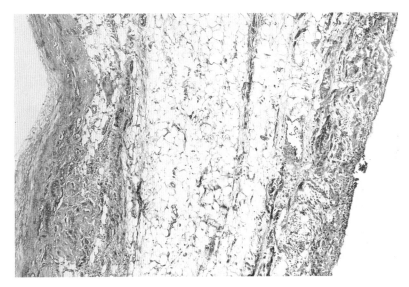

FIGURE 12-26. Right ventricular dysplasia. This condition usually presents as ventricular arrhythmia or sudden death. Morphologic findings are illustrated, including focal or multifocal infiltration of the right ventricle by mature adipocytes and fibrosis; the fibrosis involves the full thickness of right ventricular myocardium (Masson's trichrome, collagen green). This disorder must be differentiated from interstitial lipomatosis. In other cases, right ventricular dysplasia (also called arrhythmogenic right ventricular dysplasia) is associated with patchy, full-thickness loss of cardiac myocytes, which causes fusion of the endocardium and epicardium. Inflammation may be present. Diffuse involvement of the right ventricular wall by this process is termed *parchment heart* or *Uhl's anomaly* [18].

HEART TRANSPLANTATION

ENDOMYOCARDIAL BIOPSY FINDINGS FOLLOWING CARDIAC TRANSPLANTATION

Early ischemic injury and necrosis (perioperative)

Acute allograft rejection

Infection (*eg*, CMV, toxoplasmosis)

Previous biopsy site (healing or healed)

Interstitial, replacement, or endocardial fibrosis

Endocardial inflammatory infiltrate (Quilty effect)

Graft arteriosclerosis

Late ischemic myocyte vacuolization or myocyte necrosis

Posttransplant lymphoproliferative disorder

FIGURE 12-27. Endomyocardial biopsy findings after heart transplantation. Endomyocardial biopsy provides the only reliable method to diagnose acute allograft rejection at a fully reversible stage and before extensive tissue damage has occurred. In contrast, recipients of other solid organs, such as kidneys and liver, have chemical measurements of function that can be used to assist in rejection surveillance. Biopsy of a transplanted heart is done at regularly scheduled intervals and when there is a change in clinical status suggesting acute rejection. Other histologic processes are also noted in posttransplantation endomyocardial biopsies, including 1) processes that can confound the assessment of rejection, such as early ischemic injury and healing biopsy sites; 2) important pathologic processes, such as infection, late ischemic injury resulting from graft arteriosclerosis, and lymphoproliferative disease; and 3) processes of unknown significance, such as endocardial lymphoid infiltrates. CMV—cytomegalovirus. (*Adapted from* Schoen [7]; with permission.)

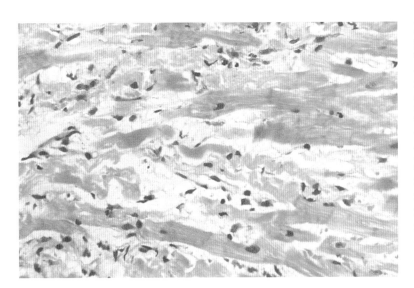

FIGURE 12-28. Perioperative ischemic myocardial injury (PIMI) noted by biopsy early (2 weeks) after heart transplantation. This disorder, which is manifested by coagulation necrosis, is prevalent in early posttransplant endomyocardial biopsies; its protracted healing phase can mimic or coexist with rejection. Myocytes that have undergone ischemic coagulation necrosis that is being cleared are shown. The inflammation associated with healing ischemic injury is characterized by a focal polymorphonuclear and histiocytic infiltrate that contains some lymphocytes and plasma cells. The infiltrate expands the interstitium but is clearly separate from viable adjacent myocytes. Fat necrosis may be present. The histologic features of healing ischemic necrosis develop and resolve more slowly than those of typical myocardial necrosis in immunocompetent patients and can be confused with rejection in some cases. Recognition of PIMI should reduce early posttransplant immunotherapy.

STANDARDIZED GRADING OF REJECTION IN HEART BIOPSIES

GRADE	DESCRIPTION	GENERIC NOMENCLATURE
0	No rejection	No rejection
1	A = Focal (perivascular/interstitial) lymphocytic infiltrate; no myocyte damage	Mild rejection
	B = Diffuse but sparse infiltrate; no myocyte damage	Mild rejection
2	One focus of aggressive infiltration with focal myocyte damage	Focal moderate rejection
3	A = Multifocal aggressive infiltrates with associated myocyte damage	Moderate rejection
	B = Diffuse inflammatory process with myocyte injury	Moderate (borderline severe) rejection
4	Diffuse, aggressive, polymorphous infiltrate (often including neutrophils), ± hemorrhage, ± vasculitis with myocyte necrosis	Severe rejection

FIGURE 12-29. Grading of cardiac allograft rejection after transplantation. The system was developed under the auspices of the International Society for Heart and Lung Transplantation (ISHLT) [19]. Five levels are established, ranging from 0 (no rejection) to 4 (severe rejection). Severe rejection is marked by diffuse, aggressive, polymorphous infiltrate. Hemorrhage and vasculitis with myocyte necrosis may or may not be present. (*Adapted from* Billingham and coworkers [19]; with permission.)

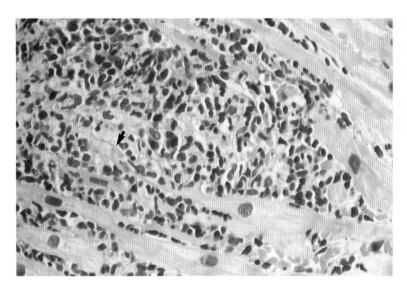

FIGURE 12-30. General histologic features of rejection with necrosis. A dense interstitial infiltrate of lymphocytes is seen, in the center of which definitive muscle fiber damage is found (*arrow*) (hematoxylin and eosin). In general, mild rejection is characterized by perivascular or interstitial lymphocytic inflammation, moderate rejection by the association of myocyte injury with the infiltrate, and severe rejection by either widespread necrosis or the superimposition of vascular injury (*eg*, edema, vasculitis, or interstitial hemorrhage).

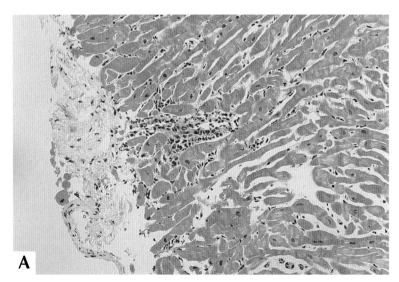

A

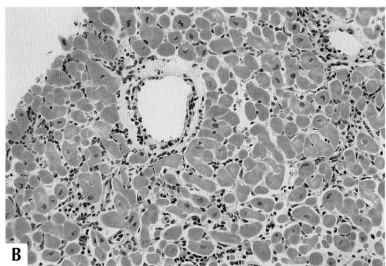

B

FIGURE 12-31. International Society for Heart and Lung Transplantation grade 1 (mild) rejection (hematoxylin and eosin). **A,** Grade 1A: a perivascular lymphoid infiltrate without muscle fiber damage. **B,** Grade 1B: diffuse interstitial inflammation without injury. This level of rejection generally receives no specific clinical response.

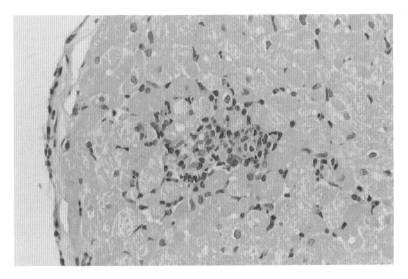

FIGURE 12-32. International Society for Heart and Lung Transplantation grade 2 (moderate) rejection. A single focus of interstitial lymphocytic infiltrate, with associated minimal muscle fiber damage (hematoxylin and eosin). The clinical response appropriate to this level is controversial. Many centers do not treat patients with grade 2 rejection; this approach is supported by recent natural history studies of this level of rejection, which suggest that progression to higher levels is unusual. Conversely, some institutions will treat this level of rejection with increased immunosuppressive therapy. An intermediate response is not to augment immunosuppression, but to take another biopsy approximately 2 weeks later.

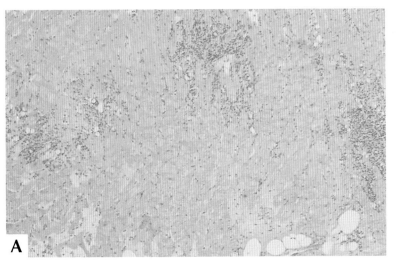

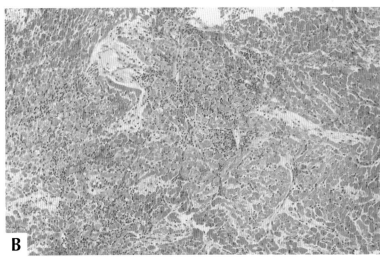

FIGURE 12-33. International Society for Heart and Lung Transplantation grade 3 (moderate) rejection (hematoxylin and eosin). A, Grade 3A: multiple foci of lymphocytic infiltrates with associated muscle fiber damage. B, Grade 3B: diffuse infiltrate with associated myocyte injury. At almost all institutions, grade 3 rejection would be treated with a bolus of immunosuppressive agents. Rejection at this level is reversible in most cases.

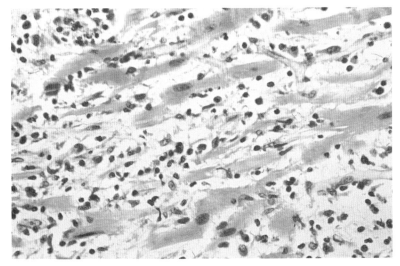

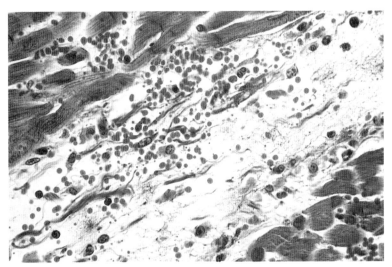

FIGURE 12-34. International Society for Heart and Lung Transplantation grade 4 (severe) rejection. Marked diffuse interstitial lymphocytic infiltrate, interstitial edema, and extensive ongoing muscle fiber loss and necrosis are shown (hematoxylin and eosin). This level of rejection is serious, although not always symptomatic. Severe rejection may be difficult to reverse; at most centers, it is treated by aggressive therapy that usually includes lymphocytolytic agents, such as OKT-3 antibodies.

FIGURE 12-35. Severe rejection with vascular changes. Interstitial edema and hemorrhage is also present; the diffuse intact and fragmented erythrocytes suggest that the hemorrhage is related to severe rejection and not to trauma caused by biopsy.

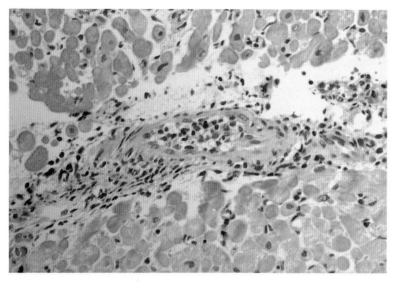

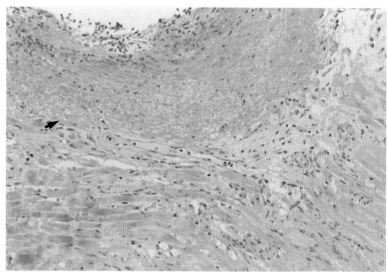

FIGURE 12-36. Vasculitis in severe rejection. A small artery with mononuclear inflammatory cells encroaching on the vessel wall and endoluminal inflammatory cell adhesion are demonstrated (hematoxylin and eosin).

FIGURE 12-37. Healing biopsy site. Repeat heart biopsies after cardiac transplantation frequently show tissue from previous biopsy sites. Healing and healed biopsy sites can show many and varied changes, from the initial superimposed rim of fibrin to later inflammatory cells and organizing thrombus and perhaps muscle fiber disarray and fibrosis (endocardial and interstitial). A fibrin cap (*arrow*) is diagnostic of a previous (recent) biopsy site. Inflammatory changes may be confused with those of important pathologic processes, such as acute rejection.

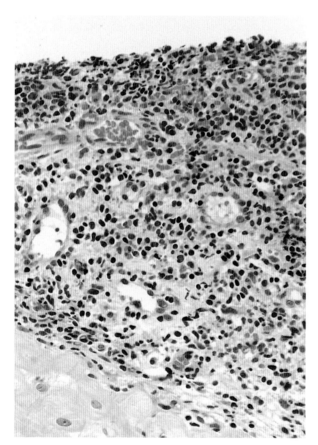

FIGURE 12-38. Quilty effect. This disorder is named after the patient in whom it was first seen (at Stanford University) and was initially (but no longer) considered to be related to cyclosporine. It now describes an endocardial infiltrate of lymphocytes. In Quilty A (shown), there is no extension into the adjoining interstitium or subendocardium and muscle fiber damage is not seen. In Quilty B (not shown), there is extension of the infiltrate into the subendocardial interstitium, often with associated muscle fiber encroachment and injury. Whether the Quilty effect is a component of rejection is unresolved. Its course is variable and resolves without enhanced immunosuppressive therapy in some patients but persists for several months in others. The Quilty effect does not appear to be related to frank lymphoproliferative disease (*see* Fig. 12-41) or otherwise portend an adverse clinical outcome [20].

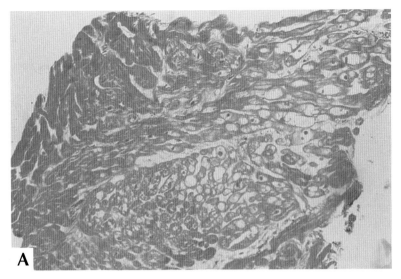

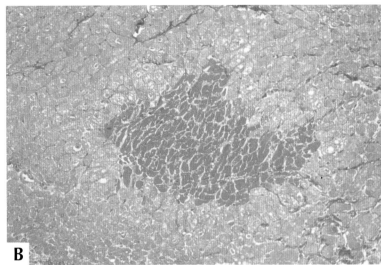

FIGURE 12-39. Myocardial sequelae of graft arteriosclerosis. The most frequent cause of late graft dysfunction is graft arteriosclerosis, a progressive luminal stenosis characterized by intimal thickening that affects both small and large epicardial vessels as well as the small intramural vessels. The internal elastic lamina is usually preserved. Small focal clusters of lymphocytoid cells may be seen in the lesion. Unlike typical atherosclerosis, lesions of graft arteriosclerosis are circumferential and diffuse (involving lengthy segments of artery), thereby rendering treatment difficult. The severe myocardial ischemia of graft arteriosclerosis has several myocardial manifestations including subendocardial myocyte vacuolization, a manifestation of severe chronic but sublethal ischemia (**A**; hematoxylin and eosin); and microinfarcts, which indicate ischemic necrosis in a microvascular distribution (**B**; Masson's trichrome, collagen blue) [21].

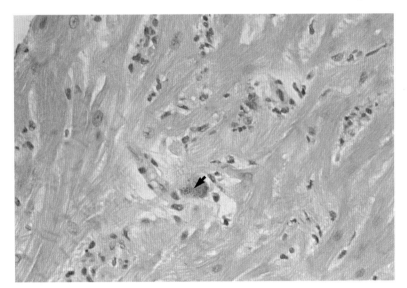

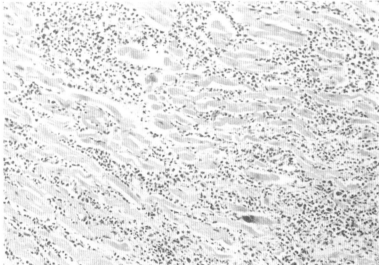

FIGURE 12-40. Cytomegalovirus infection. This biopsy shows several prominent cells with large, basophilic intranuclear inclusions surrounded by a clear space or halo (*arrow*). These findings are characteristic of cytomegalovirus infection, which is predominantly seen in immunocompromised individuals, such as organ transplant recipients and individuals with acquired immunodeficiency syndrome.

FIGURE 12-41. High-grade non-Hodgkin's lymphoma after heart transplantation, characterized by a large interstitial infiltrate of monomorphic cells, virtually all of which are atypical lymphocytes (hematoxylin and eosin). Lymphoproliferative processes, ranging from polyclonal proliferation to frank, diffuse B-cell lymphomas (immunoblastic sarcomas), sometimes occur after heart transplantation. In occasional cases, such processes may be limited to the allograft. The Epstein-Barr virus has been implicated as a frequent causal agent. Epstein-Barr virus antigen can be demonstrated by immunohistochemical methods in biopsies of transplant-related lymphoproliferative processes.

TUMORS

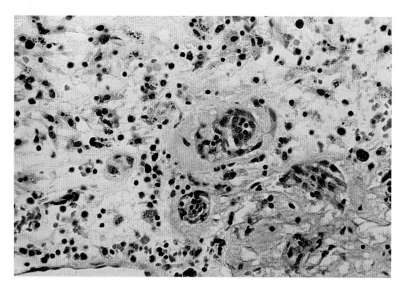

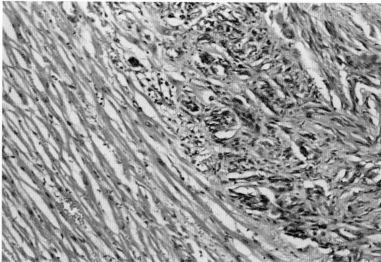

FIGURE 12-42. Primary and metastatic cardiac tumors can be diagnosed by endomyocardial biopsy [22]. The most common cardiac tumors are atrial myxoma and primary tumors of other locations that have metastasized to the heart. Atrial myxoma, the most common but generally benign cardiac tumor, occurs largely in the atria and usually arises in the region around the fossa ovalis. Extensive pale-pink areas of myxomatous material in which the typical clusters and single cells or cords of cells are illustrated.

FIGURE 12-43. Metastatic adenocarcinoma (primary renal cell carcinoma). Small clusters of metastatic adenocarcinoma, consistent with a known primary renal cell carcinoma in this patient, are shown (hematoxylin and eosin). Although primary cardiac tumors are rare, secondary cardiac involvement by malignant neoplasms is relatively common. Of these, the most frequently encountered are leukemic infiltrates, metastatic lung or breast carcinoma, and malignant melanoma. Virtually any tumor, however, may metastasize to the heart.

FUTURE CONSIDERATIONS

EXAMINATION OF ENDOMYOCARDIAL BIOPSY TISSUE: NEW TECHNIQUES

Light and electron microscopic morphometry (cell size and composition, relative composition of myocardium, characterization of vasculature)

Energy dispersive radiographic analysis (chemical analysis of inorganic deposits)

Biochemical techniques and microanalysis

Pharmacologic studies

Cell isolation techniques

Immunologic or immunohistochemical investigations

Virologic and genetic techniques

FIGURE 12-44. Modern biochemical, immunologic, and molecular techniques are increasingly being applied to human tissue. It is certain that they will be used widely in the future and will yield important data that will benefit individual patients and increase our knowledge of the mechanisms of cardiac disease in general. Examples of specific innovative approaches to biopsy include 1) biochemical measurements of enzymes, such as catecholamine-responsive adenylate cyclase, adenine nucleotides, catecholamines, and polypeptides (including actin and myosin); 2) pharmacologic studies, including tissue drug-binding assays and β-receptor quantitation and subtyping; 3) cell isolation to permit electrophysiologic studies, inflammatory cell function characterization, and cultures of myocytes and endothelium; 4) immunologic and immunohistochemical investigations, such as heart-reactive antibody and histocompatibility antigen (major histocompatibility complex) determination, lymphocyte subtyping and analysis of lymphokine production and target cell killing, amyloid subtypes, confirmation of infections (*eg*, cytomegalovirus, toxoplasmosis, and human immune deficiency virus), and determination of markers of cell activation, including endothelial cell expression of the leukocyte adhesion molecules ICAM-1 and INCAM-110 in transplant rejection; and 5) recently developed virologic and genetic techniques, including nucleic acid in situ hybridization for viral DNA genome and mRNA detection and quantitation, and gene amplification by the polymerase chain reaction, which may allow the detection of small quantities of virus. Future indications to be considered include right atrial biopsies for cardiomyopathies characterized primarily by significant ventricular arrythmias, bradycardia, or tachycardia, especially in the absence of any evidence of ischemic heart disease [23,24]. (*Data from* Fowles [2]; with permission.)

REFERENCES

1. Sakakibara S, Konno S: Endomyocardial biopsy. *Jpn Heart J* 1962, 3:537–543.

2. Fowles RE, ed. *Cardiac Biopsy*. Mt. Kisco, NY: Futura Publishing Co; 1992.

3. Hauck AJ, Edwards WD: Histopathologic examination of tissues obtained by endomyocardial biopsy. In *Cardiac Biopsy*. Edited by Fowles RE. Mt. Kisco, NY: Futura Publishing Co; 1992:95–153.

4. Billingham ME: Role of endomyocardial biopsy in diagnosis and treatment of heart disease. In *Cardiovascular Pathology*, ed 2. Edited by Silver MD. New York: Churchill Livingstone; 1991:1465–1486.

5. Mason JW, O'Connell JB: Clinical merit of endomyocardial biopsy. *Circulation* 1989, 79:971–979.

6. Tazelaar HD, Billingham ME: The surgical pathology of hypertrophic cardiomyopathy. *Arch Pathol Lab Med* 1987, 111:257–260.

7. Schoen FJ: *Interventional and Surgical Cardiovascular Pathology: Clinical Correlations and Basic Principles*. Philadelphia: WB Saunders; 1989.

8. Caves PK, Stinson EB, Billingham MA, *et al.*: Percutaneous transvenous endomyocardial biopsy in human heart recipients (experience with a new technique). *Ann Thorac Surg* 1973, 16:325–336.

9. Towbin JA, Hejtmancik JF, Brink A, *et al.*: X-linked dilated cardiomyopathy: molecular genetic evidence of linkage of the Duchenne muscular dystrophy (dystrophin) gene at the Xp21 locus. *Circulation* 1993, 87:1854–1865.

10. Schwartz F, Mall G, Zebe H, *et al.*: Quantitative morphologic findings of the myocardium in idiopathic dilated cardiomyopathy. *Am J Cardiol* 1983, 51:501–506.

11. Figulla HR, Rahlf G, Nieger M, *et al.*: Spontaneous hemodynamic improvement or stabilization and associated biopsy findings in patients with congestive cardiomyopathy. *Circulation* 1985, 71:1095.

12. Aretz HT, Billingham ME, Edwards WD, *et al.*: Myocarditis: a histopathologic definition and classification. *Am J Cardiovasc Pathol* 1986, 1:3–14.

13. Jin O, Sole MJ, Butany J, *et al.*: Detection of enterovirus RNA in myocardial biopsies from patients with myocarditis and cardiomyopathy using gene amplification by polymerase chain reaction. *Circulation* 1990, 82:8–16.

14. Fenoglio JJ Jr, Silver MD: Effects of drugs on the cardiovascular system. In *Cardiovascular Pathology*, ed 2. Edited by Silver MD. New York: Churchill Livingstone; 1991:1205–1229.

15. Sipe JD: Amyloidosis. *Ann Rev Biochem* 1992, 61:947–949.

16. Neustein HB, Lurie PR, Fujit AM: Endocardial fibroelastosis found on transvascular endomyocardial biopsy in children. *Arch Pathol Lab Med* 1979, 103:214–219.

17. Ratliff NB, Estes ML, Myles JL, *et al.*: Diagnosis of chloroquine cardiomyopathy by endomyocardial biopsy. *N Engl J Med* 1987, 316:191–193.

18. Lobo FW, Heggtveit A, Butany J, *et al.*: Right ventricular dysplasia: morphological findings in 13 cases. *Can J Cardiol* 1992, 8:3261–3268.

19. Billingham ME, Cary NRB, Hammond ME, *et al.*: A working formulation for the standardization of nomenclature in the diagnosis of heart and lung rejection: heart rejection study group. *J Heart Transplant* 1990, 9:587–593.

20. Atkinson JB, Virmani R: Pathology of heart and combined heart-lung transplantation. In *Cardiovascular Pathology*, ed 2. Edited by Virmani R, Atkinson JB, Fenoglio JJ. Philadelphia: WB Saunders Co; 1991:310–333.

21. Neish AS, Loh E, Schoen FJ: Myocardial changes in cardiac transplant–associated coronary arteriosclerosis: potential for timely diagnosis. *J Am Coll Cardiol* 1992, 19:586–592.

22. Flipse TR, Tazelaar HD, Holmes DR: Diagnosis of malignant cardiac disease by endomyocardial biopsy. *Mayo Clin Proc* 1990, 65:1415–1422.

23. Sekiguchi M, Hiroc M: Right atrial endomyocardial biopsy. In *Cardiac Biopsy*. Edited by Fowles RE. New York: Futura Publishing Co; 1993:85–93.

24. Martini B, Nava A, Thiene G, *et al.*: Ventricular fibrillation without apparent heart disease. *Am Heart J* 1989, 118:1203–1209.

PERICARDIAL DISEASE

13

CHAPTER

Noble Fowler

Pericardial disease is being recognized with increasing frequency. Among with the more common causes of pericarditis, those patients with end-stage renal disease, metastatic tumor, and connective tissue disease are living longer. Procedures or treatments that may be complicated by pericarditis include cardiac surgery, anticoagulants, immunosuppressive agents, cardiac catheterization, catheter radiofrequency bypass tract ablation, antiarrhythmic agents, and hyperalimentation catheters [1]. The widespread use of echocardiography, a sensitive diagnostic method for the recognition of pericardial effusion, has led to the recognition of more instances of pericardial disease.

This chapter is divided into three principal topics: acute pericarditis, cardiac tamponade, and constrictive pericarditis. *Acute pericarditis* refers to an acute inflammation of the pericardial sac surrounding the heart. It may be fibrinous, serous, hemorrhagic, purulent, or neoplastic. *Cardiac tamponade* is a condition in which pericardial pressure is increased because of accumulation of fluid in the pericardial sac, leading to increased venous pressure, impaired filling of the cardiac ventricles, reduced cardiac output, and falling systemic blood pressure. *Constrictive pericarditis* occurs when subacute or chronic pericardial inflammation causes a fibrous thickening leading to elevated systemic and pulmonary venous pressures, with dyspnea, fatigue, dependent edema, and often ascites. It is a relatively uncommon disease, but is important because it is usually curable by surgical resection of the pericardium.

The patient with acute pericarditis is usually hospitalized for diagnostic evaluation, observation for such complications as cardiac tamponade, and symptomatic relief [1]. Aspirin, indomethacin, or ibuprofen may be used for relief of pain. Certain cases may be treated with prednisone, starting with 20 mg orally three times a day, with a gradual tapering over a period of several weeks. Indications for prednisone may include idiopathic pericarditis not responding to the above medications, pericarditis due to connective tissue disease (*eg*, disseminated lupus erythematosus), rheumatic fever, Dressler's postmyocardial infarction syndrome, postpericardiotomy syndrome, relapsing pericarditis, and tuberculous pericarditis not responding to antituberculous triple-drug therapy (isoniazid, rifampin, and ethambutol) [2]. Certain varieties of pericarditis require specific treatment. Infectious pericarditis usually requires both antibiotics and pericardial drainage [3]. Uremic pericarditis may be treated by more frequent dialysis, adrenal steroids, and at times, pericardiectomy. Pericarditis caused by malignant disease may be treated with irradiation or chemotherapy, and at times by pericardiectomy to treat cardiac tamponade or constrictive pericarditis.

Indications for pericardiocentesis or open surgical drainage of the pericardial space include relief of cardiac tamponade, suspected infectious pericarditis, or persistent or increasing pericardial effusion in a symptomatic patient after a week or so, especially when the cause is unknown. Except in an emergency, needle pericardiocentesis should be performed in a hemodynamic laboratory and preferably under echocardiographic control.

Pericardial resection is usually indicated for constrictive pericarditis, unless the patient is in New York Heart Association functional class I. It is also indicated for recurrent cardiac tamponade not responding to specific therapy, and for some instances of purulent pericarditis that do not respond to antibiotics and surgical drainage. Uncommonly, relapsing pericarditis may require pericardial resection when it does not respond to adrenal steroids or colchicine therapy. In the United States pericardial resection is ultimately required in one fourth to three fourths of patients with tuberculous pericarditis.

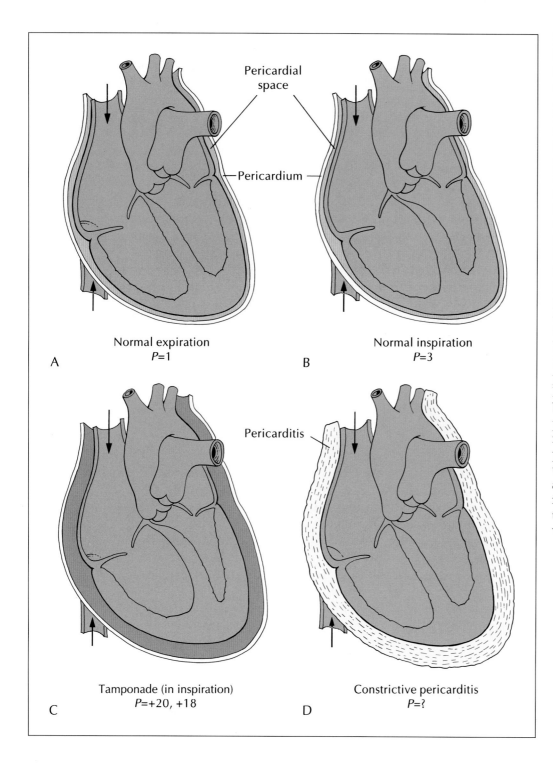

FIGURE 13-1. A comparison of the hemodynamic effects and the effects of respiration on cardiac tamponade compared with constrictive pericarditis. **A** and **B,** Normal physiology. In *A,* arrows in the venae cavae indicate systemic venous return. During inspiration, intrathoracic pressure declines, causing the pericardial pressure to fall from 1 to -3 mm Hg. Venous return increases (*arrows* in *B*), causing an increase in the size of the right heart at the expense of the left ventricle, which becomes smaller. The latter effect is caused in part by bowing of the interventricular septum from right to left. The upper lead lines indicate the parietal pericardium; the lower ones indicate the pericardial space, which normally may contain up to 25 mL of pericardial fluid. **C** and **D,** Compressive cardiac disorders. During inspiration in cardiac tamponade (*C*), venous return increases (*arrows*) and pericardial pressure falls from 20 to 18 mm Hg. Right heart volume increases slightly because of septal bulging. In constrictive pericarditis (*D*), inspiration does not increase venous return (*arrows*). The pericardial space is obliterated and therefore intrathoracic pressure changes are not transmitted to the heart. During inspiration the septum does not bow toward the left. (*Adapted from* Shabetai [4]; with permission.)

Labels in figure:
Pericardial space
Pericardium
Pericarditis

Normal expiration
P=1
A

Normal inspiration
P=3
B

Tamponade (in inspiration)
P=+20, +18
C

Constrictive pericarditis
P=?
D

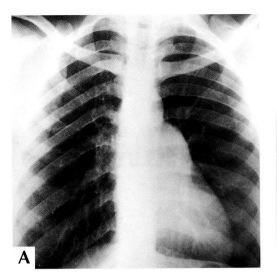

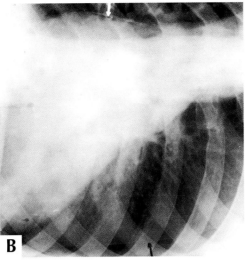

A **B**

FIGURE 13-2. Congenital defect of the parietal pericardium. **A,** Chest radiograph demonstrates displacement of the heart to the left and the prominent pulmonary artery (*black arrow*). **B,** Radiograph with patient lying on her left side, showing that the left-sided pneumothorax has been induced (*black arrow*). Air has entered the pericardial space through the pericardial defect (*white arrow*). Because of the prominent pulmonary artery segment that results from the left shift of the heart, pulmonary hypertension or right heart enlargement may be suggested. Computed tomography or magnetic resonance imaging may aid in the diagnosis [5]. (*Adapted from* Fowler [6]; with permission.)

ACUTE PERICARDITIS

A. CAUSES OF ACUTE PERICARDITIS

Malignant tumor
Idiopathic pericarditis
Uremia
Bacterial infection
Anticoagulant therapy
Dissecting aortic aneurysm
Diagnostic procedures
Connective tissue disease
Postpericardiotomy syndrome
Trauma
Tuberculosis
Others
  Radiation
  Drugs inducing lupuslike syndrome
  Myxedema
  Chylopericardium
  Postmyocardial infarction syndrome
   (Dressler's)
  Fungal infections
  AIDS-related pericarditis

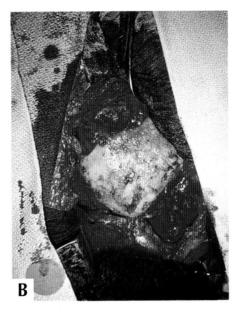

B

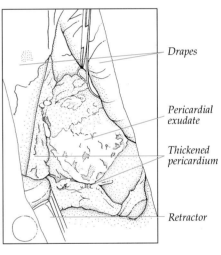

Drapes

Pericardial exudate

Thickened pericardium

Retractor

FIGURE 13-3. **A,** In most hospital series, malignant tumors are the most common cause of acute pericarditis, and idiopathic pericarditis is the second most common. These two causes, together with chronic renal failure, infection, and connective tissue disease, comprise about 50% of cases. In some inner-city hospitals, acquired immunodeficiency syndrome (AIDS)–related pericarditis has become one of the most common causes. **B,** The exposed heart of a patient with pneumococcal pericarditis, showing purulent exudate and thickened pericardium. (Part A *adapted from* Fowler [1]; with permission.)

PRESENTING FEATURES OF ACUTE PERICARDITIS

Chest pain of pleuropericardial quality
Dull, oppressive chest pain
Pericardial rub
Dyspnea or tachycardia
Unexplained fever or toxicity

Cardiac tamponade with elevated venous pressure
Incidental finding on electrocardiogram, echocardiogram, or chest radiogram

FIGURE 13-4. Acute pericarditis is usually recognized by the presenting findings of chest pain or pericardial rub, but may be first recognized by echocardiographic evidence of pericardial effusion or changes on the chest radiogram or electrocardiogram. Some cases present with cardiac tamponade, dyspnea, tachycardia, and elevated venous pressure, simulating congestive heart failure.

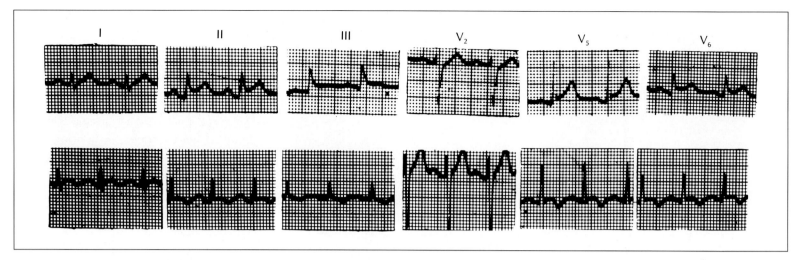

FIGURE 13-5. Electrocardiographic changes in acute pericarditis. The upper tracing shows elevated ST segments in leads II, III, V_5, and V_6. The lower tracing (2 days later) shows return of ST segments to baseline, with negative T waves in leads II, III, V_5, and V_6. A distinction from myocardial infarction is that pathologic Q waves are not present, and T waves did not become negative until ST segments returned to baseline. Usually in acute pericarditis there is sinus rhythm. The ST segment changes must be distinguished from those of normal early repolarization, acute myocardial injury, or hyperkalemia (*see* Fig. 13-6). Spodick [7] described four stages of electrocardiographic changes in acute pericarditis. In stage I there are elevated ST segments with isoelectric or depressed PR segments. Stage II involves isoelectric ST segments with isoelectric or depressed PR segments. In stage III there are inverted T waves. Stage IV involves isoelectric ST segments with upright T waves.

ELECTROCARDIOGRAPHIC CHANGES IN ACUTE PERICARDITIS

Concordant ST-segment elevation in most leads except aVR and V_1
Absence of ST-segment depression except in lead aVR, and occasionally in lead V_1
PR segment depression
Sinus rhythm (usually); occasional atrial fibrillation or flutter
T waves become negative only after ST segments return to baseline
QRS voltage decreases if there is considerable pericardial effusion
Occasional electrical alternans (more common in cardiac tamponade)

FIGURE 13-6. Typical electrocardiographic changes are found in 50% to 70% or fewer of patients with acute pericarditis, depending on the stage of the disease, the frequency with which electrocardiograms are made, and the presence or absence of preexisting electrocardiographic changes. (*Adapted from* Fowler [1]; with permission.)

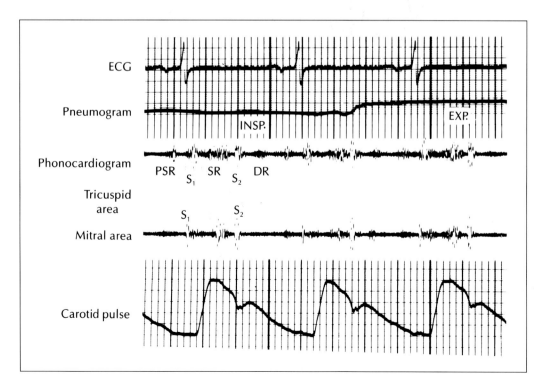

FIGURE 13-7. Phonocardiogram of a 24-year-old woman demonstrating the three phases of a typical pericardial friction rub. S_1 and S_2 are the first and second heart sounds, respectively. The rub is usually most intense just to the left of the center of the sternum. Spodick [8] found that it may be limited to systole or presystole. DR—diastolic component of the rub; ECG—electrocardiogram; EXP—expiration; INSP—inspiration; PSR—presystolic component; SR—systolic component.

ETIOLOGY OF INFECTIOUS PERICARDITIS

Viral diseases (coxsackie A and B viruses, echovirus, influenza, adenovirus, Epstein-Barr virus, chicken pox, psittacosis, AIDS, mumps, infectious mononucleosis)

Mycobacterial infections (*Myobacterium tuberculosis, M. avium, M. intracellulare*)

Protozoa (toxoplasmosis, *Entamoeba histolytica, Trypanosoma cruzi*)

Fungal infections (histoplasma, coccidioides, blastomycosis, candida, aspergillus)

Bacterial infections (staphylococcus, streptococcus, gram-negative bacilli, meningococcus, pneumococcus, salmonella species, brucella, Legionella, Campylobacter, *Hemophilus influenzae*, Lyme disease)

Rickettsial infections

Parasitic infections (trichinosis, microfilaria, echinococcus disease)

Anaerobic organisms (clostridium, anaerobic streptococcus)

Miscellaneous infections (Nocardia, Actinomyces, Mycoplasma, psittacosis-lymphophatia venereum group)

FIGURE 13-8. Pericardial infections may arise from septicemia, infectious endocarditis, contiguous pleuropulmonary infections, penetrating trauma, cardiac surgery, rupture of a hepatic abscess, or needling esophageal varices. (*Adapted from* Fowler [1]; with permission.)

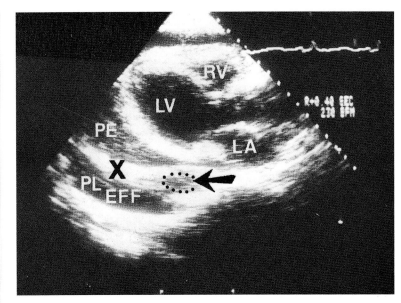

FIGURE 13-9. Two-dimensional echocardiogram (parasternal long-axis view) in a patient with pericardial and pleural effusions. A large pericardial effusion (PE) is present posterior to the left ventricle (LV) and left atrium (LA). A left pleural effusion (PL EFF) is seen as an echo-free space posterior to the pericardial effusion and partitioned from it by a linear echo (X) representing the pericardium. The most important landmark in distinguishing pleural from pericardial effusions is the descending thoracic aorta (*outlined, arrow*). Pericardial fluid accumulates anterior to the pericardial effusion, insinuating itself between the aorta and the heart; the left pleural effusion, conversely, resides exclusively posterior to the descending aorta. RV—right ventricle. (*Adapted from* Fowler [9]; with permission.)

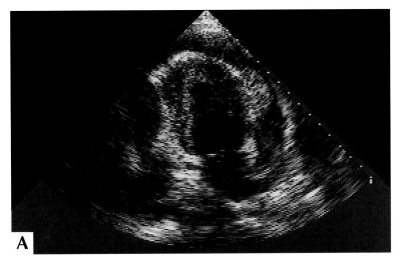

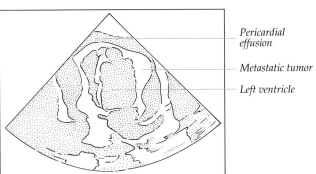

Pericardial effusion

Metastatic tumor

Left ventricle

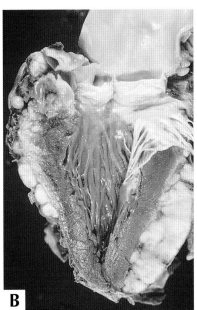

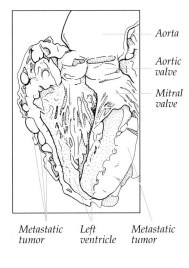

Aorta

Aortic valve

Mitral valve

Metastatic tumor   Left ventricle   Metastatic tumor

FIGURE 13-10. A, Echocardiogram of a patient with a pericardial effusion caused by metastatic carcinoma. The most common cause of metastatic pericardial tumor is lung cancer; the second most common is breast cancer; the third most common is leukemia and lymphoma [10,11]. Melanoma, sarcoma, and gastrointestinal carcinoma also occur. Primary malignant mesothelioma is rare. **B,** Postmortem specimen of adenocarcinoma of the lung metastatic to the pericardium. (Part A courtesy of Dr. Brian Hoit, University of Cincinnati.)

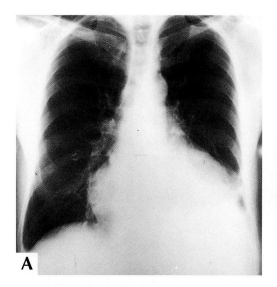

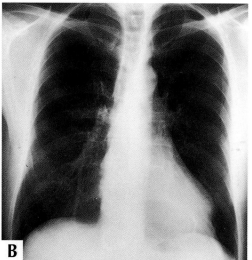

FIGURE 13-11. Chest radiographs of a patient with relapsing idiopathic pericarditis [12]. **A,** Enlarged cardiopericardial silhouette with a left pleural effusion. **B,** Essentially normal radiograph made during a remission following prednisone therapy. Pleural effusions occur commonly in idiopathic pericarditis and usually are either on the left or bilateral.

PERICARDITIS RELATED TO THERAPEUTIC PROCEDURES AND DRUGS

Lupuslike syndrome: procainamide, diphenylhydantoin, hydralazine, isonicotinic acid hydrazide
X-irradiation
Anticoagulants
Methysergide
Cyclosporine (after cardiac transplant) [14]
Minoxidil [15]
Streptokinase [16]
Endoscopic sclerotherapy of esophageal varices [17]
Central venous catheter placement [18–20]
Automatic defibrillator placement [21]
Complicating pacemaker catheter placement [22]
Complicating cardiac transplantation [23]

FIGURE 13-12. Procainamide is probably the most common agent that may produce pericarditis accompanying a lupuslike syndrome. Mediastinal x-irradiation may produce acute pericardial effusion, and later, constrictive pericarditis, often with a delay of months or years. Central venous catheter placement, especially for hyperalimentation, may be complicated by cardiac tamponade owing to right atrial or caval perforation. (*Adapted from* Fowler [13]; with permission.)

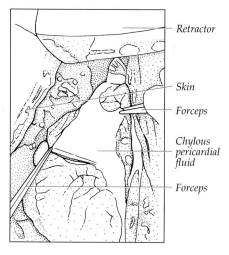

FIGURE 13-13. Chylopericardium at operation, showing creamy white pericardial fluid. Chylopericardium may result from surgical or traumatic rupture of the thoracic duct or from neoplasm, tuberculosis, or congenital lymphangiomatosis. The fluid has a high fat and cholesterol content, and the protein content usually exceeds 3.5 g/100 mL. It rarely produces cardiac tamponade, but did in this case. (Courtesy of Dr. Eli Roth, Christ Hospital, Cincinnati, OH.)

FIGURE 13-14. In most patients with a pericardial effusion associated with acquired immunodeficiency syndrome (AIDS), the effusion is not due to infection or neoplasm. In some large inner-city hospitals, AIDS is becoming one of the most common causes of acute pericarditis. (*Adapted from* Fowler [13]; with permission.)

CAUSES OF PERICARDIAL COMPLICATIONS IN AIDS

Unrelated to infection or neoplasm
Lymphoma
Kaposi's sarcoma
Mycobacterium tuberculosis
Mycobacterium avium intracellulare
Nonspecific pericarditis
Herpes simplex type II
Cytomegalovirus
Cryptococcus neoformans
Nocardia asteroides

TUBERCULOUS PERICARDITIS

Occurs in 1%–2% of patients with pulmonary tuberculosis

Prior to 1953, it was found in 0.4%–1.1% of autopsies and 7.3%–11% of acute pericarditis in the US [2]

Currently constitutes 4% of acute pericarditis and 7% of tamponade in developed countries

Most common cause of acute pericarditis in India and Transkei (Africa) (240 cases in one hospital in 1 year)

Caused 2% of recent cases of constrictive pericarditis [24]

Caused 72 of 118 cases of constrictive pericarditis in India [25]

At least 25% of patients have no radiographic evidence of pulmonary tuberculosis (72% in our series)

Approximately one third require pericardiectomy (varies from 7%–67%)

Found in 11 of 643 patients with AIDS [26]

FIGURE 13-15. Although tuberculous pericarditis is relatively uncommon in the United States, its prevalence is increasing because of the acquired immunodeficiency syndrome (AIDS) epidemic. It is the most common cause of acute pericarditis in India and Transkei, Africa [2].

POSTPERICARDIOTOMY SYNDROME

Occurs in 10%–40% of patients following cardiac operations [9]

Uncommon in children <2 y of age

Usually found 1 wk to 2 mo postoperatively

Characterized by chest pain, fever, increased sedimentation rate, pericardial effusion, pleural effusion, and at times, pulmonary infiltrates

Radiographs showed pleural effusion in 26 of 38 patients; pericardial effusion in 18 of 38; and no change in 8 of 38 [27]

Pericardial fluid is often serosanguineous; leukocyte count 3300–7500/mm^3 [28]

May be associated with a rise in antiviral antibody titers

Cardiac tamponade may develop in almost 1% of patients after cardiac surgery

Constrictive pericarditis develops in about 0.2% of patients after cardiac surgery

Electrocardiographic changes of acute pericarditis are found in approximately 50%

FIGURE 13-16. The postpericardiotomy syndrome must be distinguished from the common finding of a pericardial rub, elevated sedimentation rate, and low-grade fever following cardiac operations. Cardiac tamponade may occur, especially in patients who receive anticoagulants following prosthetic valve insertion.

PERICARDITIS IN ACUTE MYOCARDIAL INFARCTION

Pericardial rub reported in 5%–15% of patients

Associated with a larger number of asynergic myocardial segments and reduced left ventricular ejection fraction

Greater prevalance in anterior infarction

Greater in-hospital mortality

Higher prevalence in three-vessel disease

Cardiac tamponade is rare in patients receiving thrombolysis

FIGURE 13-17. In patients with acute cardiac infarction, the pericardial rub usually appears during the first 10 days [29]. In Dressler's postmyocardial infarction syndrome, the rub usually appears between 11 days and 2 to 3 months postinfarction, is more often accompanied by pericardial pain, and is more often associated with tamponade and recurrences [30]. Dressler's syndrome has become uncommon, and complicates no more than 1% to 3% of acute infarctions. (*Adapted from* the TAMI Study Group [31]; with permission.)

CARDIAC TAMPONADE

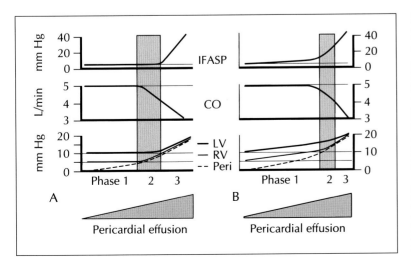

FIGURE 13-18. Hemodynamic changes in cardiac tamponade, including pericardial (Peri), right ventricular (RV), and left ventricular (LV) pressures and the inspiratory fall in arterial systolic pressure (IFASP) and cardiac output (CO), with increasing pericardial effusion in any given patient depicted by the increasing height of the triangle from left to right. *Shaded vertical area* indicates phase 2. **A,** The original concept. **B,** The revised concept, in which LV diastolic pressure does not equilibrate with RV diastolic pressure and pericardial pressure until phase 3. In phase 1, pericardial pressure rises but does not equilibrate with RV and LV diastolic pressures. There is no pulsus paradoxus. In phase 2, RV diastolic pressures equilibrate but not with LV diastolic pressure, which remains higher. Pulsus paradoxus is often present. In phase 3, left and right diastolic pressures equilibrate with pericardial pressure, and pulsus paradoxus is nearly always present. (*Adapted from* Reddy and coworkers [32]; with permission.)

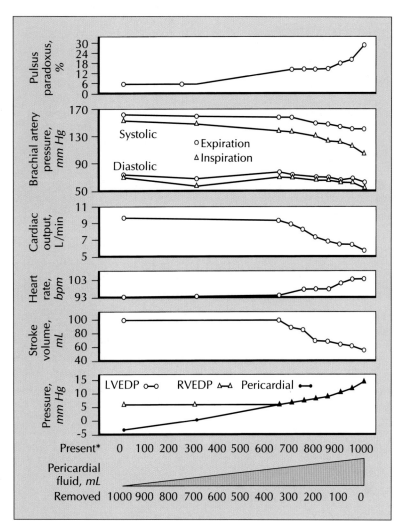

FIGURE 13-19. Hemodynamic changes during serial fluid withdrawals in a 22-year-old man with tamponade due to uremic pericarditis. Pulsus paradoxus is expressed as a percentage fall in systolic arterial pressure with inspiration. Note that significant pulsus paradoxus (>9% inspiratory fall in systolic blood pressure) and changes in cardiac output, heart rate, and stroke volume occur at the point of equilibrium of right ventricular diastolic pressure (RVEDP) and pericardial pressure. *Asterisk* indicates the predicted values assuming complete withdrawal. (*Adapted from* Reddy [33]; with permission.)

CAUSES OF PULSUS PARADOXUS

Cardiac tamponade	Pulmonary embolism
Acute or chronic airway disease	Right ventricular infarction
Constrictive pericarditis	Circulatory shock
Restrictive cardiomyopathy	

FIGURE 13-20. Causes of pulsus paradoxus. Pulsus paradoxus may be absent in cardiac tamponade with left ventricular dysfunction, regional tamponade, pulmonary arterial obstruction, hypovolemia, positive pressure breathing, atrial septal defect, or aortic incompetence. (*Adapted from* Fowler [9]; with permission.)

CAUSES OF CARDIAC TAMPONADE

CAUSE	CASES, n
Malignant tumor	28
Idiopathic pericarditis	10
Uremia	7
Bacterial infections	7
Anticoagulant therapies	6
Dissecting aneurysm	5
Diagnostic procedures	4
Tuberculosis	3
Postpericardiotomy	3
Trauma	3
Connective tissue disease	3
Radiation	2
Myxedema	2
Cardiac rupture postinfarction	2
Primary chylopericardium	1

FIGURE 13-21. Causes of cardiac tamponade in 86 cases at the University of Cincinnati Medical Center from 1963 to 1986. The most common cause of cardiac tamponade in most hospital series is metastatic neoplasm, followed by nonspecific pericarditis, renal failure, infections, and connective tissue disease. (*Adapted from* Fowler [34]; with permission.)

PHYSICAL FINDINGS IN CARDIAC TAMPONADE

FINDING	n(%)
Elevated systemic venous pressure	56(100)
Paradoxical pulse	55(98)
Respiratory rate >20/min	45(80)
Heart rate ≥100/min	43(77)
Systolic blood pressure ≥100 mm Hg	36(64)
Diminished heart sounds	19(34)
Pericardial friction rub	16(29)
Rapidly declining blood pressure	14(25)

FIGURE 13-22. Physical findings in 56 cases of cardiac tamponade [35]. The percentage of patients with pulsus paradoxus (inspiratory systolic arterial pressure decline >10 mm Hg) is high in this group because cardiac tamponade was defined by clinical criteria. If it is defined by echocardiographic criteria, the percentage with pulsus paradoxus is lower [36].

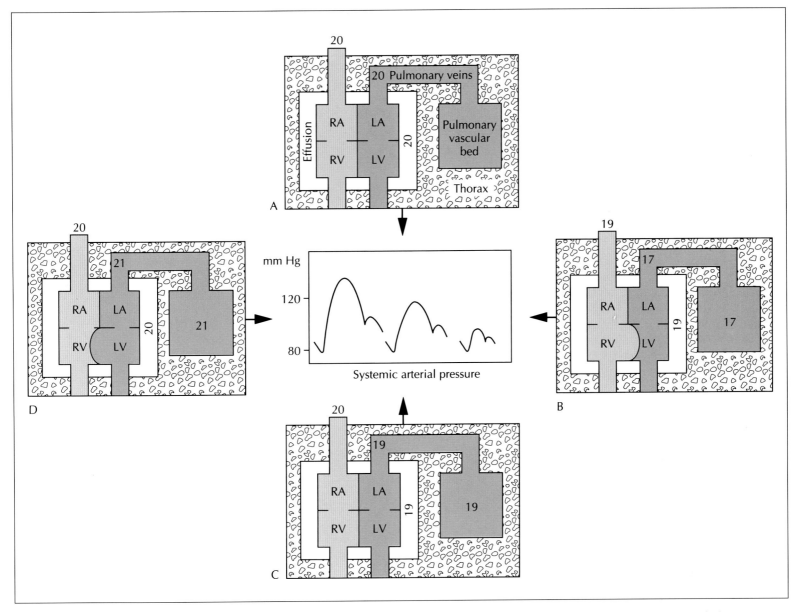

FIGURE 13-23. Mechanism of pulsus paradoxus at midexpiration (**A**), early inspiration (**B**), midinspiration (**C**), and early expiration (**D**). Note that the left atrial (LA) pressure of 21 mm Hg exceeds the intrapericardial pressure of 20 mm Hg during early expiration, facilitating left ventricular (LV) filling. In early inspiration, LA pressure is 17 mm Hg, falling below the intrapericardial pressure of 19 mm Hg. This impairs LV filling, leading to decreased stroke volume and a fall in systolic arterial pressure. All values are mm Hg. RA—right atrial; RV—right ventricle. (*Adapted from* Reddy [33]; with permission.)

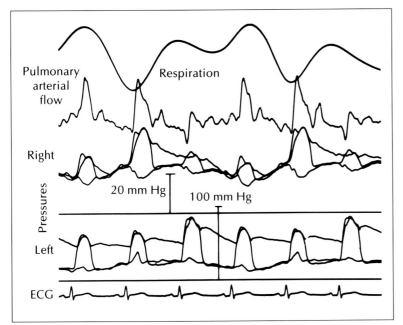

FIGURE 13-24. Physiologic signals in a patient with pericardial tamponade prepericardiocentesis. The additional pressure associated with the diastolic portion of the left ventricle is intrapericardial pressure. Marked elevation of diastolic pressures in the right ventricle, right atrium, left ventricle, and pericardial cavity is evident. The right atrial pressure displays a loss of the Y descent. Marked variations in the pulmonary artery and aortic pressure are present, which is consistent with pulsus paradoxus. When diastole occurs during active inspiration, the subsequent pulmonary artery pulse pressure and pulmonary artery flow are augmented dramatically. Simultaneously, aortic pulse pressure and aortic flow (not illustrated) achieve a minimal value. In the subsequent beat, these relationships are reversed. ECG—electrocardiogram; Left—aortic and left ventricular pressures; Right—right ventricular and atrial pressures. (*Adapted from* Murgo and coworkers [37]; with permission.)

ECHOCARDIOGRAPHIC FINDINGS IN CARDIAC TAMPONADE

RA diastolic collapse

RV early diastolic collapse

LA collapse

Abnormal inspiratory increase in tricuspid valve flow and >15% inspiratory decrease of mitral valve flow

Abnormal inspiratory increase of RV dimension with abnormal inspiratory decrease of LV dimension

Inspiratory decrease of mitral valve DE excursion and EF slope

Inferior vena caval plethora (failure to decrease proximal diameter by ≥50% on sniff or deep inspiration)

LV pseudohypertrophy

Swinging heart

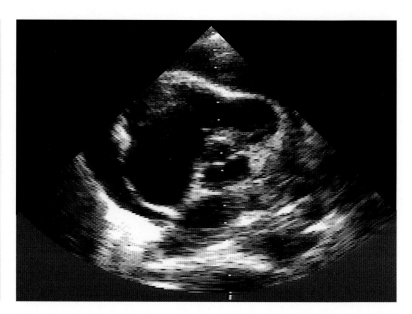

FIGURE 13-25. Right atrial (RA) collapse and right ventricular (RV) diastolic collapse are the most sensitive echocardiographic signs of cardiac tamponade. However, these signs may be absent when there is elevation of right heart pressures, RV or RA hypertrophy with reduced compliance, or with regional tamponade of the left heart. LA—left atrial; LV—left ventricular.

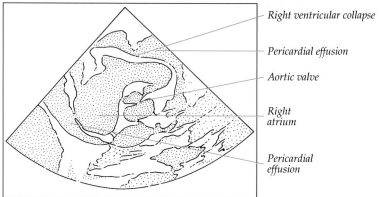

FIGURE 13-26. Two-dimensional echocardiogram, parasternal short-axis view, showing right ventricular diastolic collapse in a patient with a large pericardial effusion and cardiac tamponade. (Courtesy of Dr. Brian Hoit.)

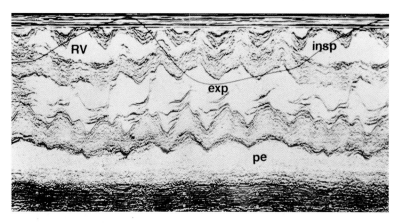

FIGURE 13-27. M-mode echocardiogram of a patient with cardiac tamponade showing the inspiratory (insp) increase of right ventricular (RV) dimension and the inspiratory decrease of left ventricular (LV) dimension. exp—expiration; pe—pericardial effusion. (*Adapted from* Fowler [9]; with permission.)

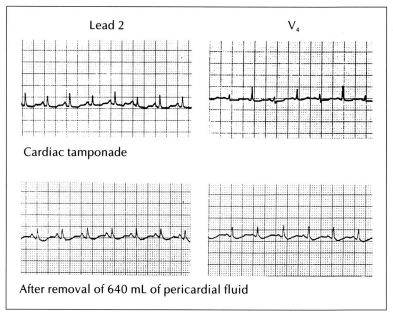

FIGURE 13-28. Electrical alternans of the QRS complex in a patient with cardiac tamponade. We found electrical alternans of the QRS complex in 11 of 54 cases of cardiac tamponade [35]. Electrical alternans of the QRS complex may also occur with pericarditis without tamponade, with supraventricular or ventricular tachycardia, and with coronary artery disease. Total alternans, involving P, QRS, and T complexes, is almost diagnostic of cardiac tamponade.

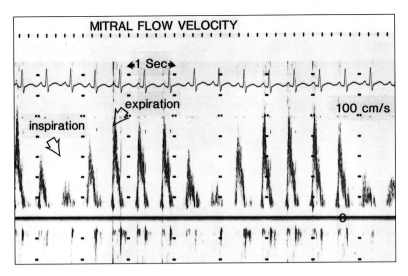

FIGURE 13-29. Doppler echocardiogram demonstrating abnormal inspiratory decrease in mitral flow velocity in cardiac tamponade. The normal decrease is less than 15%. Abnormal inspiratory decreases in mitral flow velocity also occur in constrictive pericarditis, right ventricular infarction, and chronic obstructive airway disease. (*Adapted from* Hoit [5]; with permission.)

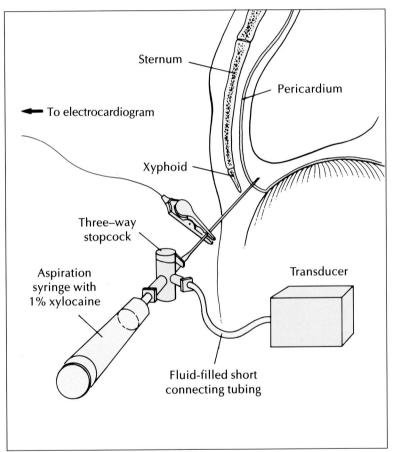

FIGURE 13-30. Pericardiocentesis using the subxiphoid approach, which avoids the major epicardial vessels. A hollow needle, which is attached via a stopcock to an aspiration syringe and a short length of connecting tubing to a transducer, is used to enter the pericardial space. When fluid is aspirated initially, the pressure waveform at the needle tip should be examined briefly to confirm that the needle tip is in the pericardial space. A floppy-tipped guidewire is then passed through the hollow needle, and the needle is exchanged for a soft flexible catheter with end and side holes to facilitate safe and thorough drainage of the pericardial sac. (*Adapted from* Lorell and Grossman [38]; with permission.)

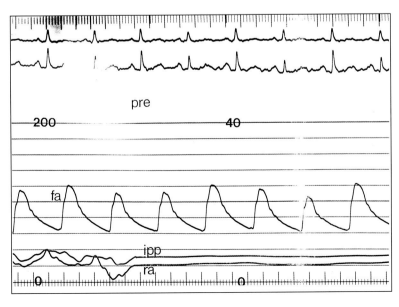

FIGURE 13-31. Low-pressure cardiac tamponade. This hemodynamic study was made prior to drainage of 800 mL of intrapericardial fluid (indicated by "pre" in figure). Intrapericardial pressure (ipp) is only 6 mm Hg. Right atrial (ra) pressure is 4 mm Hg. Systolic arterial pressure is approximately 110 mm Hg with a paradoxical pulse of 16 to 18 mm Hg. After drainage of 800 mL of pericardial fluid, right atrial pressure fell to 0 and intrapericardial pressure was subatmospheric. The inspiratory fall in systolic atrial pressure was reduced to approximately 8 mm Hg. Low pressure cardiac tamponade is diagnosed when cardiac tamponade is present with right atrial and right ventricular end-diastolic pressures below the usual tamponade values of 12 to 32 mm Hg. It generally occurs with dehydration, after diuretics, or with other causes of the low blood volumes [39]. fa—femoral artery; 200—pressure scale for femoral artery; 40—pressure scale for intrapericardial and right atrial pressure.

ETIOLOGY OF CONSTRICTIVE PERICARDITIS

Unknown	Connective tissue disease
Irradiation	Uremia
After nonspecific pericarditis	Sarcoidosis
Postsurgical	Trauma
Neoplasm	Tuberculosis
Postinfective	

FIGURE 13-32. More cases of constrictive pericarditis are of unknown cause than are of any known etiology. Mediastinal irradiation may be the most common known cause in areas where it is commonly used. Most causes of acute pericarditis are capable of producing constrictive pericarditis. Tuberculous pericarditis is no longer a common cause in the United States, but has been reported as the most common cause in some areas in India. In a Stanford University study of 95 cases [40], 42% were idiopathic, 31% were caused by x-irradiation, 6% followed infections, 4% were due to a connective tissue disorder, 3% were neoplastic, 2% followed dialysis, and 1% were due to sarcoidosis. (*Adapted from* Fowler [1]; with permission.)

A. CLINICAL FEATURES ASSOCIATED WITH CONSTRICTIVE PERICARDITIS

SYMPTOMS	SIGNS
Effort dyspnea	Elevated venous pressure
Fatigue	Edema
Abdominal swelling	Hepatomegaly
Abdominal discomfort	Ascites
Orthopnea	Pleural effusion
Cough	Kussmaul's sign
	Pericardial knock
	Pulsus paradoxus
	Decreased precordial activity

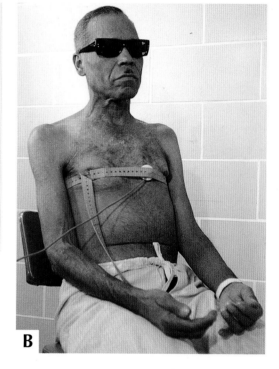

B

FIGURE 13-33. A, Of the clinical features associated with constrictive pericarditis, exertional fatigue and dyspnea are the most common complaints. Abnormally distended neck veins, dependent edema, and hepatic engorgement are almost universally present, and ascites is found in 15% to 50% or more. Pulsus paradoxus is present in the minority. **B,** Distended neck veins in a seated patient with effusive-constrictive pericarditis. Right atrial pressure was 20 mm Hg. (Part A *adapted from* Fowler [1]; with permission.)

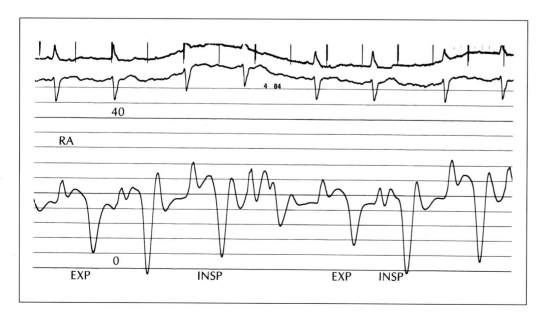

FIGURE 13-34. Kussmaul's sign in a patient with proven constrictive pericarditis. The upper two tracings are electrocardiograms showing atrial fibrillation. The right atrial pressure (RA) record shows an increase during inspiration (INSP) to 22 mm Hg compared with the mean expiratory pressure (EXP) of 18 mm Hg. Normally, RA pressure falls 3 to 7 mm Hg during inspiration. There is a prominent Y descent. Kussmaul's sign is actually inspiratory swelling of the neck veins, as would be seen in this case because of the inspiratory rise in RA pressure. Kussmaul's sign also occurs with right ventricular (RV) infarction, restrictive cardiomyopathy, and tricuspid stenosis, and may occur with RV failure. It does not occur with cardiac tamponade.

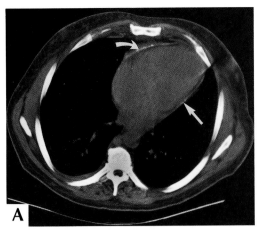 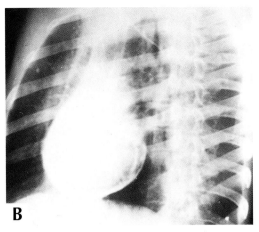 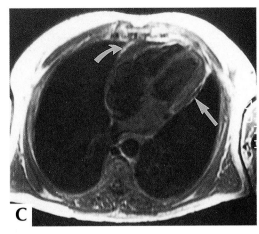

FIGURE 13-35. A, Computed tomography of the chest showing thickened pericardium and calcification (*arrows*) in a patient with constrictive pericarditis. **B,** Extensive pericardial calcification may occur with chronic pericarditis without constriction. The typical hemodynamic pattern must also be present to make the diagnosis of constrictive pericarditis. **C,** Magnetic resonance imaging from a patient with constrictive pericarditis. Note a dark area of thickened pericardium over the left ventricle (*straight arrow*) and a light area of pericardial fat over the right ventricle (*curved arrow*). (Part A *adapted from* Fowler [1]; with permission.)

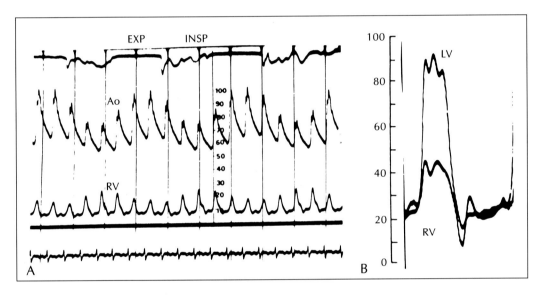

FIGURE 13-36. Contrasting pattern of a ventricular pressure pulse recording in cardiac tamponade (**A**) and in constrictive pericarditis (**B**) [41]. In constrictive pericarditis, there is a dip and plateau pattern (square-root sign) in both ventricular pressure pulse tracings with equalization of right (RV) and left ventricular (LV) end-diastolic pressures. In cardiac tamponade, there is no pronounced diastolic dip in the RV pressure pulse. The patient with cardiac tamponade demonstrates a pronounced inspiratory decline of aortic pressure (Ao). Pressure scale is in mm Hg. EXP—expiration; INSP—inspiration. (*Adapted from* Shabetai and coworkers [41]; with permission.)

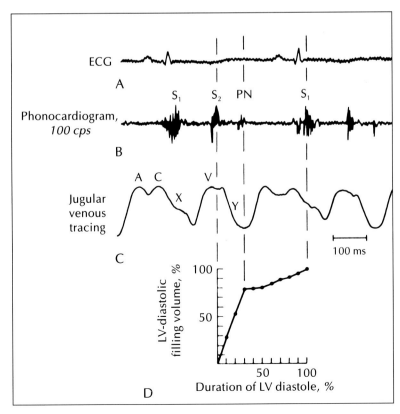

FIGURE 13-37. Electrocardiogram (**A**), phonocardiogram with a 100-Hz filter (**B**), jugular venous pulse tracing (**C**), and left ventricular diastolic filling curve (**D**, expressed as percentages of left ventricular diastolic filling volume and duration of left ventricular diastole) in a patient with constrictive pericarditis and pericardial knock (PN). The knock coincides with the trough of the Y descent and with the end of rapid ventricular filling. Early diastolic ventricular filling is more rapid than normal in constrictive pericarditis. A—A wave; C—C wave; S_1—first heart sound; S_2—second heart sound; V—V wave; X—X descent; Y—Y descent. (*Adapted from* Tyberg and coworkers [42]; with permission.)

A. ELECTROCARDIOGRAPHIC CHANGES IN CONSTRICTIVE PERICARDITIS

Nonspecific T-wave abnormalities
Low-voltage QRS complex
Intra-atrial conduction defect
Atrial fibrillation in 20%–25%

Atrial flutter in ≤5%
Right ventricular hypertrophy in 5%–6%
Bundle branch block and left ventricular hypertrophy are rare

FIGURE 13-38. A, Electrocardiographic changes in constrictive pericarditis. **B,** Electrocardiogram of a patient with constrictive pericarditis, showing low-voltage QRS in limb and precordial leads, with minor nonspecific T-wave changes. The diagnosis was confirmed by autopsy. (Part A *adapted from* Fowler [9]; with permission.)

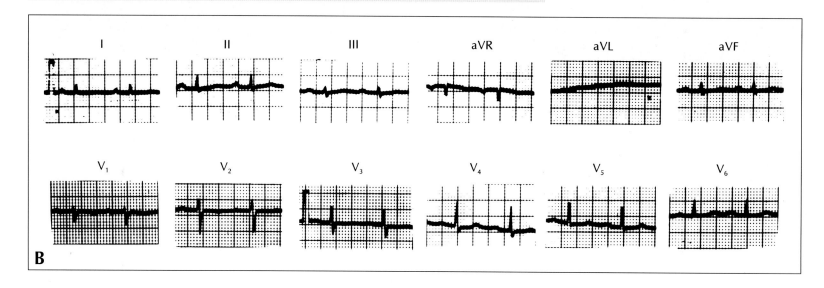

B

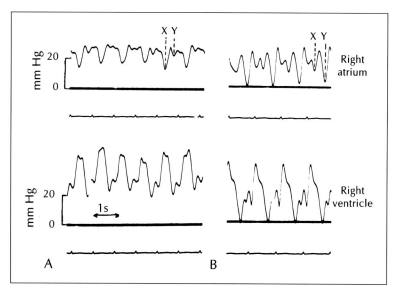

FIGURE 13-39. Right atrial and right ventricular pressure pulses before and after removal of pericardial fluid in a patient with subacute effusive-constrictive pericarditis following radiotherapy. The right atrial pulse shows a prominent systolic descent (X>Y) initially (**A**) and a predominant diastolic descent (X<Y) after removal of fluid (**B**). The diastolic dip-plateau pattern in the right ventricular pulse is prominent only after removal of fluid, in association with X<Y right atrial pulse. Effusive-constrictive pericarditis is most commonly caused by neoplastic disease, connective tissue disease, radiation, idiopathic pericarditis, purulent bacterial infection, or tuberculosis, but may result from any of the causes of constrictive pericarditis. (*Adapted from* Hancock [43]; with permission.)

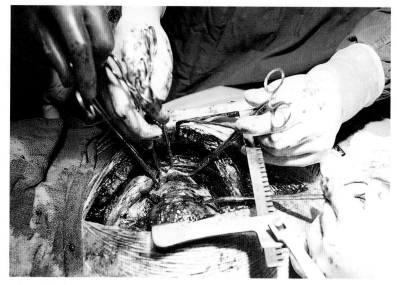

FIGURE 13-40. Exposed heart at operation of a patient with effusive-constrictive pericarditis associated with rheumatoid arthritis. Both parietal and visceral pericardium were thickened, with several hundred milliliters of serosanguineous fluid between the two.

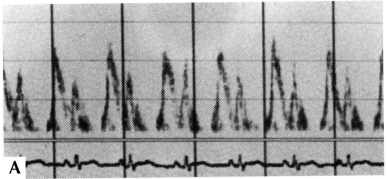

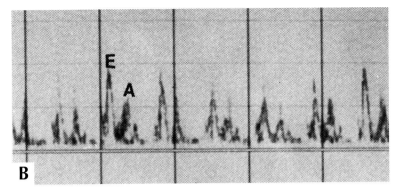

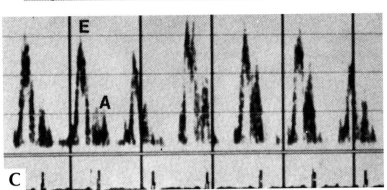

FIGURE 13-41. Mitral flow velocity from a normal subject (**A**) and from two patients with constrictive pericarditis (**B** and **C**). Compared with the normal individual, there is exaggerated respiratory variation in the mitral flow velocity in the patients with constrictive pericarditis. Typically early mitral flow velocity decreases less than 15% during inspiration in normal subjects, and decreases more than 25% in constrictive pericarditis [44]. A—late diastolic filling wave; E—early diastolic filling wave. (*Adapted from* Brockington and coworkers [45]; with permission.)

CONSTRICTIVE PERICARDITIS VS RESTRICTIVE CARDIOMYOPATHY

	CONSTRICTIVE PERICARDITIS	RESTRICTIVE CARDIOMYOPATHY
Hemodynamic pattern	RAP=PWP; RVEDP=LVEDP (within 4 mm Hg); dip and plateau pattern in ventricular diastole	Same, but PWP and LVEDP may exceed RAP and RVEDP by >4 mm Hg
RVSP	<50 mm Hg	May exceed 50 mm Hg
LVEF	>0.50	>0.50
Pericardial calcification	<50%	Absent
Right ventricular endomyocardial biopsy	Usually normal; may show fibrosis postradiation or in connective tissue disease	May show fibrosis, amyloidosis, or other specific pattern; not specific in 23% in one study
Left ventricular filling	Rapid: >60% first half diastole	Variable
Respiratory variations in early mitral valve flow velocity by Echo-Doppler	>25% inspiratory decrease	≤15% inspiratory decrease
Pericardial thickness by CT scan or MR image	Increased (>3 mm) (may be normal in postsurgical constriction)	Normal

FIGURE 13-42. The hemodynamic findings in restrictive cardiomyopathy and constrictive pericarditis may be similar. However, left ventricular end-diastolic pressure (LVEDP) commonly exceeds right ventricular end-diastolic pressure (RVEDP) by more than 4 mm Hg in restrictive cardiomyopathy, and usually does not in constrictive pericarditis [46]. As a rule computed tomography (CT) scans or magnetic resonance (MR) imaging studies show abnormal pericardial thickening in constrictive pericarditis, and not in restrictive cardiomyopathy, but there are exceptions. LVEF—left ventricular ejection fraction; PWP—pulmonary artery wedge pressure; RAP—right atrial pressure; RVSP—right ventricular systolic pressure.

REFERENCES

1. Fowler NO: Pericardial disease. *Heart Dis Stroke* 1992, 1:85–94.
2. Fowler NO: Tuberculous pericarditis. *JAMA* 1991, 266:99–103.
3. Soler-Soler J, Permanyer-Miralda G, Sagristà-Sauleda J: A systematic diagnostic approach to primary acute pericardial disease. In *Diseases of the Pericardium: Cardiology Clinics*, vol. 8. Edited by Shabetai R. Philadelphia: WB Saunders; 1990:609–620.
4. Shabetai R: *The Pericardium*. New York: Grune and Stratton; 1981.
5. Hoit BD: Imaging the pericardium. In *Diseases of the Pericardium: Cardiology Clinics*, vol. 8. Philadelphia: WB Saunders; 1990:587–600.
6. Fowler NO: Congenital defect of the pericardium: its resemblance to pulmonary artery enlargement. *Circulation* 1962, 26:114–120.
7. Spodick DH: Electrocardiographic changes in acute pericarditis. In *The Pericardium in Health and Disease*. Edited by Fowler NO. Mount Kisco, NY: Futura Publishing Company; 1985:79–98.
8. Spodick DH: Acoustic phenomena in pericardial disease. *Am Heart J* 1971, 81:114–124.
9. Fowler NO: *The Pericardium in Health and Disease*. Mount Kisco, NY: Futura Publishing Co; 1985.
10. Goodie RB: Secondary tumors of the heart and pericardium. *Br Heart J* 1955, 17:183–188.
11. Scott RW, Garvin CF: Tumors of the heart and pericardium. *Am Heart J* 1939; 17:431–436.

12. Fowler NO: Recurrent pericarditis. In *Diseases of the Pericardium: Cardiology Clinics*, vol. 8. Edited by Shabetai R. Philadelphia: WB Saunders; 1990:621–626.

13. Fowler NO: Update in pericarditis. In *Progress in Cardiology*, vol. 5, number 2. Edited by Zipes DP, Rowlands DJ. Philadelphia: Lea & Febiger; 1992:199–211.

14. Hastillo A, Thompson JA, Lower RR, *et al.*: Cyclosporine-induced pericardial effusion after cardiac transplantation. *Am J Cardiol* 1987, 59:1220–1222.

15. Hovsepian PG, Coto H, Joseph A, *et al.*: Minoxidil induced pericardial effusion. *J KY Med Assoc* 1988, 86:235–237.

16. Giles PJ, D'Cruz IA, Killam HAW: Tamponade due to hemo-pericardium after streptokinase therapy for pulmonary embolism. *South Med J* 1988, 81:912–914.

17. Brown DL, Luchi RJ: Cardiac tamponade and constrictive peri-carditis complicating endoscopic sclerotherapy. *Arch Intern Med* 1987, 147:2169–2170.

18. Coe AJ: Complications of central venous cannulation [letter]. *BMJ* 1988, 297:1126.

19. Chabanier A, Dany F, Brutus P, *et al.*: Iatrogenic cardiac tamponade after central venous catheter. *Clin Cardiol* 1988, 11:91–99.

20. Hunt R, Hunter TB: Cardiac tamponade and death from perforation of the right atrium by a central venous catheter [letter]. *AJR Am J Roentgenol* 1988, 151:1250.

21. Almassi GH, Chapman PD, Troup PJ, *et al.*: Constrictive peri-carditis associated with patch electrodes of the automatic implantable cardioverter-defibrillator. *Chest* 1987, 92:369–371.

22. Sandler MA, Wertheimer JH, Kotler MN: Pericardial tamponade associated with pacemaker catheter manipulation. *PACE Pacing Clin Electrophysiol* 1989, 12:1085–1088.

23. Vandenberg BF, Mohanty PK, Craddock KJ, *et al.*: Clinical significance of pericardial effusion after heart transplantation. *J Heart Transplant* 1988, 7:128–134.

24. Tuna IC, Danielson GK: Surgical management of pericardial diseases. In *Diseases of the Pericardium: Cardiology Clinics*. Edited by Shabetai R. Philadelphia: WB Saunders; 1990:683–696.

25. Bashi VV, John S, Ravikumar E, *et al.*: Early and later results of pericardiectomy in 118 cases of constrictive pericarditis. *Thorax* 1988, 43:637–641.

26. Anderson DW, Virmani R: Emerging patterns of heart disease in human immunodeficiency virus infection. *Prog Pathol* 1990, 21:253.

27. Kaminsky ME, Rodan BA, Osborne DR. *et al.*: Postpericardiotomy syndrome. *AJR Am J Roentgenol* 1982, 138:503–508.

28. Ofori-Krakye SK, Tyberg TI, Geha AS, *et al.*: Late cardiac tamponade after open heart surgery: incidence, role of antico-agulants in its pathogenesis and its relationship to the postperi-cardiotomy syndrome. *Circulation* 1981, 63:1323–1328.

29. Wall TC, Califf RM, Harrelson-Woodlief L, *et al.*: Usefulness of a pericardial friction rub after thrombolytic therapy during acute myocardial infarction in predicting amount of myocardial damage. *Am J Cardiol* 1990, 66:1418–1421.

30. Dressler WH: The post-myocardial infarction syndrome. *Arch Intern Med* 1959, 103:28–42.

31. TAMI Study Group: Usefulness of a pericardial friction rub after thrombolytic therapy during acute myocardial infarction in predicting the amount of myocardial damage. *Am J Cardiol* 1990, 66:1418–1421.

32. Reddy PS, Curtiss EI, Uritsky BF: Spectrum of hemodynamic changes in cardiac tamponade. *Am J Cardiol* 1990, 66:1487–1491.

33. Reddy PS: Hemodynamics of cardiac tamponade in man. In *Pericardial Disease*. Edited by Reddy PS, Leon DF, Shaver JA. New York: Raven Press; 1982:161–177.

34. Fowler NO: Pericarditis. *New Dev Med* 1988, 3:41–47.

35. Guberman BA, Fowler NO, Engel PJ, *et al.*: Cardiac tamponade in medical patients. *Circulation* 1981, 64:633–640.

36. Levine MJ, Lorell BH, Diver DJ, *et al.*: Implications of electrocardio-graphically assisted diagnosis of pericardial tamponade in contemporary medical patients: detection before hemodynamic embarrassment. *J Am Coll Cardiol* 1991, 17:59–65.

37. Murgo JP, Uhl GS, Felter HG: Right and left heart ejection dynamics during pericardial tamponade in man. In *Pericardial Disease*. Edited by Reddy PS, Leon DF, Shaver JA. New York: Raven Press; 1982:189–201.

38. Lorell BH, Grossman W: Profiles in constrictive pericarditis, restrictive cardiomyopathy, and cardiac tamponade. In *Cardiac Catheterization, Angiography, and Intervention*. Edited by Grossman W, Baim DS. Philadelphia: Lea and Febiger; 1991:643.

39. Antman EM, Cargill V, Grossman W: Low-pressure cardiac tamponade. *Ann Intern Med* 1979, 91:403–406.

40. Cameron J, Oesterle SN, Baldwin JC, *et al.*: The etiologic spectrum of constrictive pericarditis. *Am Heart J* 1987, 113:354–360.

41. Shabetai R, Fowler NO, Guntheroth WG: The hemodynamics of cardiac tamponade and constrictive pericarditis. *Am J Cardiol* 1970, 26:480–489.

42. Tyberg TI, Goodyer AVN, Langou RA: Genesis of pericardial knock in constrictive pericarditis. *Am J Cardiol* 1980, 46:570–575.

43. Hancock EW: Subacute effusive-constrictive pericarditis. *Circulation* 1971, 43:183–192.

44. Hatle LK, Appleton CP, Popp RL: Differentiation of constrictive pericarditis and restrictive cardiomyopathy by Doppler echocar-diography. *Circulation* 1989, 79:357–370.

45. Brockington CM, Zebedi J, Pandian NG: Constrictive pericarditis. In *Diseases of the Pericardium*. Edited by Shabetai R. Philadelphia: WB Saunders; 1990:655.

46. Vaitkus PT, Kussmaul WG: Constrictive pericarditis versus restrictive cardiomyopathy: a reappraisal and update of diagnostic criteria. *Am Heart J* 1991, 122:1431–1441.

INDEX